Musculoskeletal Radiology for Residents

Pawel Szaro

Musculoskeletal Radiology for Residents

Self-Assessment Questions

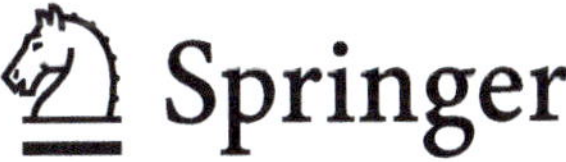

Pawel Szaro
Musculoskeletal Radiology
Sahlgrenska University Hospital Göteborg
Västra Götalands Län, Sweden

Department of Descriptive and Clinical Anatomy
Medical University of Warsaw
Warsaw, Poland

ISBN 978-3-030-85184-2 ISBN 978-3-030-85182-8 (eBook)
https://doi.org/10.1007/978-3-030-85182-8

This Springer imprint is published by the registered company Springer Nature Switzerland AG
The registered company address is: Gewerbestrasse 11, 6330 Cham, Switzerland

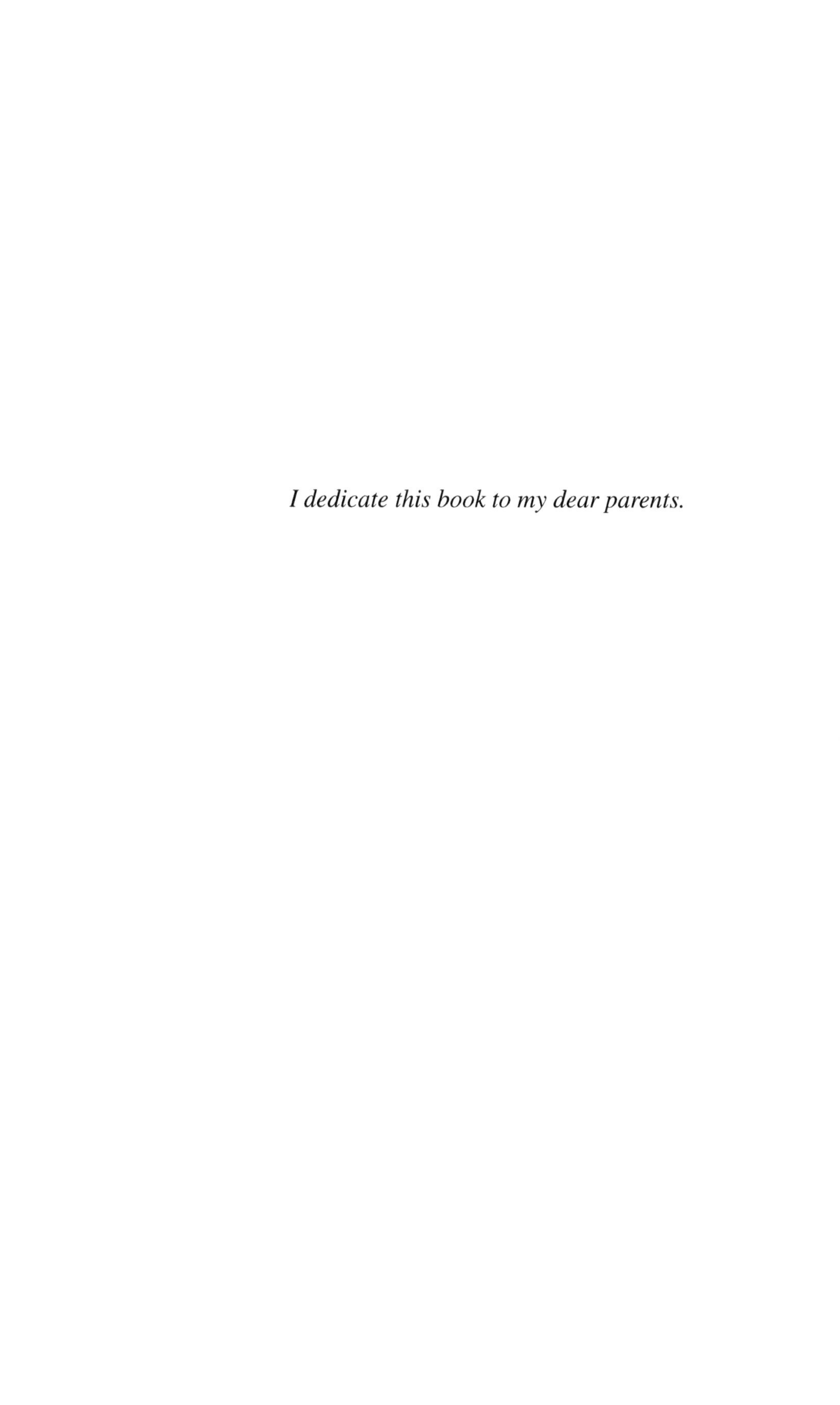

I dedicate this book to my dear parents.

How to Use this Book?

This book includes 1060 questions from all parts of the radiology of the musculoskeletal system. The book aims to present essential issues of the basics of orthopaedic radiology. In the first seven parts (Parts I–VIII), the questions are arranged thematically, and the key to more complex questions include short comments and references to the literature. The purpose of these chapters is to show essential issues and highlight the differences between often similar conditions. These questions cover problems that, in my opinion, are essential and sometimes misunderstood. In radiology, we deal daily with debatable issues; hence in many places, I refer to contemporary literature. The first seven parts aim to teach a reader by solving problems. In some questions, there is more than one correct answer.

In the Part VIII are examples of the three exam sets. I recommend that you use these parts after going through the first seven parts. The purpose of the Part VIII is to test the knowledge. For each question in these sections, only one answer is correct.

I will be very grateful for any comments from readers that will help improve the subsequent editions of the book.

Good luck!

Acknowledgements

I would not have written this book without the help of many people. I would like to thank a few of them. I owe my interest in the musculoskeletal system to Professor Bogdan Ciszek, MD, PhD (Head of the Department of Clinical and Descriptive Anatomy of the Medical University of Warsaw, Poland). I would like to thank him for awakening my scientific ambitions, mentoring, and requirements motivating me to continuous improvement.

I would also like to thank Dr. Nektarios Solidakis, MD (Head of the Department of Musculoskeletal Radiology at Sahlgrenska University Hospital in Gothenburg, Sweden). Thank you for enabling me to continue my research and development and work on this book. Special thanks to my colleagues from the Department of Musculoskeletal Radiology at Sahlgrenska University Hospital in Gothenburg, Sweden, for compelling cases and inspiring questions that were the direct inspiration for writing this book.

Contents

Part I

Anatomy

Clinical Anatomy and Developmental Variants

1

1. Which of these structures inserts on the coracoid process?
   A. The short head of the biceps brachii muscle
   B. The coracohumeral ligament
   C. The superior glenohumeral ligament
   D. The pectoralis minor muscle
   E. The biceps pulley
2. What is the difference between a Hill-Sachs lesion and a flattening or concavity of the normally round contour of the humeral head?
   A. Normal variant is usually located more lateral than a Hill-Sachs lesion.
   B. Normal variant is usually located more medial than a Hill-Sachs lesion.
   C. Normal variant is favoured when the deformity is identified at or above the level of the coracoid process.
   D. Anatomical variant is usually accompanied by round T2-hyperintense structures in the posterior, superior, and lateral aspect of the humeral head.
   E. Normal variant is usually located more inferior than a Hill-Sachs lesion.
3. Choose the correct statement(s) regarding the rotator cable:
   A. It runs along the articular surface of the supraspinatus tendon.
   B. It runs from the coracohumeral ligament.
   C. Retraction of the ruptured supraspinatus tendon is more prominent when the cable is larger.
   D. It is located medially to the rotator crescent.
   E. The cable is seen in about 50% of cases.

P. Szaro, *Musculoskeletal Radiology for Residents*,
https://doi.org/10.1007/978-3-030-85182-8_1

4. Choose the correct statement(s) about anatomical variants of the shoulder labrum:
   A. It can be absent between 6 and 9 o'clock, and it is called the Buford complex.
   B. The Buford complex is seen in about 1–5% of patients.
   C. The incomplete Buford complex is a developmental defect between the labrum and the underlying bone.
   D. The Buford complex may be confused with a superior labral anterior to posterior (SLAP) lesion.
   E. The Buford complex is often associated with the absence of the medial glenohumeral ligament.
5. Choose the correct statement(s) concerning the biceps pulley:
   A. The C-shaped sling-formed structure that runs below the biceps tendon is the coracohumeral ligament.
   B. It is formed by the coracohumeral ligament, superior glenohumeral ligament, and superior fibres from the subscapularis tendon, which blend in relation to the lesser tubercle.
   C. The anterior band of the inferior glenohumeral ligament is an essential contributor to the biceps pulley.
   D. Its apex and base are formed by the transverse humeral ligament.
   E. It is in the space limited by the subscapularis tendon and supraspinatus tendon.
6. Choose the correct statement(s) regarding elbow anatomy:
   A. The synovial plica is often seen in the humeroulnar joint.
   B. A pseudodefect in the cartilage may be seen in the posterior outline of the capitellum or anteriorly to the articular surface of the olecranon.
   C. The anterior bundle of the ulnar collateral ligament is the primary restraint factor against valgus forces.
   D. The anterior bundle of the ulnar collateral ligament complex is more solid than the posterior bundle.
   E. The floor of the cubital tunnel is formed by a transverse bundle of the ulnar collateral ligament.
7. Choose the correct statement(s) regarding the distal insertion of the biceps brachii muscle:
   A. The lacertus fibrosus ascends from the distal biceps myotendinous junction and runs to the antebrachial fascia.
   B. The biceps tendon inserts onto the radial tuberosity.
   C. At the level of the articular rim of the elbow, the brachialis tendon is located anterior to the biceps brachii tendon.
   D. "The cobra position" on ultrasound is a good method for assessing the lacertus fibrosus.
   E. The biceps brachii tendon is situated lateral to the brachial artery.
8. What values are normal with regard to lateral wrist projection?
   A. scapholunate angle 25°
   B. capitolunate angle 42°
   C. scapholunate angle 92°
   D. capitolunate angle 61°
   E. capitolunate angle 10°

9. Choose the correct statement(s) regarding the scapholunate ligament (SL):
   A. The most proximal component of the SL is the most significant functionally.
   B. The anterior part of the SL is the strongest.
   C. It decreases the scapholunate angle.
   D. The primary stabilizers of the scaphoid and lunate are the anterior and posterior capsular (extrinsic) wrist ligaments.
   E. The SL is considered ruptured if the scapholunate interval on posterior anterior projection is more than 4 mm.
10. Choose the structures that are included in the triangular fibrocartilage complex:
    A. the ulnar styloid process
    B. the ulnolunate ligament
    C. the meniscal homologue
    D. the ulnar collateral ligament
    E. the volar radioulnar ligament
11. Choose the correct statement(s) regarding the tendons of the finger:
    A. The flexor pollicis longus inserts onto the proximal phalanx.
    B. The extensor pollicis longus inserts onto the distal phalanx.
    C. The extensor digiti minimi is located in the fourth extensor compartment.
    D. The abductor pollicis brevis inserts onto the lateral part of the base of the proximal phalanx.
    E. The third metacarpal bone is an origin of the adductor pollicis muscle.
12. What structures run separately from the compartment in the carpal tunnel where the median nerve is located?
    A. the flexor digitorum superficialis
    B. the flexor digitorum profundus
    C. the flexor carpi ulnaris
    D. the flexor carpi radialis
    E. the flexor pollicis longus
13. What structure can be palpated?
    A. the scaphoid tubercle
    B. the radial styloid process
    C. the ulnar styloid process
    D. the coracoid process
    E. the coronoid process
14. What nerves arise from the posterior cord of the brachial plexus?
    A. the ulnar nerve
    B. the axillary nerve
    C. the median nerve
    D. the thoracic longus nerve
    E. the thoracodorsal nerve
15. What structures are located in the quadrilateral space?
    A. a. axillaris
    B. n. axillaris
    C. n. thoracodorsalis
    D. n. subscapularis
    E. n. radialis

16. The normal variant of ossification in the knee is seen most often in:
    A. the anterior part of the medial femoral condyle
    B. the anterior part of the lateral femoral condyle
    C. the posterior part of the medial femoral condyle
    D. the posterior part of the lateral femoral condyle
    E. on the lateral part of the articular surface of the patella
17. The os cuneiforme intermedium is related to:
    A. the medial and lateral cuneiform bones
    B. the navicular bone
    C. the cuboid bone
    D. the calcaneus
    E. the third metatarsal bone
18. What structures insert onto the lateral malleolus?
    A. the flexor retinaculum
    B. the anterior talofibular ligament
    C. the posterior talofibular ligament
    D. the calcaneofibular ligament
    E. the superior peroneal retinaculum
19. Choose the correct tendon and its insertion:
    A. the peroneus longus—the first metatarsal and medial cuneiform bone
    B. the tibialis posterior—the navicular and medial cuneiform bone
    C. the popliteus—the posterior surface of the tibial shaft, distal to the soleus line
    D. the biceps femoris—the head of the fibula
    E. the adductor longus—the superior third of the linea aspera
20. What nerve is located directly to the biceps femoris tendon?
    A. n. ischiadicus
    B. n. tibialis
    C. n. peroneus profundus
    D. n. peroneus communis
    E. n. peroneus superficialis
21. Choose the correct statement(s) regarding the dorsal defect of the patella:
    A. X-ray revealed a rounded focal radiolucent lesion surrounded by a sclerotic margin; the lesion is located on the lateral part of the patella.
    B. On MRI, the dorsal defect of the patella is filled by cartilage.
    C. It is located more often in the inferior part of the lateral half of the patella.
    D. It usually occurs if the patella is luxated.
    E. Osteochondritis dissecans is in the differential diagnosis.
22. What statements are correct regarding the ligaments of the knee?
    A. The medial patellofemoral ligament is a part of the medial patellar retinaculum.
    B. The anterior cruciate ligament inserts on the medial surface of the lateral condyle.
    C. The popliteofibular ligament inserts on the apex fibulae.

   D. The medial collateral ligament originates anteroinferior to the adductor tubercle.
   E. The arcuate ligament merges with the articular capsule and the medial collateral ligament.
23. What statements are correct regarding the meniscus?
   A. The ring meniscus or discoid meniscus is a rare variant of the medial meniscus.
   B. The discoid meniscus is less prone to degeneration compared to the normal meniscus.
   C. If the meniscal body is larger than 15 mm on the coronal plane, the discoid meniscus may be considered.
   D. The posterior root of the lateral meniscus is more posterior than the posterior root of the medial meniscus.
   E. Secondary to flexion of the knee, meniscal flounce can be seen.
24. What structures are involved in Shenton's line?
   A. the inferior pubic ramus
   B. the ramus ossis ischii
   C. the lateral edge of the femoral neck
   D. the medial edge of the femoral neck
   E. the trochanter major
25. Choose the muscle and its origin:
   A. the sartorius muscle—the anterior superior iliac spine
   B. the tensor fasciae latae—the anterior inferior iliac spine
   C. the rectus femoris muscle—the anterior inferior iliac spine
   D. the piriformis muscle—the sacrum
   E. the adductor longus muscle—the pubic tubercle
26. Choose the abnormal value of the caput-collum-diaphyseal femoral angle:
   A. 126°
   B. 130°
   C. 150°
   D. 100°
   E. 170°
27. Choose the correct statement(s) regarding the calf muscles:
   A. The extensor hallucis longus tendon is located between the tibialis anterior and extensor digitorum longus.
   B. The plantaris tendon runs between the soleus and gastrocnemius in the upper half of the calf.
   C. The soleus muscle is related anteriorly to the flexor hallucis longus muscle.
   D. The Achilles tendon is a common tendon of the soleus, gastrocnemius, and plantaris.
   E. Kager's fat pad is interposed between the popliteus muscle and the Achilles tendon.

28. What structure(s) are located in the tarsal tunnel?
    A. the flexor digitorum longus
    B. the posterior tibial artery
    C. the deep fibular nerve
    D. the tibial nerve
    E. the interosseous talocalcaneal ligament
29. Which ligament(s) run in the axial plane?
    A. the spring ligament
    B. the anterior talofibular ligament
    C. the posterior talofibular ligament
    D. the calcaneofibular ligament
    E. the deltoid ligament
30. The tarsal sinus contains:
    A. the spring ligament
    B. the talocalcaneal interosseous ligament
    C. the tibial nerve
    D. the talonavicular ligament
    E. the posterior tibiofibular ligament
31. Choose the correct statement(s) regarding levels of the vertebrae:
    A. The coeliac trunk is located on the Th12/L1 level.
    B. The superior mesenteric artery runs on the L1 level.
    C. The iliolumbar ligament joins with the transverse process of L3.
    D. The posterior inferior iliac spine is located at the L3/L4 level.
    E. The inferior mesenteric artery runs on the L4 level.
32. What structure limits the intervertebral foramen?
    A. the spinal process
    B. the facet joint
    C. the superior vertebral notch
    D. the transverse process
    E. the intervertebral disc
33. The ligamenta flava:
    A. It connects the laminae of adjacent vertebrae.
    B. The most superior is located between C1 and C2.
    C. The most inferior is located between L5 and the sacrum.
    D. It limits the posterior part of the vertebral canal.
    E. It is thickest in the cervical part.
34. Choose the correct statement(s) regarding facet joints:
    A. In the cervical part, the joint surface is orientated in the sagittal plane.
    B. In the thoracic part, the joint surface is located in the coronal plane.
    C. A strong articular capsule is present on the anterior and posterior parts.
    D. In the lumbar part, the joint surface is located between the sagittal and coronal planes.
    E. The fat pad protrudes to the superior and inferior parts.

35. Choose the correct statement(s) regarding the craniocervical junction:
    A. The atlantooccipital ligament runs between the occipital bone and C1.
    B. The ligamentum nuchae runs from the occipital bone down to the spinal process of the whole cervical vertebrae.
    C. The alar ligaments run between the anterior arch of C1 and the occipital condyles.
    D. The most significant ligament for stabilizing the craniocervical junction is the transverse ligament.
    E. The posterior longitudinal ligament originates from the posterior surface of the anterior arch of C1.
36. Which of the following is the biggest subarachnoid cistern?
    A. cisterna magna
    B. cisterna ambiens
    C. cisterna sacralis
    D. cisterna lumbalis
    E. cisterna thoracalis
37. What is located in the epidural space of the spine?
    A. the sympathetic trunk
    B. the external venous plexus
    C. the internal venous plexus
    D. the spinal nerves
    E. the cerebrospinal fluid
38. Choose the correct statement(s) regarding topography:
    A. In the cervical part, the transverse process is anterior to the articular process.
    B. In the thoracic part, the transverse process is anterior to the articular process.
    C. In the cervical part, the transverse process is posterior to the articular process.
    D. In the thoracic part, the transverse process is posterior to the articular process.
    E. In the lumbar part, the transverse process is posterior to the articular process.
39. Choose the contents of the suboccipital triangle:
    A. the greater occipital nerve
    B. the internal carotid artery
    C. the lesser occipital nerve
    D. the vertebral artery
    E. the suboccipital nerve
40. Choose the correct combination of the muscle and its insertion:
    A. the splenius capitis—the mastoid process of the temporal bone
    B. the levator scapulae—the superior part of the medial border of the scapula
    C. the rhomboideus major—the lateral border of the scapula
    D. the latissimus dorsi muscle—the intertubercular groove of the humerus
    E. the trapezius muscle—the clavicle, spine of the scapula and acromion

41. Choose the correct combination of nerve and level:
    A. The C5 nerve passes via the intervertebral foramen of C5/C6.
    B. The L3 nerve is located in the intervertebral foramen of L3/L4.
    C. The L4 nerve is located in the lateral recess at the level of L3/L4.
    D. The S1 nerve passes via the intervertebral foramen of L5/S1.
    E. The C1 nerve passes via the intervertebral foramen of C1/C2.
42. Disc protrusion at the level the L1/L2 disc to the right lateral recess may compress:
    A. the conus medullaris
    B. the right L1 nerve
    C. the right L2 nerve
    D. the right L1 and L2 nerves
    E. the artery of Adamkiewicz
43. Choose the correct statement(s) regarding C2 or axis:
    A. The body of C2 fuses with the odontoid process by 10 years of age.
    B. A secondary ossification centre at the apex of the odontoid process may not be fused and is called the os terminale.
    C. The following ossification centrum for C2 are seen one for each neural arch, one for the body, and one for the odontoid process.
    D. The fusion line between the odontoid process and body may be confused with a fracture until age 16 years.
    E. The ossification centrum in neural arches fuse by 2–3 years of age.
44. The limbus vertebrae occur most often:
    A. on the anterosuperior corner of the vertebral body
    B. on the posterosuperior corner of the vertebral body
    C. on the anteroinferior corner of the vertebral body
    D. on the posteroinferior corner of the vertebral body
    E. in the anterior part of the intervertebral disc
45. Where are the most common limbus vertebrae seen?
    A. in the cervical spine
    B. in the thoracic spine
    C. in the lumbar spine
    D. in the sacrum
    E. in C1 and C2
46. Anatomical variation of insertion of the meniscofemoral ligament to the posterior horn of the lateral meniscus may lead to an incorrect diagnosis of a tear. What indicates that it is an anatomical variant?
    A. association with PCL tears
    B. absence of subchondral bone marrow oedema
    C. fluid cleft located between the meniscofemoral ligament of Wrisberg
    D. fracture of the lateral tibial condyle
    E. meniscal tears and ACL tears

47. A 14-year-old patient presented with knee pain. A thin strip of high signal on proton density with fat suppression in the subcortical posterior part of the distal femur enhances intensely after the gadolinium injection. What is your opinion about this finding?
    A. It is suspicious for osteosarcoma.
    B. It is unclear; I would recommend bone core biopsy.
    C. It is probably cortical desmoid.
    D. It is probably a posterior metaphyseal stripe.
    E. It is probably hematopoietic marrow.
48. You find multiple small bone fragments in relation to the patellar apex. What is your differential diagnosis?
    A. Sinding-Larsen-Johansson disease
    B. patella multipartite
    C. variant of the accessory ossification centre
    D. synovial chondromatosis
    E. jumper's knee
49. A 19-year-old patient presented with a painful foot after a football match. X-ray of the foot showed a small fragment in relation to the basis of the fifth metatarsal bone. What would you include in the differential diagnosis?
    A. avulsion of the peroneus longus
    B. avulsion of the peroneus brevis
    C. apophysis of the fifth metatarsal bone
    D. os peroneum
    E. os trigonum
50. A 35-year-old patient presented with painful and limited hip motion. X-ray revealed the ossicle in direct relation to the lateral outline of the acetabulum. What is the differential diagnosis?
    A. calcification in the labrum
    B. fabella
    C. os acetabuli
    D. acetabular fracture
    E. avulsion of the rectus femoris
51. Choose two most common types of tarsal coalition:
    A. the talocalcaneonavicular coalition
    B. the talocuboid coalition
    C. the talonavicular coalition
    D. the talocalcaneal coalition
    E. the calcaneonavicular coalition
52. What structure passes through the cubital tunnel?
    A. the median nerve
    B. the ulnar nerve
    C. the radial nerve
    D. the brachial artery
    E. the cubital nerve

53. The medial boundary of the anatomical snuffbox is:
    A. the abductor pollicis longus
    B. the abductor pollicis brevis
    C. the extensor pollicis longus
    D. the extensor pollicis brevis
    E. the extensor pollicis communis
54. Choose the correct statement(s) regarding Guyon's canal or the ulnar tunnel:
    A. The floor is formed by the transverse carpal ligament.
    B. It contains the flexor digiti minimi.
    C. The hook of the hamate forms the lateral boundary.
    D. It contains the median nerve.
    E. The flexor digitorum superficialis forms the medial boundary.
55. Choose the correct statement(s) regarding the triceps brachii:
    A. The long head originates from the infraglenoid tubercle.
    B. The radial nerve passes between the medial and lateral heads.
    C. Only the long head may act in the shoulder joint.
    D. It is located in the posterior compartment of the arm.
    E. The ulnar nerve provides innervation.
56. The most common place for compression of the posterior interosseus nerve is located:
    A. in the radial groove of the humerus
    B. under the lacertus fibrosus
    C. in the supinator muscle
    D. in the cubital tunnel
    E. in Guyon's canal
57. Which of the following is correct regarding the lumbar vertebrae?
    A. L1 and L2 are often atypical because of the orientation of the superior articular processes.
    B. Sacralization is more common than lumbarization.
    C. The iliolumbar ligament originates from the transverse process of L5.
    D. L2 has the longest transverse processes.
    E. The longest spine process is in L5.
58. The persistence of the notochord during vertebrae formation may cause:
    A. lumbarization
    B. sacralization
    C. hemivertebrae
    D. block vertebrae
    E. butterfly vertebrae
59. The spinal epidural space is located between:
    A. The dura mater and arachnoid mater.
    B. The periosteal layer and dura mater.
    C. The arachnoid mater and pia mater.
    D. The dura mater and pia mater.
    E. The spinal epidural space is a potential space.

60. The bases of the denticulate ligaments arise in the:
    A. dura mater
    B. arachnoid mater
    C. pia mater
    D. dura mater and pia mater
    E. arachnoid mater and pia mater
61. The arrow shows (Fig. 1.1) the:

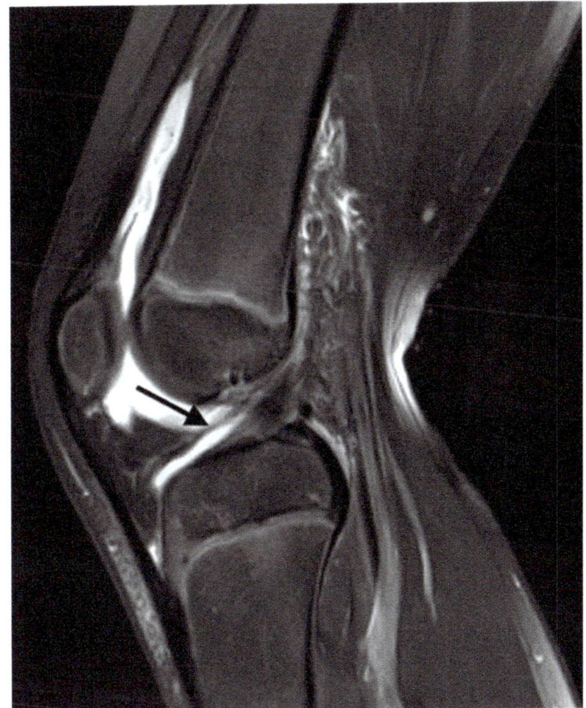

Fig. 1.1 Fat-suppressed proton density-weighted image, sagittal section

    A. anterior cruciate ligament
    B. ligamentum mucosum
    C. infrapatellar plica
    D. subpatellar plica
    E. synovitis

62. Choose the correct answer(s) regarding the structure marked with the arrow (Fig. 1.2):

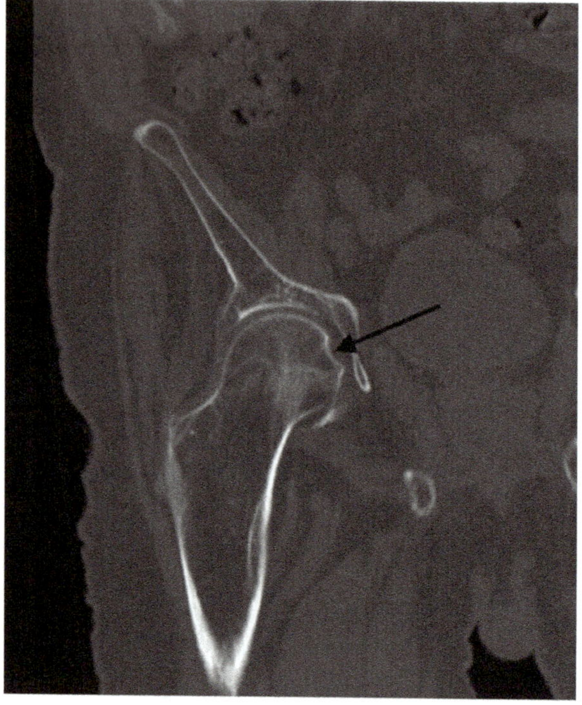

Fig. 1.2 Computed tomography of the right hip, coronal section

A. Its insertion is the round ligament of the hip.
B. It is a variably occurring structure called the fovea capitis femoris.
C. It is a constantly occurring structure called the fovea capitis femoris.
D. It is deformation that may be an early sign of avascular necrosis, MRI is recommended.
E. It is deformation that may be an early sign of avascular necrosis, scintigraphy is recommended.

63. A 10-year-old boy presents with knee pain after a football match. Choose the correct answer regarding the structure that is marked with the arrow in the lateral compartment (Fig. 1.3):

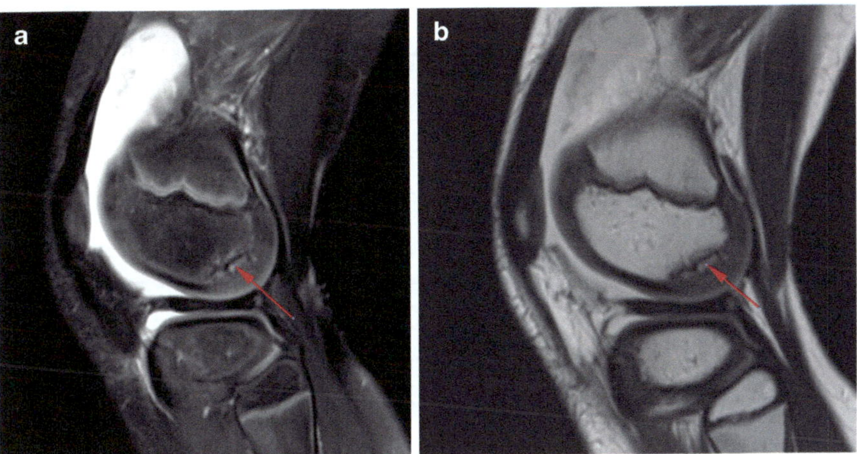

Fig. 1.3 (**a**) Fat-suppressed proton density-weighted image, (**b**) non-fat-suppressed proton density-weighted image, sagittal sections

A. It is probably a developmental variant, X-ray is recommended after 2 months.
B. It is probably a developmental variant, MRI is recommended after 2 months.
C. It is a developmental variant, no further diagnostic imaging is recommended.
D. It is probably osteochondritis dissecans, MRI is recommended.
E. It is probably osteochondritis dissecans, CT is recommended.

64. With regard to the patient from the previous question, choose the correct answer(s) regarding the structure that is marked with the arrow (Fig. 1.4):

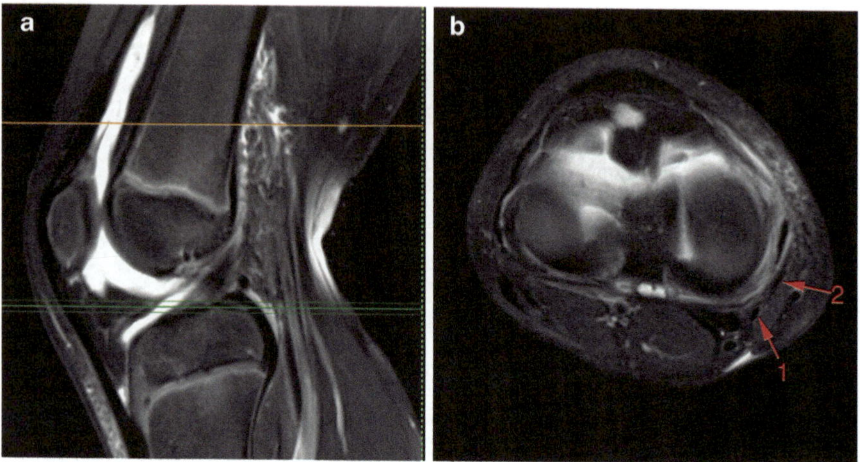

Fig. 1.4 Fat-suppressed proton density-weighted images. (**a**) Sagittal section; (**b**) axial section

A. An aggressive cortical and periosteal process is seen.
B. It is an abnormal finding, CT is recommended.
C. It is a "do not touch" lesion.
D. It is the cortical desmoid.
E. It is a stress fracture.

65. Choose the correct names for the tendons marked in Fig. 1.4:
A. 1—semitendinosus, 2—semimembranosus
B. 1—sartorius, 2—semimembranosus
C. 1—sartorius, 2—semitendinosus
D. 1—gracilis, 2—sartorius
E. 1—sartorius, 2—gracilis

66. What structure is marked with the arrow in Fig. 1.5?

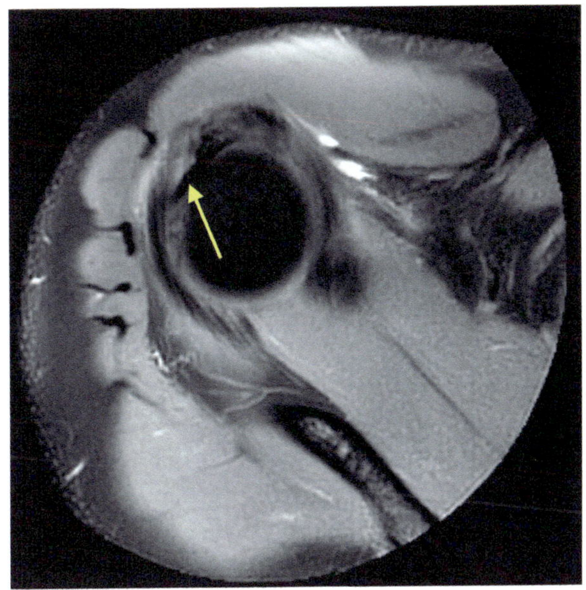

Fig. 1.5 MRI of the shoulder, proton density-weighted image with fat suppression, axial section

A. diffuse calcification
B. focal tendinopathy
C. long delamination
D. normal structure
E. focal fibrosis

67. Choose the correct answer regarding the structure marked with the letter "a" in Fig. 1.6:

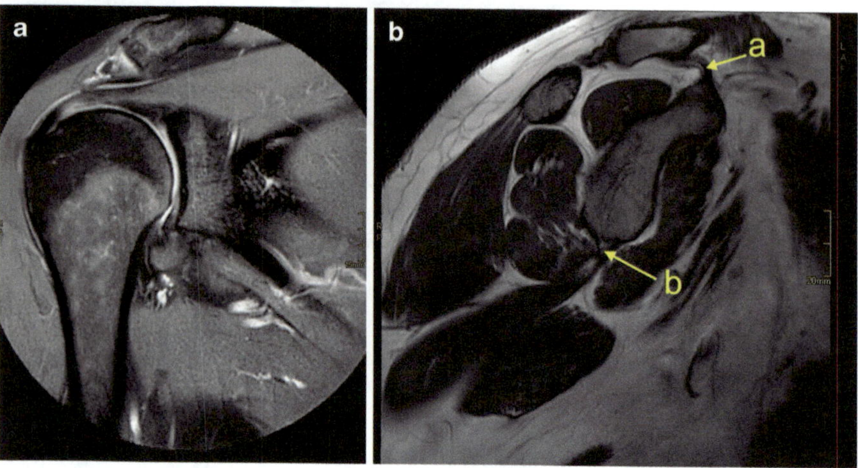

Fig. 1.6 MRI of the shoulder. (**a**) T2-weighted image with spectral adiabatic inversion recovery, coronal section; (**b**) T1-weighted image, sagittal section

A. coracohumeral ligament
B. coracoacromial ligament
C. coracoacromial ligament
D. coracoclavicular ligament
E. superior glenohumeral ligament

68. Choose the correct answer regarding the structure marked with the letter "b" in Fig. 1.6:

A. medial head of triceps brachii
B. long head of triceps brachii
C. latissimus dorsi
D. teres major
E. teres minor

69. The rotator cuff tendon is composed of layers. Which of the marked parts belong to the supraspinatus tendon (Fig. 1.7)?

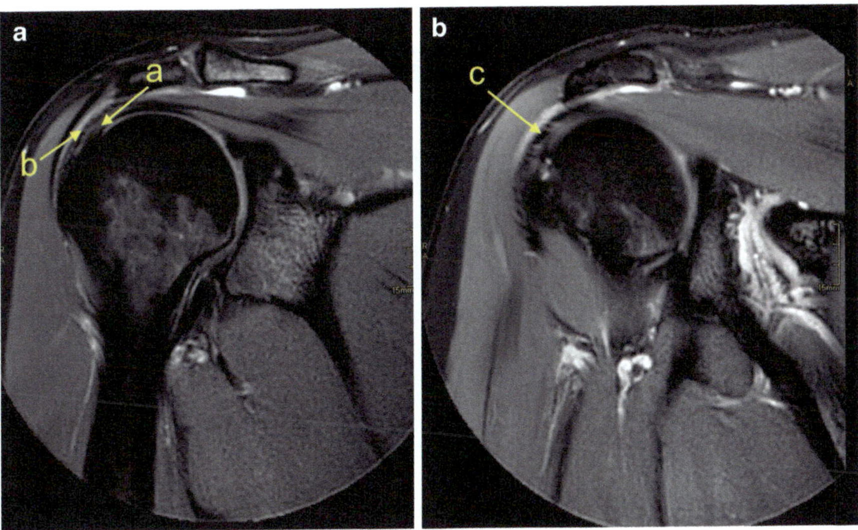

Fig. 1.7 MRI of the shoulder. (**a** and **b**) T2-weighted image with spectral adiabatic inversion recovery, coronal sections

A. a, b, c
B. a, c
C. b, c
D. a
E. b

70. What is the name of the structure marked in Fig. 1.8?

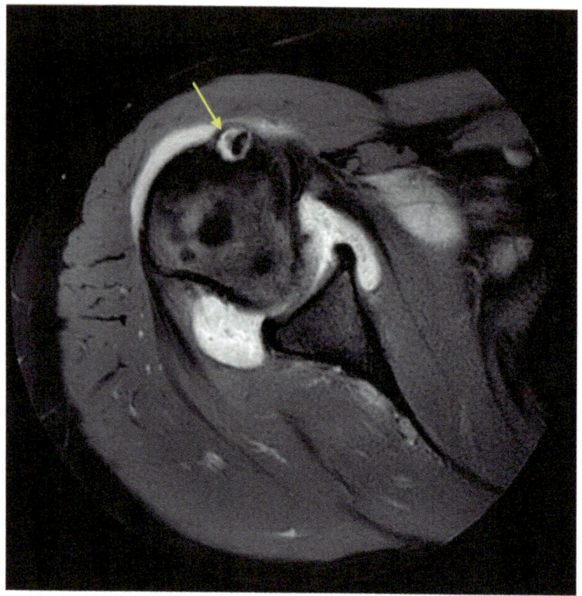

Fig. 1.8 MRI of the shoulder, proton density-weighted image with fat suppression, axial section

A. superior glenohumeral ligament
B. middle glenohumeral ligament
C. transverse humeral ligament
D. coracohumeral ligament
E. biceps pulley

71. Choose the correct answer regarding the structures marked on the sagittal arthrography MRI picture (Fig. 1.9):

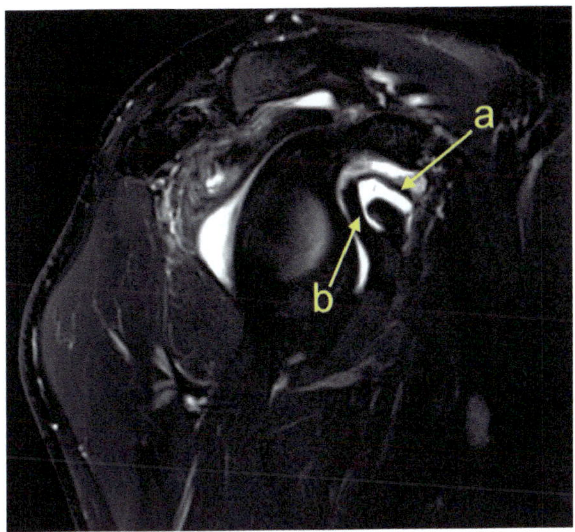

Fig. 1.9 MRI arthrography of the shoulder, sagittal section

A. a—middle glenohumeral ligament, b—anterior bundle of inferior glenohumeral ligament
B. a—superior glenohumeral ligament, b—middle glenohumeral ligament
C. a—coracohumeral ligament, b—superior glenohumeral ligament
D. a—coracohumeral ligament, b—inferior glenohumeral ligament
E. a—supraspinatus tendon, b—superior glenohumeral ligament

72. What letters mark the middle glenohumeral ligament on the MR arthrography presented in Fig. 1.10?

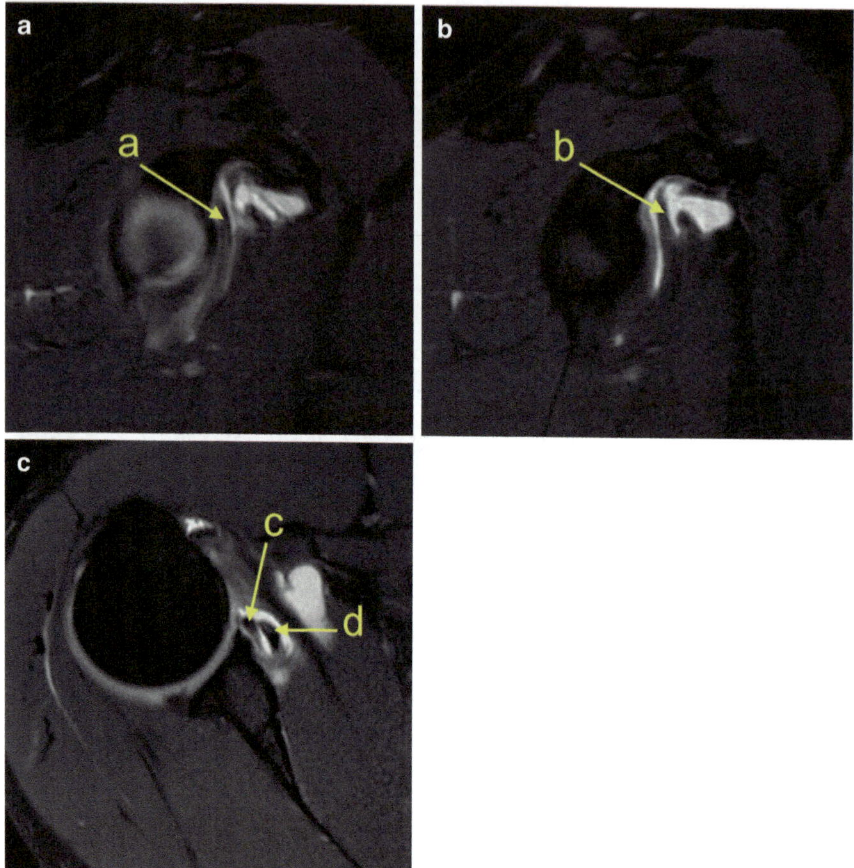

Fig. 1.10 MRI arthrography of the shoulder. (**a** and **b**) Sagittal section, (**c**) axial section

A. a, c
B. a, d
C. b, c
D. b, d
E. a, b, c

73. Match the letters with the names of the anatomical structures shown on this elbow MRI (Fig. 1.11):
    (1) biceps brachii
    (2) brachialis
    (3) brachioradialis
    (4) supinator
    (5) ulnar nerve
    (6) median nerve
    (7) ulnar collateral ligament

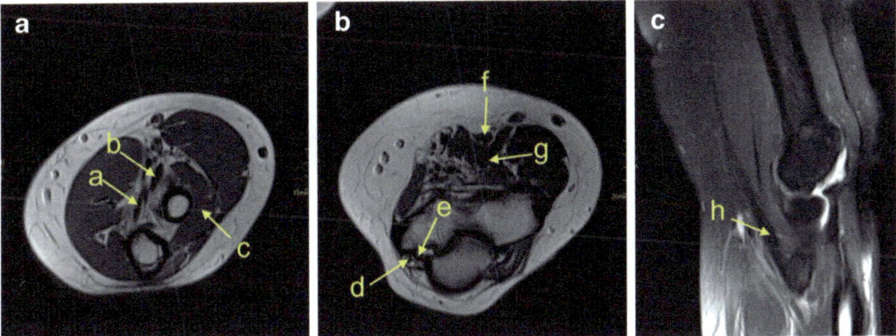

Fig. 1.11 MRI of the elbow. (**a** and **b**) T2-weighted images, axial sections; (**c**) proton density-weighted image with fat suppression, sagittal section

A. 1—b, f, h; 2—a, g; 3—none, 4—c; 5—d; 6—none, 7—e
B. 1—a, g, h; 2—b, f; 3—none, 4—c; 5—d; 6—none, 7—e
C. 1—b, f; 2—a, g, h; 3—none, 4—c; 5—e; 6—f; 7—e
D. 1—a, g; 2—b, h; 3—none, 4—c; 5—d; 6—f, 7—e
E. 1—b; 2—a, h; 3—c; 4—g; 5—e; 6—f; 7—d

74. Which letter indicates the extensor pollicis brevis in Fig. 1.12?

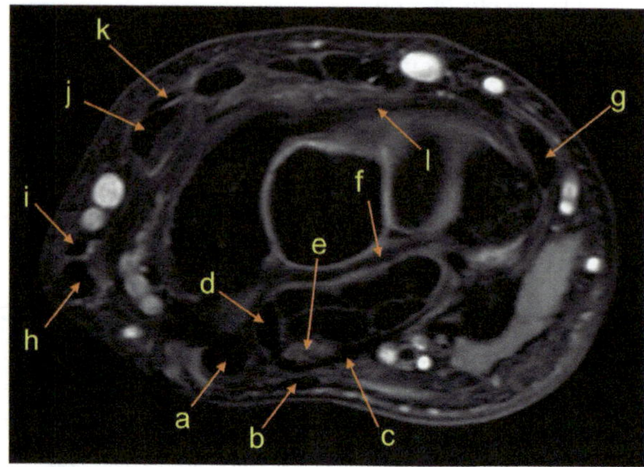

Fig. 1.12 MRI of the wrist, T2-weighted image, spectral adiabatic inversion recovery, coronal section

   A. h
   B. i
   C. j
   D. k
   E. extensor pollicis brevis is not marked.

75. Which letter indicates the flexor carpi radialis in Fig. 1.12?
   A. a
   B. b
   C. d
   D. e
   E. flexor carpi radialis is not marked.

76. What is the structure indicated by the letter "g" in Fig. 1.12?
   A. extensor digiti minimi
   B. extensor carpi ulnaris
   C. flexor carpi ulnaris
   D. ulnar collateral ligament
   E. v. basilica

77. Which letter indicates the flexor retinaculum in Fig. 1.12?
   A. b
   B. c
   C. d
   D. f
   E. l

78. Letter "a" in Fig. 1.13 indicates:

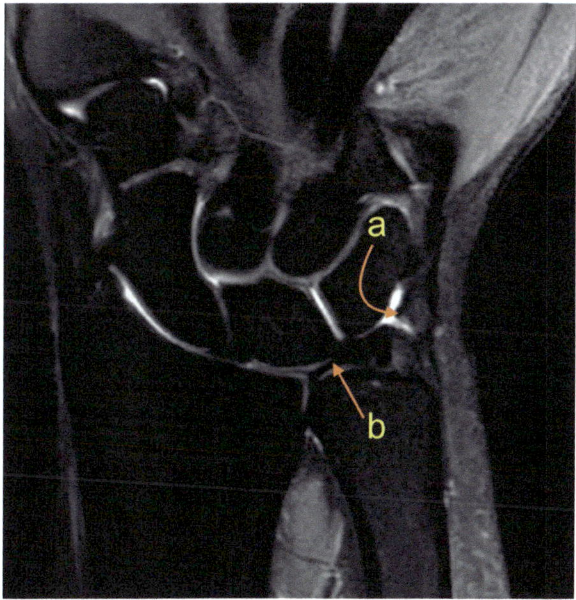

Fig. 1.13 MRI of the wrist, proton density-weighted image, spectral adiabatic inversion recovery, axial section

A. meniscal homologue
B. ulnotriquetral ligament
C. extensor carpi ulnaris subsheath
D. triangular fibrocartilage complex
E. the same structure as the arrow marked with the letter "b"

79. Which letter indicates the lateral band of the extensor digitorum in Fig. 1.14?

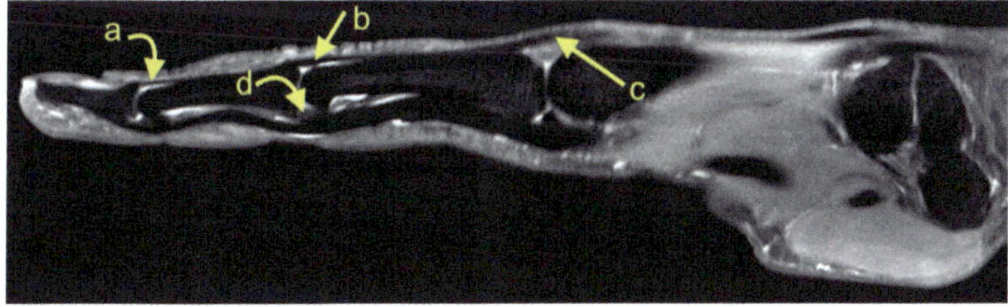

Fig. 1.14 MRI of the third finger of the hand. Proton density-weighted image with fat suppression, sagittal section

A. a, b, c, d
B. a, b, c
C. a, b
D. a
E. b

80. Choose the correct option regarding the structures in Fig. 1.15:
    (1) anterior talofibular ligament
    (2) calcaneofibular ligament
    (3) posterior talofibular ligament
    (4) superior peroneal retinaculum
    (5) inferior peroneal retinaculum

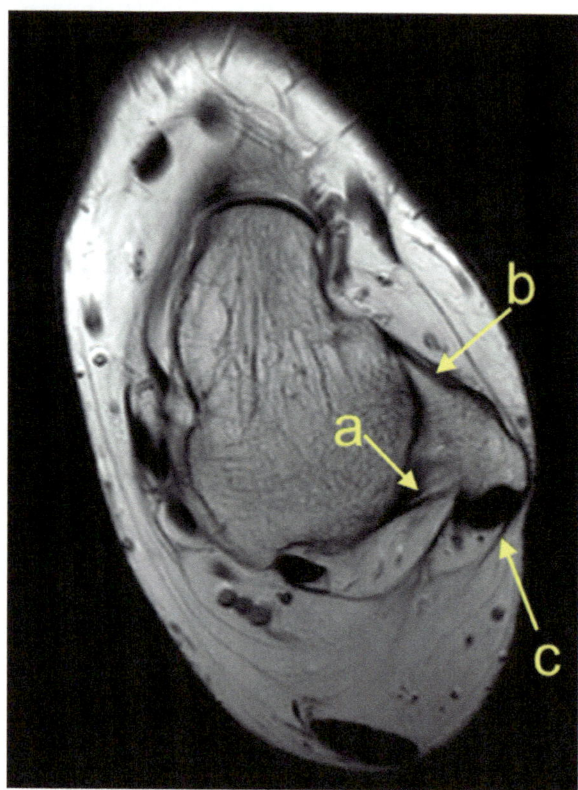

Fig. 1.15 MRI of the ankle. Proton density-weighted, axial section

A. a—2, b—5, c—4
B. a—2, b—1, c—5
C. a—3, b—1, c—4
D. a—3, b—1, c—5
E. a—4, b—4, c—2

81. What is the structure indicated by the arrow in Fig. 1.16?

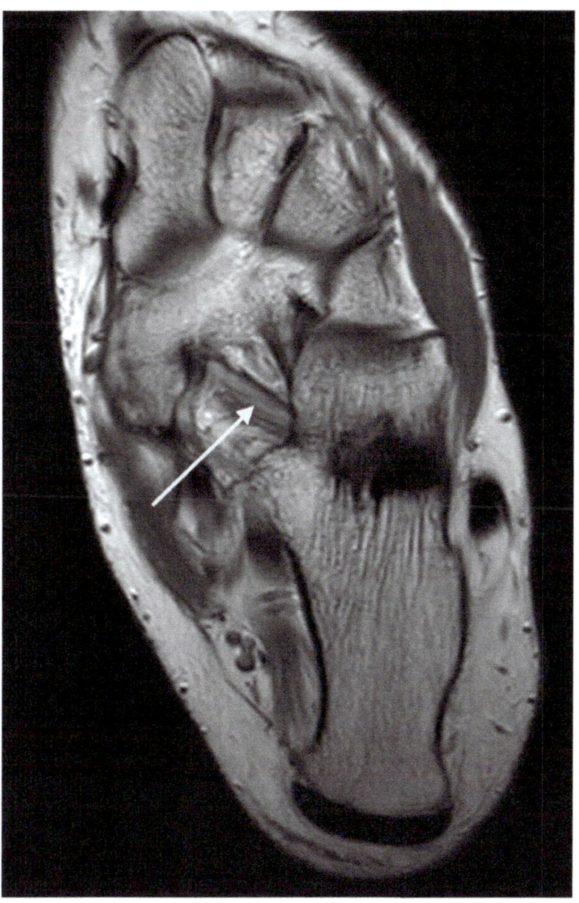

Fig. 1.16 MRI of the foot. Proton density-weighted, axial section

A. superomedial ligament
B. medioplantar oblique ligament
C. lateroplantar oblique ligament
D. inferoplantar longitudinal ligament
E. medioplantar longitudinal ligament

82. What structure is indicated by the arrow in Fig. 1.17?

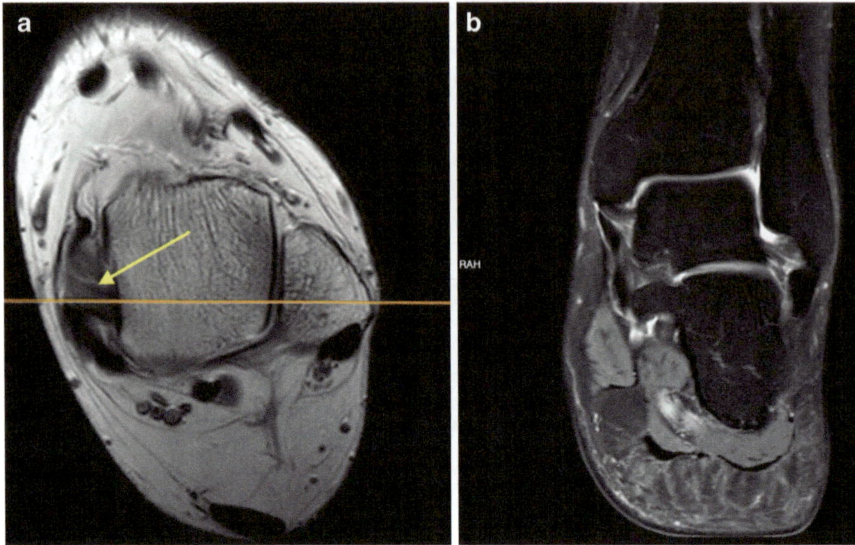

Fig. 1.17 MRI of the ankle. (**a**) Proton density-weighted, axial section; (**b**) proton density-weighted with fat suppression, coronal section

A. tibiospring ligament
B. tibionavicular ligament
C. tibiocalcaneal ligament
D. spring ligament complex
E. deep posterior tibiotalar ligament

83. What muscles attach on the structure that is indicated by the arrow in Fig. 1.18?
    - a. gluteus maximus
    - b. gluteus medius
    - c. gluteus minimus

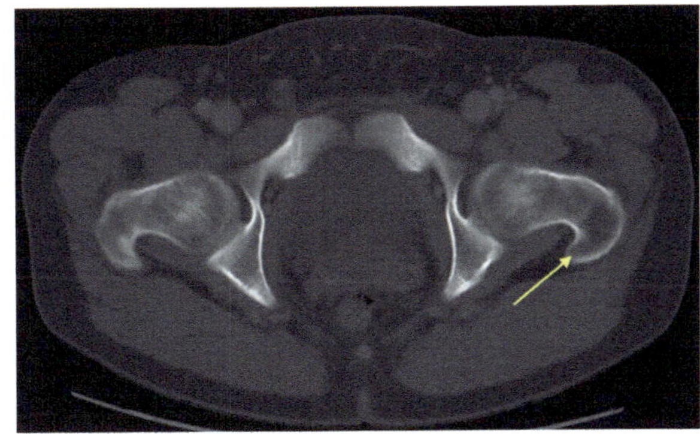

Fig. 1.18 Computed tomography of the pelvis, axial section

- A. a, b, c
- B. a, b
- C. a, c
- D. b, c
- E. a

84. What structure is indicated by the arrow in Fig. 1.19?

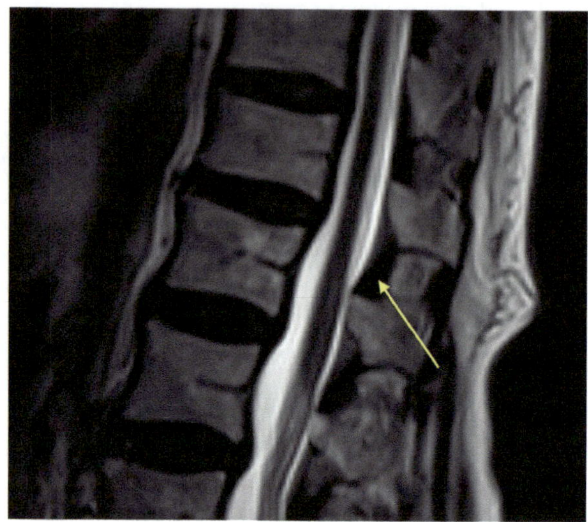

Fig. 1.19 MRI of the spine. T2-weighted image, sagittal section

A. posterior longitudinal ligament
B. supraspinous ligament
C. interspinous ligament
D. ligamentum flavum
E. articular capsule

85. What structure is indicated by the arrow in Fig. 1.20?

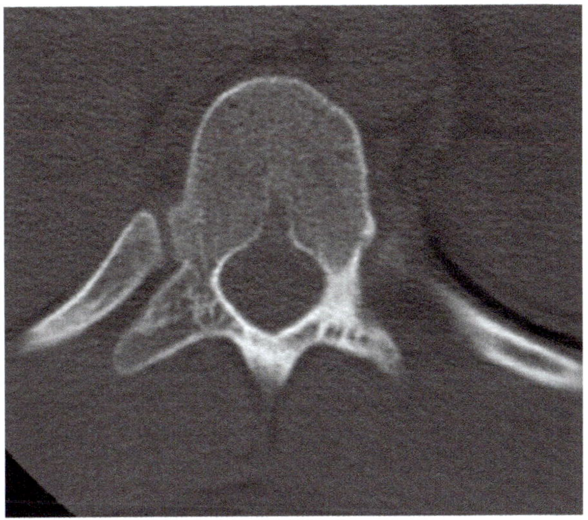

Fig. 1.20 Computed tomography of the thoracic spine, axial section

A. posterior external venous plexus
B. anterior external venous plexus
C. internal vertebral vein
D. central vertebral vein
E. basivertebral vein

Key to Chapter 1

1. A, B, C, D.
2. B, C, E. Small round T2-hyperintense pseudocyst in the posterior, superior, and lateral aspects of the humeral head may be confused with cysts related to internal impingement but probably have got a developmental background [1].
3. A, B, D. Rotator cable is located on the inferior surface of the rotator cuff. It runs from the coracohumeral ligament in the posterior direction, medially to the rotator crescent. It unites the coracohumeral ligament, supraspinatus and infraspinatus tendon [1].
4. B. Defect between labrum and glenoid is called sublabral foramen which may be confused with SLAP.
5. A, B, D, E [2].
6. B, C, D. The floor of the cubital tunnel where the ulnar nerve runs is formed by the posterior bundle of the ulnar collateral ligament [3].
7. A, B, D, E.
8. A, E. Capitolunate angle is considered abnormal if it is more than 30°, while the scapholunate angle if it is more than 80°. The scapholunate angle is normal between 30° and 60° in the neutral position, clear abnormality is considered more than 80° [4].

9. E.
10. B, C, D, E.
11. B, C, D, E.
12. D, E.
13. A, B, C, D.
14. B, E.
15. B.
16. D.
17. A, B.
18. B, C, D, E.
19. A, B, D.
20. D.
21. A, B, E.
22. A, B, C, D.
23. B, C, E [5].
24. A, D.
25. A, C, D, E.
26. C, D, E. The normal range of this angle is 125°–135°. Coxa vara is considered if angle is less than 120°, while coxa valga if the angle is more than 140°.
27. A, B, C.
28. A, B, D [6].
29. A, B, C [6].
30. B.
31. A, B.
32. B, C, E.
33. A, C, D. The thickest ligamentum flavum is in the lumbar part of spine, and thus hypertrophy may cause the spinal stenosis.
34. B, D, E.
35. A, B, D.
36. D.
37. C.
38. A, D.
39. D, E.
40. A, B, D, E.
41. B, C.
42. C.
43. B, C, E. The body of C2 fuses with the odontoid process by 3–6 years of age, but the fusion line may be seen until age 11 years which may be a potential pitfall [7].
44. A.
45. C [8].
46. C [9].
47. D. Cortical desmoid or avulsive cortical irregularity changes cortex. Hematopoietic marrow is present usually more central in metaphysis in relation to the epiphyseal line [10].

48. A, E.
49. B, D.
50. A, C. Fabella is the accessory bone lateral to the lateral femoral condyle.
51. D, E.
52. B.
53. C.
54. A, C.
55. A, B, C, D.
56. C. Mostly in the arcade of Frohse compress the posterior interosseus nerve when radial nerve enters the supinator.
57. B, C. The longest transverse process is present in L3 [11].
58. E.
59. B.
60. C.
61. B, C.
62. A, C.
63. C.
64. C, D.
65. D.
66. D.
67. D.
68. B.
69. D.
70. C.
71. B.
72. D.
73. A.
74. B.
75. A.
76. B.
77. B.
78. A.
79. D.
80. C.
81. B.
82. E.
83. D.
84. D.
85. E.

References

1. Motamedi D, Everist BM, Mahanty SR, Steinbach LS. Pitfalls in shoulder MRI: Part 1—Normal anatomy and anatomic variants. AJR Am J Roentgenol. 2014;203(3):501–7. https://doi.org/10.2214/AJR.14.12848.
2. Nakata W, Katou S, Fujita A, Nakata M, Lefor AT, Sugimoto H. Biceps pulley: normal anatomy and associated lesions at MR arthrography. Radiographics. 2011;31(3):791–810. https://doi.org/10.1148/rg.313105507.
3. Acosta Batlle J, Cerezal L, Marquez MV, Lopez Parra MD, Soteras C, Resano S, et al. MRI of the normal elbow and common pathologic conditions. Radiographics. 2020;40(2):468–9. https://doi.org/10.1148/rg.2020190134.
4. Goldfarb CA, Yin Y, Gilula LA, Fisher AJ, Boyer MI. Wrist fractures: what the clinician wants to know. Radiology. 2001;219(1):11–28. https://doi.org/10.1148/radiology.219.1.r01ap1311.
5. Nguyen JC, De Smet AA, Graf BK, Rosas HG. MR imaging-based diagnosis and classification of meniscal tears. Radiographics. 2014;34(4):981–99. https://doi.org/10.1148/rg.344125202.
6. Rosenberg ZS, Beltran J, Bencardino JT. From the RSNA Refresher Courses. Radiological Society of North America. MR imaging of the ankle and foot. Radiographics. 2000;20 Spec No:S153–79. https://doi.org/10.1148/radiographics.20.suppl_1.g00oc26s153.
7. Lustrin ES, Karakas SP, Ortiz AO, Cinnamon J, Castillo M, Vaheesan K, et al. Pediatric cervical spine: normal anatomy, variants, and trauma. Radiographics. 2003;23(3):539–60. https://doi.org/10.1148/rg.233025121.
8. Carr RB, Fink KR, Gross JA. Imaging of trauma: Part 1, Pseudotrauma of the spine—osseous variants that may simulate injury. AJR Am J Roentgenol. 2012;199(6):1200–6. https://doi.org/10.2214/AJR.12.9083.
9. Mohankumar R, White LM, Naraghi A. Pitfalls and pearls in MRI of the knee. AJR Am J Roentgenol. 2014;203(3):516–30. https://doi.org/10.2214/AJR.14.12969.
10. Laor T, Chun GF, Dardzinski BJ, Bean JA, Witte DP. Posterior distal femoral and proximal tibial metaphyseal stripes at MR imaging in children and young adults. Radiology. 2002;224(3):669–74. https://doi.org/10.1148/radiol.2243011259.
11. Ucar D, Ucar BY, Cosar Y, Emrem K, Gumussuyu G, Mutlu S, et al. Retrospective cohort study of the prevalence of lumbosacral transitional vertebra in a wide and well-represented population. Arthritis. 2013;2013:461425. https://doi.org/10.1155/2013/461425.

Part II

Appendicular Skeleton Trauma

Upper Extremity Trauma

2

1. A displaced fat pad in the elbow may indicate:
   A. Fracture.
   B. Arthritis.
   C. Pigmented villonodular synovitis.
   D. Unclear findings, CT is always indicated.
   E. Unclear findings, MRI is always indicated.
2. An 87-year-old patient fell from a chair. There was a clinical suspicion of fracture, but the X-ray was normal. What would you do next?
   A. CT with contrast
   B. CT without contrast
   C. MRI
   D. scintigraphy
   E. ultrasound
3. What examination is unnecessary?
   A. coccyx after trauma
   B. acute back pain after lifting a heavy object
   C. X-ray of the hand in a patient with hyperparathyroidism
   D. X-ray of the cervical spine in the unconscious patient
   E. ankle X-ray in the patient who is not able to walk after the injury
4. Choose the correct statement(s) regarding a clavicle fracture:
   A. It is uncommon in children.
   B. It associated with pneumothorax.
   C. In a majority, fracture non-union is seen.
   D. There is a risk of brachial plexus injury.
   E. Often indirect trauma is a cause of the fracture.

P. Szaro, *Musculoskeletal Radiology for Residents*,
https://doi.org/10.1007/978-3-030-85182-8_2

5. Choose the differential diagnosis of post-traumatic distal clavicle osteolysis:
   A. septic arthritis
   B. coracoclavicular ligament injury
   C. acromioclavicular arthrosis
   D. rheumatic arthritis
   E. os acromiale
6. Avulsion of the greater tubercle of the humerus:
   A. It needs to be differenced from a supraspinatus tear.
   B. It is usually associated with a direct impact.
   C. it is common, especially after an anterior dislocation.
   D. It may be related to a Bankart lesion.
   E. It represents about 25% of proximal humerus fractures.
7. Choose the correct statement(s) regarding scapular fractures:
   A. They often require high-energy direct trauma.
   B. Fracture of the glenoid should be differentiated from fracture of the accessory ossicle.
   C. They may be associated with injury of the brachial plexus.
   D. It is usually avulsive in character.
   E. It is associated with clavicle fractures.
8. The Neer classification of clavicle fractures is based on the relation of the fracture to:
   A. the acromioclavicular joint
   B. the trapezoid ligament
   C. the sternoclavicular joint
   D. the conoid ligament
   E. the subclavius muscle
9. Sternoclavicular dislocation:
   A. It may occur without trauma when laxity of the ligaments is seen.
   B. It occurs mostly in sport-related trauma as compared to that in a car accident.
   C. X-ray is the preferred imaging tool.
   D. Anterior dislocation is more common than posterior dislocation.
   E. It may be associated with a pneumothorax.
10. A 35-year-old patient presenting with ankylosis of the first costosternal articulation and hyperostosis of the sternal end of the clavicle with erosion, osteophyte, and capsular thickening. What is the differential diagnosis?
    A. osteomyelitis
    B. arthritis
    C. SAPHO (synovitis, acne, pustulosis, hyperostosis, osteitis)
    D. callus
    E. dislocation

11. What value is considered abnormal when assessing the diameter of the acromioclavicular joint space on ultrasound?
    A. 4 mm
    B. 5.5 mm
    C. 8 mm
    D. 12 mm
    E. 14.5 mm
12. Choose the correct statement(s) regarding post-traumatic osteolysis of the clavicle:
    A. Osteolysis may include up to 3 cm of clavicle.
    B. Most of the acromion is included in the osteolysis.
    C. Rheumatic arthritis is a differential diagnosis.
    D. Resorption starts about 6 months after trauma.
    E. CT is the best imaging tool.
13. What MRI feature(s) are more typical for rheumatoid arthritis than post-traumatic osteolysis of the clavicle?
    A. presence of bone marrow oedema
    B. presence of contrast enhancement
    C. presence of subchondral line on the clavicle
    D. presence of thickening of the articular capsule
    E. presence of erosions also on the acromion
14. Scapular fractures:
    A. They often occur in the acromion.
    B. They are associated with lung contusions.
    C. They coexist with rib fractures.
    D. Glenoid fracture is associated with shoulder dislocation.
    E. CT is the best imaging tool.
15. What fracture is typical for children?
    A. scaphoid fracture
    B. tuberculum majus fracture
    C. distal radius fracture
    D. supracondylar humeral fracture
    E. lateral epicondyle fracture
16. Choose the correct name of the fracture with its fracture localization:
    A. gamekeeper's thumb—avulsion of the ulnar collateral ligament on MCP 1
    B. Jersey finger—avulsion of the flexor digitorum superficialis
    C. mallet finger—the base of the distal phalanx
    D. Rolando fracture—the base of the first metacarpal bone
    E. Bennett fracture—the base of the proximal phalanx

17. Choose the correct statement(s) regarding perilunate dislocation:
    A. Similarly to lunate dislocations, the lunate shows normal alignment in the radiolunate joint.
    B. In most cases, it is associated with a scaphoid fracture.
    C. More overlap of the lunate and capitate may indicate perilunate dislocation.
    D. On the lateral view, the capitate bone is located dorsally to the line drawn up to the radius.
    E. Ligament ruptures are associated with this injury.
18. Choose the correct statement(s) regarding scaphoid fractures:
    A. The scaphoid is the most commonly fractured carpal bone.
    B. Falling on an outstretched hand is the most common cause.
    C. Articular fracture of the distal radius is commonly associated.
    D. Slight sclerosis of the proximal fragment suggests avascular necrosis.
    E. Non-union is the least common in distal pole fractures.
19. Choose the correct statement(s) regarding distal radius fractures:
    A. Volar angulated fracture is more common than dorsal angulated.
    B. Fall on the outstretched arm is a common mechanism.
    C. Smith fracture is more common than Colles fracture.
    D. It may be accompanied by ulnar styloid fracture.
    E. Colles fracture is not more frequent in younger than older patients.
20. Which variant of forearm fractures is the most common?
    A. fractures of the ulna and radius in their shafts
    B. fracture of the ulna and dislocation of the radius
    C. fracture of the radius and dislocation of the ulna
    D. fracture of the caput radii and dislocation of the radioulnar joint
    E. fracture of the caput ulnae and dislocation of the radius
21. Choose the correct statement(s):
    A. Galeazzi fracture-dislocations are more common than Monteggia fracture-dislocations.
    B. Fracture of the distal ulna and dislocation of the proximal radius is more common than fracture of the distal radius and dislocation of the distal ulna.
    C. Fracture of the distal radius and dislocation of the distal ulna is more common than fracture of the distal ulna and dislocation of the proximal radius.
    D. A Monteggia fracture-dislocation is the fracture of the distal radius and dislocation of the distal ulna.
    E. A Galeazzi fracture is the fracture of the ulnar shaft and dislocation of the radial head.

22. The sail sign in the elbow corresponds to:
    A. a joint effusion
    B. synovitis
    C. occult caput radii fracture
    D. coronoid process fracture
    E. supracondylar fracture
23. Choose the correct statement(s) regarding shoulder luxation:
    A. Posterior luxation accounts for about 30% of cases
    B. Posterior luxation is usually associated with a Hill-Sachs deformity.
    C. Anterior luxation occurs when the arm is externally rotated and abducted.
    D. Electrocution is the most common cause.
    E. Humeral avulsion of the glenohumeral ligament is associated with posterior luxation.
24. What radiologic sign can be seen in posterior shoulder dislocation?
    A. Glenohumeral joint is widened more than 6 mm.
    B. AP view shows two parallel lines in the superomedial part of the caput humeri.
    C. Light bulb sign.
    D. McLaughlin lesion.
    E. Hill-Sachs deformity
25. Choose the correct statement(s) regarding anterior shoulder dislocation:
    A. Anterior inferior labral tear is common.
    B. Tear of the posterior limb of the inferior glenohumeral ligament is common.
    C. MRI arthrography in abduction and external rotation increases the diagnostic accuracy.
    D. CT arthrography may be considered as an alternative to MRI after bone fragment fixation.
    E. Most Hill-Sachs lesions are unstable.
26. What is the role of CT in the preoperative assessment of anterior shoulder dislocation?
    A. assessing the type of acromion
    B. assessing the glenoid
    C. evaluating the Hill-Sachs deformity
    D. evaluating the size of the humeral head
    E. evaluating the brachial plexus
27. Choose the correct statement(s) regarding posterior shoulder dislocation:
    A. Joint space is less than 5 mm on AP view
    B. Light bulb sign is present.
    C. Loss of overlay of humeral head and glenoid.
    D. Vertical sclerosis in the medial part of the humeral head.
    E. Osteolysis of the humeral head.

28. Choose the features of luxatio erecta:
    A. It occurs mainly with epileptic seizures.
    B. It coexists with inferior articular capsule tears.
    C. Sensory deficits are common.
    D. It may be associated with greater tuberculum fractures.
    E. It occurs usually when muscles are weaker.
29. Little Leaguer's shoulder:
    A. It occurs mostly medially in the humeral epiphyseal line.
    B. It is grade 2 according to Salter-Harris classification.
    C. It is most common in ages 11–16 years.
    D. Surgical fixation is gold standard of treatment.
    E. The best imaging tool is X-ray.
30. A 34-year-old patient presented with arm pain after trauma during a handball match. Irregular focal cortical thickening with radiolucent components is seen in the anterolateral part of the humeral shaft; no soft tissue mass is present. What is the differential diagnosis?
    A. chronic osteomyelitis
    B. tug lesion
    C. classic osteosarcoma
    D. Ewing sarcoma
    E. deltoid tuberosity
31. Choose the correct statement(s) regarding distal humerus fractures:
    A. Ligaments are usually intact.
    B. "Drop wrist" sign may be seen.
    C. "Hand of benediction" may be seen.
    D. Floating elbow may occur.
    E. It is seen mainly in adolescents.
32. You noticed a defect in the posterolateral capitellum. What is the most probable diagnosis?
    A. osteochondral lesion
    B. chondral lesion
    C. fracture
    D. avascular necrosis
    E. normal finding
33. Choose the correct statement(s) regarding elbow dislocation:
    A. It is the most common dislocation in adults
    B. In adults, it is related to chronic dislocation of the radial head.
    C. It is usually associated with a tear of the radial collateral ligament.
    D. It is usually associated with coronoid and caput radii fractures.
    E. Posterior dislocation is most common.

34. Essex-Lopresti fracture includes:
    A. comminuted olecranon fracture
    B. comminuted caput radii fracture
    C. proximal migration of the radial shaft
    D. proximal migration of the ulnar shaft
    E. disruption of the scapholunate joint
35. An intra-articular radial styloid process fracture is called a:
    A. Colles fracture
    B. Smith fracture
    C. Barton fracture
    D. Chauffeur fracture
    E. die-punch fracture
36. A fracture that occurs because of carpal impaction is called a:
    A. Colles fracture
    B. Smith fracture
    C. Barton fracture
    D. Chauffeur fracture
    E. die-punch fracture
37. What fracture is most commonly associated with osteoporosis?
    A. Colles fracture
    B. Smith fracture
    C. Barton fracture
    D. Chauffeur fracture
    E. die-punch fracture
38. A 53-year-old female fell on a dorsal surface with her wrist bent volarly. What fracture is the most probable (choose one)?
    A. Colles fracture
    B. Smith fracture
    C. Barton fracture
    D. Chauffeur fracture
    E. die-punch fracture
39. Why information about the fracture of the styloid process of the ulna should be included in the radiological report of a distal radius fracture?
    A. higher risk for caput ulnae necrosis
    B. higher risk of non-union of the distal radius fracture
    C. risk of a tear of the triangular fibrocartilage
    D. risk of ulnar nerve injury
    E. risk of intra-articular involvement
40. Choose an early complication of distal radius fixation:
    A. lucent zone around screws
    B. infection
    C. fusion between the ulna and radius
    D. hardware limits the movement of the joint
    E. complex regional pain

41. A 34-year-old patient presented after fall on an outstretched hand. No distinct pathology was seen on X-ray, but MRI showed a non-displaced scaphoid fracture in the waist with bone marrow oedema only in the distal fragment. How would you explain this finding?
    A. It is nothing dangerous; bone marrow oedema is often present only in the distal fragment.
    B. It is a sign of ischaemia in the proximal fragment.
    C. It is a typical sign of osteochondritis dissecans.
    D. It is a sign of scaphoid dislocation.
    E. It is a sign of sclerosis in the proximal fragment.
42. A 56-year-old patient presented with chronic wrist pain 4 months after a previous scaphoid fracture. CT revealed a humpback deformity and sclerosis in the proximal part. Choose the correct statement(s) regarding this patient:
    A. It is a sign of osteonecrosis in the proximal part.
    B. Vascularity in the sclerotic part may be normal.
    C. There is a higher risk of arthrosis.
    D. There is a sign of an osteochondral lesion.
    E. There is a sign of a TFCC tear.
43. Choose the correct statement(s) regarding carpal dislocation:
    A. Triquetrum fracture is associated more often than scaphoid fracture.
    B. Volar perilunate dislocation is seen less often than dorsal perilunate dislocation.
    C. In lunate dislocation, the lunate-capitate dislocate dorsally.
    D. In perilunate dislocation, the capitate dislocates volarly.
    E. Scaphoid waist fracture is associated.
44. Choose the correct statement(s) regarding ulnar impaction syndrome:
    A. The ulnar styloid process may conflict with the triquetrum.
    B. Ulna plus variant conflicts with the lunate.
    C. Kienböck disease is in the differential diagnosis of ulnar impaction syndrome.
    D. Avascular necrosis of the scaphoid may mimic ulnar impaction syndrome.
    E. Malunion of the distal radius is a predisposing factor.
45. Choose the correct statement(s) regarding ulnar impingement syndrome:
    A. It is a synonym for ulnar impaction syndrome
    B. The triangular fibrocartilage complex is usually not affected.
    C. Ulna minus variant is often present.
    D. Radial cortex scalloping is seen.
    E. Ulnar plus variant is often present.

46. Choose the correct statement(s) regarding scaphoid fractures:
    A. Lack of contrast enhancement on MRI indicates infection.
    B. If the fracture callus is not seen 5 months after fracture, a deleted union may be recognized.
    C. A radiolucent line in the fracture indicates osteonecrosis.
    D. Anterior angulation is one of the most often seen deformations.
    E. A higher risk of osteonecrosis is noticed when the fracture is located more distally.
47. What is the second most common carpal fracture?
    A. os lunatum fracture
    B. triquetrum fracture
    C. os trapezium fracture
    D. os trapezoideum
    E. os capitatum
48. The thickened and inhomogeneous tendon of the supraspinatus:
    A. It probably shows a higher signal on pulse sequences.
    B. It is a sign of tendinosis.
    C. It represents an intratendinous ganglion.
    D. It may coexist with impingement.
    E. It may be related to the magic angle artefact.
49. Which sequence is most useful to assess supraspinatus tendinopathy?
    A. T1-weighted
    B. PD-weighted
    C. PD-weighted with fat suppression
    D. T2-weighted
    E. MRI arthrography
50. Choose the correct statement(s) regarding painful conditions of the shoulder:
    A. Surrounding is visible in direct relation to tendon calcifications
    B. Full-thickness rotator cuff tears usually show no communication between the subacromial bursa and joint space.
    C. Rotator cuff tendinopathy usually coexists with subacromial impingement.
    D. An intratendinous cyst is usually flattened and coexists with a partial tear.
    E. Deposition of calcium hydroxyapatite shows a high signal on pulse sequences
51. Which tendons are usually changed in posterosuperior glenoid impingement?
    A. subscapularis
    B. supraspinatus
    C. infraspinatus
    D. teres minor
    E. teres major

52. What features other than a partial rotator cuff tear are typical signs for posterosuperior glenoid impingement?
    A. posterosuperior humeral head deformation
    B. anterior labrum tear
    C. posterior labrum tear
    D. denervation of the supraspinatus
    E. denervation of the subscapularis
53. The double cortex sign in ultrasonography of the shoulder refers to:
    A. septic arthritis
    B. gout
    C. non-dislocated fracture
    D. osteochondritis dissecans
    E. total supraspinatus rupture
54. The magic angle artefact occurs in the supraspinatus:
    A. in the bony insertion
    B. at the myotendinous junction
    C. at the level of the acromion
    D. slightly proximal to the insertion
    E. in the intramuscular tendon
55. Which sequence is least susceptible to the magic angle artefact?
    A. proton density weighted
    B. gradient echo
    C. T2*-weighted
    D. T2-weighted
    E. T1-weighted
56. What is the most common type of acromion, according to Bigliani?
    A. type 1
    B. type 2
    C. type 3
    D. type 4
    E. type 3 and 4
57. What type of acromion, according to Bigliani, is a risk factor for impingement?
    A. type 1
    B. type 2
    C. type 3
    D. type 4
    E. type 1 and 2

58. What is the cause of impingement?
    A. muscle overgrowth
    B. acromial lateral tilt
    C. partial rotator cuff tear
    D. os acromiale
    E. thick coracoacromial ligament
59. Acromial slope:
    A. It may cause subacromial impingement.
    B. It occurs when the anterior part of the acromion is more inferior than the posterior part of the acromion in the sagittal plane.
    C. It occurs when the anterior part of the acromion is more superior than the posterior part of the acromion in the sagittal plane.
    D. It occurs when the acromion is more inferior than the clavicle in the coronal plane.
    E. It occurs when the acromion is more superior than the clavicle in the coronal plane.
60. Subcoracoid impingement usually affects the:
    A. subscapularis tendon
    B. supraspinatus tendon
    C. infraspinatus tendon
    D. long head of the biceps brachii tendon
    E. inferior glenohumeral ligament
61. A fluid collection located between the coracoid process, short head of the biceps, and the coracobrachialis and subscapularis tendons is:
    A. a synovial cyst of the acromioclavicular joint
    B. subacromial bursitis
    C. subcoracoid bursitis
    D. subdeltoid bursitis
    E. paralabral cyst
62. Os acromiale is:
    A. usually symptomatic
    B. seen in about 25% of the population
    C. may cause subacromial impingement
    D. usually immobile
    E. represents fracture of the edge of the acromion
63. What is the most common site of supraspinatus tear?
    A. bursal side
    B. intrasubstance
    C. articular side
    D. avulsion fracture
    E. myotendinous junction

64. Choose the correct statement(s) regarding rotator cuff tear:
    A. it is more common in athletes than in the elderly population
    B. The supraspinatus muscle is most commonly affected in partial and total ruptures.
    C. The infraspinatus muscle is most commonly involved in myotendinous junction tears.
    D. The infraspinatus muscle is the most frequently affected in avulsion.
    E. A tear of the tendon insertion is often related to degeneration.
65. The critical zone of the supraspinatus tendon is located:
    A. in the bony insertion
    B. about 1–7 mm proximal to the insertion
    C. about 8–16 mm proximal to the insertion
    D. about 17–25 mm proximal to the insertion
    E. in the myotendinous junction
66. Massive rotator cuff rupture:
    A. It is present when the geyser sign is visible.
    B. It is a partial tear that extends in the sagittal section more than 2 cm.
    C. It is a full-thickness tear of more than one tendon.
    D. It is a full-thickness tear of the supraspinatus and infraspinatus tendons.
    E. It is a full-thickness tear of the supraspinatus and superior part of the subscapularis tendons.
67. Choose the radiological features of a total rotator cuff rupture:
    A. superior subluxation of the humerus on X-ray
    B. highlight articular cartilage on ultrasound
    C. synovial proliferation in the tendon
    D. high signal on the sequences with long TR and long TE
    E. high signal on the sequences with long TR and short TE
68. Tendon delamination:
    A. It is the longitudinal split of the supraspinatus.
    B. It may be a full-thickness or partial tear.
    C. It usually occurs vertically.
    D. It usually occurs horizontally.
    E. It is an intratendinous cleft.
69. What information is mandatory in the rotator cuff report?
    A. localization of the tear with a 2D description
    B. if there is muscle atrophy
    C. localization of the rupture in relation to the rotator cable
    D. what tendons are involved
    E. type of acromion

70. Grade 2 partial rotator cuff rupture means that the defect of the tendon is:
    A. less than 10%
    B. 10–20%
    C. 25–50%
    D. 50–75%
    E. 75–90%
71. Choose the correct statement(s) regarding partial supraspinatus tears:
    A. Rim rent is an articular side tear with insertion involvement.
    B. CID is an articular side tear with insertion involvement.
    C. A PASTA tear is a rim rent tear.
    D. A rim rent tear is a PITA tear.
    E. A rim rent tear with intratendinous involvement is called a PAINT tear.
72. What structure is located in the rotator interval?
    A. supraspinatus tendon
    B. long head of the biceps tendon
    C. coracohumeral ligament
    D. infraspinatus tendon
    E. inferior glenohumeral ligament
73. What is the incorrect information regarding the boundaries of the rotator interval?
    A. anterior—subscapularis tendon
    B. roof—coracohumeral ligament
    C. posterior—supraspinatus tendon
    D. medial—rotator cable
    E. anterior—superior glenohumeral ligament
74. What type of glenohumeral instability is the most common?
    A. anterior
    B. posterior
    C. superior
    D. inferior
    E. multidirectional
75. Choose what may cause anterior shoulder instability:
    A. Bankart and bony Bankart lesions
    B. GLAD
    C. HAGL
    D. POLPSA
    E. Kim lesion
76. Bankart lesions:
    A. They often coexist with a Hill-Sachs deformity.
    B. They occur when the humerus compresses the posterior labrum.
    C. They are the most common cause of anterior instability.
    D. If the bony variant is seen, it is present between 3 and 6 o'clock.
    E. Deformation of the labrum may be a sign of a Bankart lesion.

77. What are congenital anomalies that may result in shoulder instability?
    A. shallow glenoid cavity
    B. lateral capsular insertion
    C. increased capsular laxity
    D. increased rotator tendon laxity
    E. increased ligament laxity
78. Choose the correct statement(s) regarding the middle glenohumeral ligament:
    A. Insertion is on the superior aspect of the minor tubercle.
    B. Origin is slightly inferior to the superior glenohumeral ligament.
    C. Runs obliquely, down, and lateral.
    D. It is an essential stabilizer of the shoulder.
    E. It is absent in 50–60% of the population.
79. What ligament runs between the inferior two-thirds of the labrum to the surgical neck of the humerus?
    A. coracohumeral ligament
    B. superior glenohumeral ligament
    C. middle glenohumeral ligament
    D. inferior glenohumeral ligament
    E. transverse humeral ligament
80. What ligament is the most variable?
    A. coracoacromial ligament
    B. superior glenohumeral ligament
    C. middle glenohumeral ligament
    D. inferior glenohumeral ligament
    E. coracohumeral ligament
81. What ligament runs in the same plane as the coracoid process?
    A. coracoacromial ligament
    B. superior glenohumeral ligament
    C. middle glenohumeral ligament
    D. inferior glenohumeral ligament
    E. transverse humeral ligament
82. What ligament is the tautest when the arm is abducted and externally rotated?
    A. superior glenohumeral ligament
    B. middle glenohumeral ligament
    C. anterior limb of the inferior glenohumeral ligament
    D. posterior limb of the inferior glenohumeral ligament
    E. transverse humeral ligament
83. Choose the correct statement(s) regarding a sublabral recess:
    A. It is a defect between the cartilage and labrum.
    B. It is present between "10 and 2 o'clock."
    C. It is at the level of the insertion of the long head of biceps brachii.
    D. It is related to shoulder instability.
    E. It is an asymptomatic labral variant.

84. Choose the correct statement(s) regarding the Buford complex:
    A. It is labrum hypertrophy in the 1–3 o'clock position.
    B. The inferior glenohumeral ligament is often thickened.
    C. The labrum is more round.
    D. The middle glenohumeral ligament is often thickened.
    E. The middle glenohumeral ligament is absent.
85. What is Bennett's lesion regarding the shoulder?
    A. extra-articular posterior capsular avulsion
    B. intra-articular posterior capsular avulsion
    C. extra-articular anterior capsular avulsion
    D. intra-articular anterior capsular avulsion
    E. reverse Bankart lesion
86. What lesions suggest shoulder dislocation?
    A. bony Bankart lesion
    B. Hill-Sachs deformity
    C. reverse Bankart lesion
    D. McLaughlin lesion
    E. thickened articular capsule
87. Choose the variant of the Bankart lesion:
    A. GLAD
    B. HAGL
    C. ALPSA
    D. SLAP
    E. POLPSA
88. What two labral lesions are significantly associated with shoulder instability?
    A. SLAP
    B. Bankart
    C. POLPSA
    D. ALPSA
    E. GLAD
89. Choose the correct statement(s) regarding SLAP lesions:
    A. It occurs when the labrum is interposed between the humeral head and glenoid.
    B. Joint is usually stable in clinical examination.
    C. Intact LHB is the difference between type 2 and 3.
    D. Type 2 is a bucket handle without extension to the LHB.
    E. It occurs in position 10–2 o'clock.
90. What feature is more typical for a sublabral recess rather than a SLAP lesion?
    A. High T2 signal or contrast follows the cartilage.
    B. High T2 signal or contrast is more than 2 mm.
    C. High T2 signal or contrast is visible posterior to the biceps insertion.
    D. High T2 signal or contrast in the labrum is visible as one line.
    E. High T2 signal or contrast is visible in position 11–1 o'clock.

91. Choose the features of frozen shoulder on MRI:
    A. T1-weighted images show lower signal in the subcoracoid space.
    B. Thickening of synovium in the rotator interval.
    C. Medial insertion of the articular capsule.
    D. Thickening of the inferior glenohumeral ligament.
    E. Oedema of the articular capsule.
92. Cyst in the spinoglenoid notch:
    A. is often related to SLAP
    B. may compress the dorsal scapular nerve
    C. is often less than 5 mm
    D. may cause atrophy of the infraspinatus muscle
    E. may cause atrophy of the teres minor muscle
93. Diffuse higher signal on T2-weighted with fat suppression in the supraspinatus, infraspinatus, and deltoid muscles with some atrophy may indicate:
    A. muscle atrophy
    B. quadrilateral space syndrome
    C. compression of the supraspinatus nerve
    D. compression of the infraspinatus nerve
    E. acute idiopathic brachial neuritis
94. What nerve is compressed in quadrilateral space syndrome?
    A. subscapular
    B. axillary
    C. thoracodorsal
    D. dorsal scapular
    E. ulnaris
95. Choose the correct statement(s) regarding ulnar impaction syndrome:
    A. Bone marrow oedema is visible in the entire os lunatum.
    B. Positive ulnar variance is a risk factor.
    C. Subchondral sclerosis in the lunate and triquetrum.
    D. It may be caused by distal radius fracture.
    E. It is related to the TFCC tear.
96. Choose the correct statement(s) regarding TFCC tears:
    A. Ulnar styloid avulsion may cause TFCC tears.
    B. Ulnar-sided pain is a common clinical manifestation.
    C. TFCC perforation is a common finding in patients who are older than 50 years of age.
    D. Most partial injuries are present along the medial part.
    E. MRI arthrography is the imaging tool.

97. The volar plate is located at the level of pulley:
    A. A1
    B. A2
    C. A3
    D. A4
    E. A5
98. Choose the correct statement(s) regarding a wrist ganglion:
    A. Rim contrast enhancement is usually present.
    B. Homogenic low signal on T1-weighted imaging is usually present.
    C. It may be associated with a ligament tear.
    D. Communication with the articular space can be seen.
    E. All ganglia are symptomatic.
99. A 34-year-old patient presented with shoulder pain. MRI was performed (Fig. 2.1). What is your diagnosis?

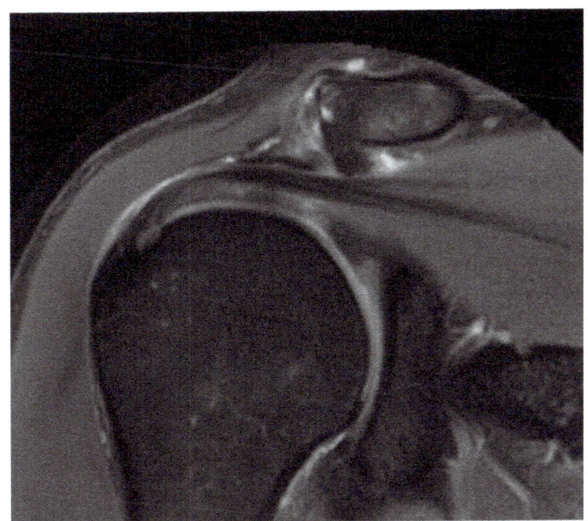

Fig. 2.1 T2-weighted image with fat suppression, the coronal section

    A. pita bread rupture
    B. rim rent rupture
    C. reverse PASTA
    D. PASTA
    E. PAINT

100. A 54-year-old patient presented with chronic shoulder pain. MRI was done (Fig. 2.2). Choose the correct statement(s) regarding the lesion seen on MRI:

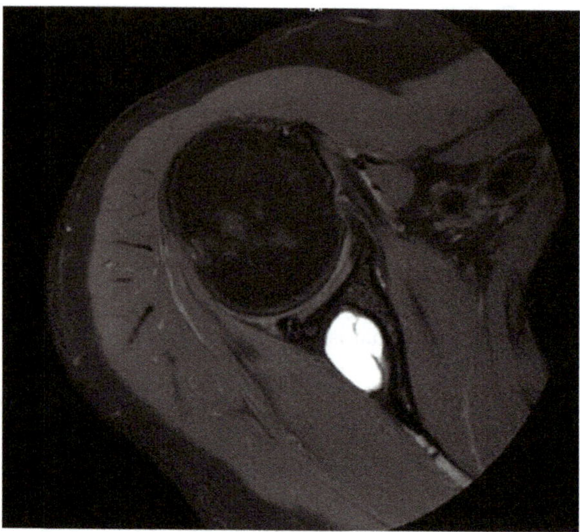

Fig. 2.2 Proton density image with fat suppression, the axial section

A. It is associated with SLAP.
B. It may compress the dorsal scapular nerve.
C. Infraspinatus atrophy may be seen.
D. Posterior shoulder tenderness can occur.
E. Contrast injection is indicated because a defect in the scapula is seen.

101. Patient presented after shoulder trauma during a basketball match. Choose the correct statement(s) regarding the MRI, which was performed 3 weeks after trauma (Fig. 2.3a–e):

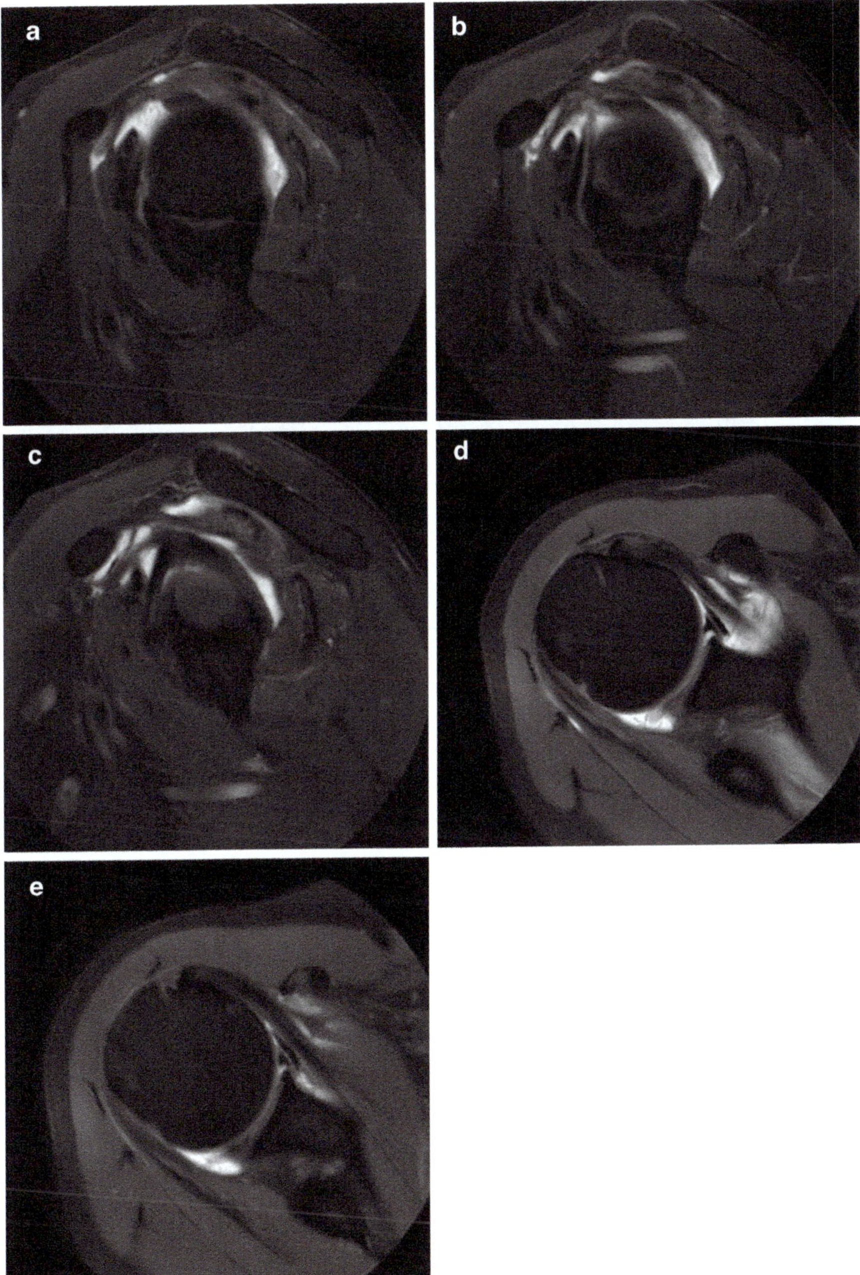

Fig. 2.3 (**a**–**c**) T2-weighted images with fat suppression, coronal sections; (**d**, **e**) proton density-weighted image with fat suppression, axial sections

A. There is a soft tissue Bankart lesion.
B. There is a Buford complex.
C. High insertion of the inferior glenohumeral ligament is seen.
D. Joint effusion is seen.
E. Joint synovitis is visible.

102. A 69-year-old patient presented with chronic shoulder pain. MRI was performed (Fig. 2.4a–c). Choose the correct statement(s) regarding this patient:

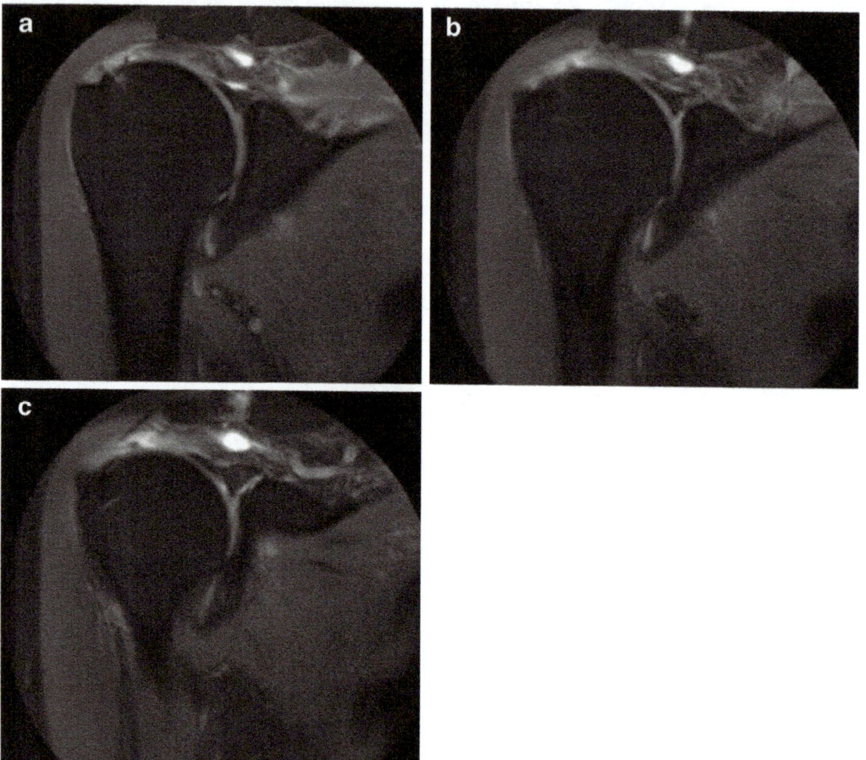

Fig. 2.4 (**a**–**c**) T2-weighted images with fat suppression, coronal sections

A. Total rupture of the supraspinatus is visible.
B. Partial rupture of the supraspinatus is visible.
C. The supraspinatus is normal.
D. SLAP is visible.
E. The labrum is intact.

103. A 56-year-old patient presented with shoulder pain. MRI was performed (Fig. 2.5a–c). What is the correct statement regarding MRI?

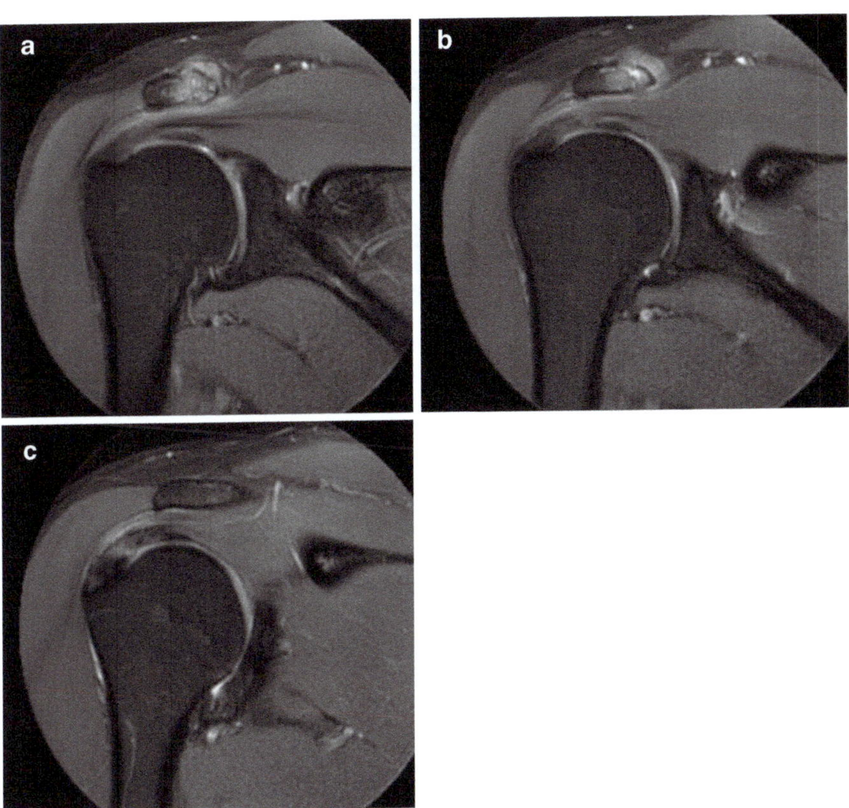

Fig. 2.5 (**a–c**) T2-weighted images with fat suppression, coronal sections

A. total supraspinatus rupture
B. supraspinatus tendinopathy
C. enthesitis of the supraspinatus
D. bursal side rupture of supraspinatus
E. articular side rupture of supraspinatus

104. A 56-year-old patient presented with shoulder pain. MRI was performed (Fig. 2.6a–d). Choose the correct statement(s) regarding this patient:

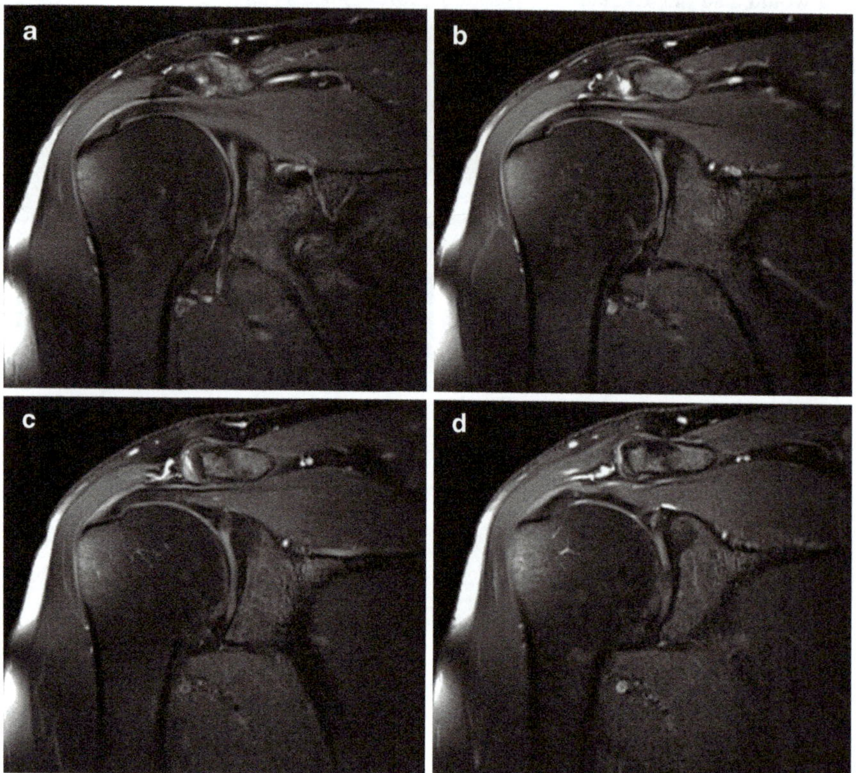

Fig. 2.6 (**a–d**) Proton density-weighted images with fat suppression, coronal sections

A. Supraspinatus total rupture.
B. Supraspinatus partial rupture.
C. Supraspinatus tendinopathy.
D. Labrum is normal.
E. SLAP is visible.

105. A 34-year-old patient presented with shoulder pain and limitation of abduction. MRI was done (Fig. 2.7a–e). Choose the correct statement(s) regarding this patient:

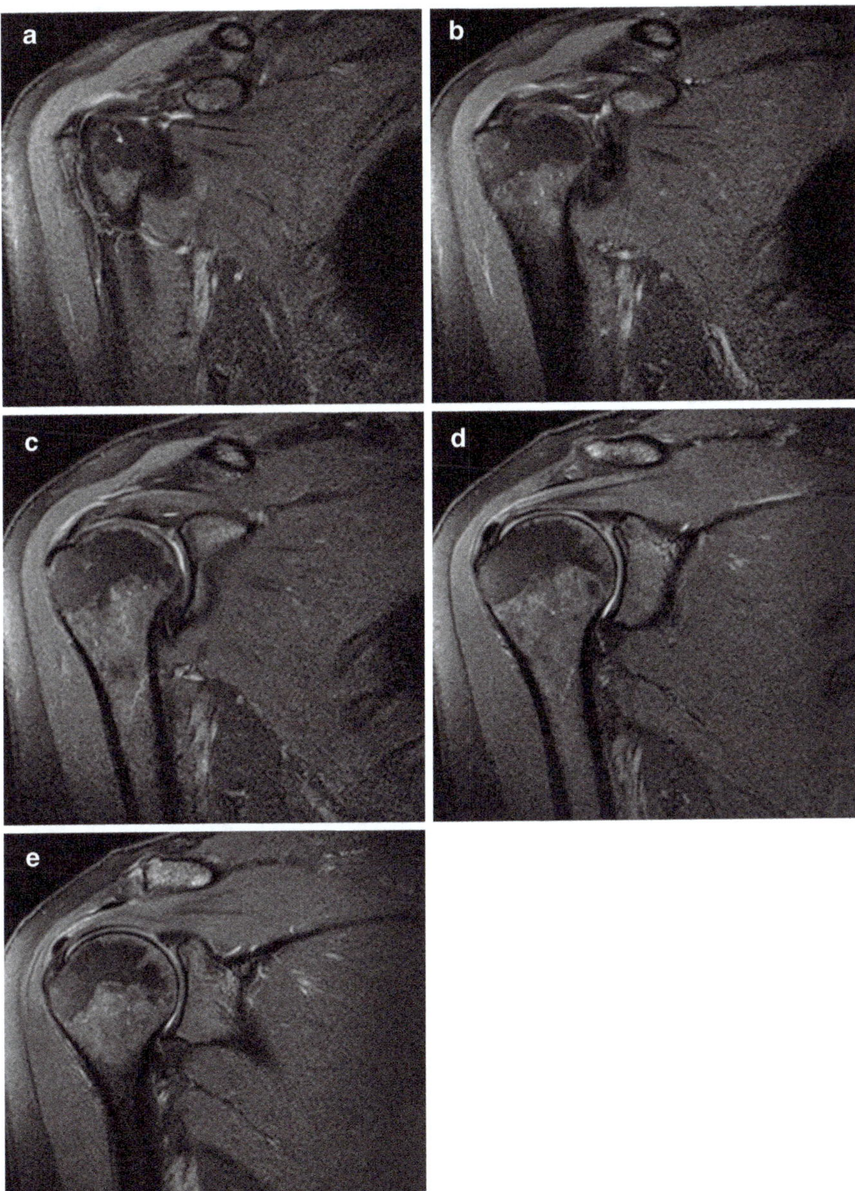

Fig. 2.7 (**a**–**e**) Proton density-weighted images with fat suppression, coronal sections

A. Supraspinatus showed PASTA rupture.
B. Supraspinatus showed rim rent rupture.
C. Supraspinatus showed calcific tendinopathy.
D. Supraspinatus is normal.
E. SLAP is visible.

106. Choose the correct statement(s) regarding the MRI (Fig. 2.8a, b):

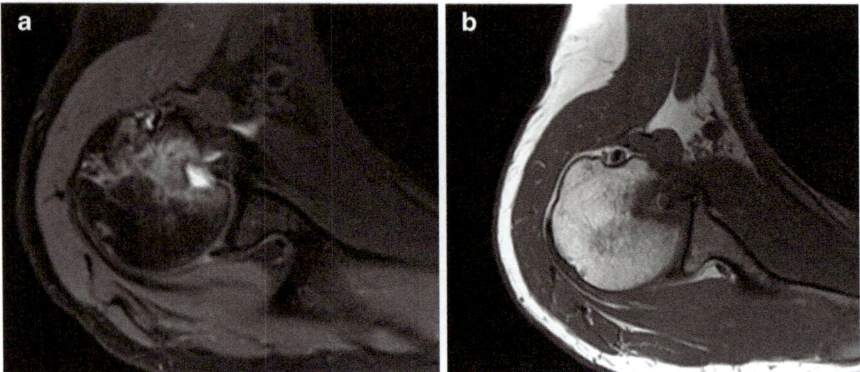

Fig. 2.8 (**a**) Proton density-weighted images with fat suppression, axial section; (**b**) T1-weighted axial section

A. Intraosseous ganglion in caput humeri.
B. McLaughlin lesion is seen.
C. Reverse Hill-Sachs deformity.
D. Hill-Sachs deformity.
E. Hatchet sign is visible.

107. Choose the correct statement(s) regarding the MRI (Fig. 2.9):

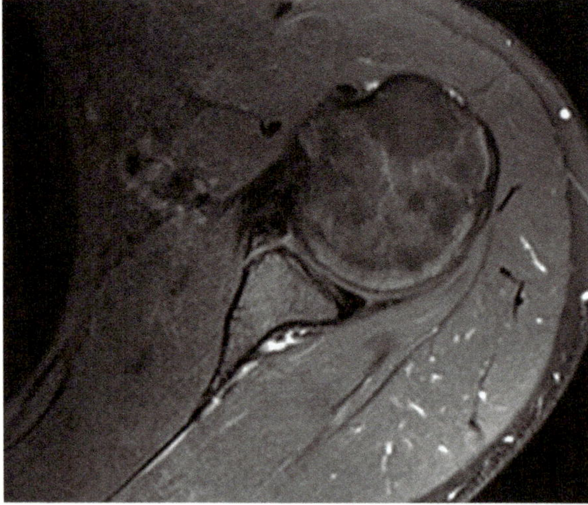

Fig. 2.9 Proton density image with fat suppression, axial section

A. Acute bony Bankart lesion.
B. Chronic bony Bankart lesion.
C. Acute soft tissue Bankart lesion.
D. Chronic soft tissue Bankart lesion.
E. Glenoid cavity is normal.

108. A 45-year-old patient presented with diffuse shoulder pain. MRI was performed (Fig. 2.10). Choose the correct statement(s) regarding the deltoid muscle:

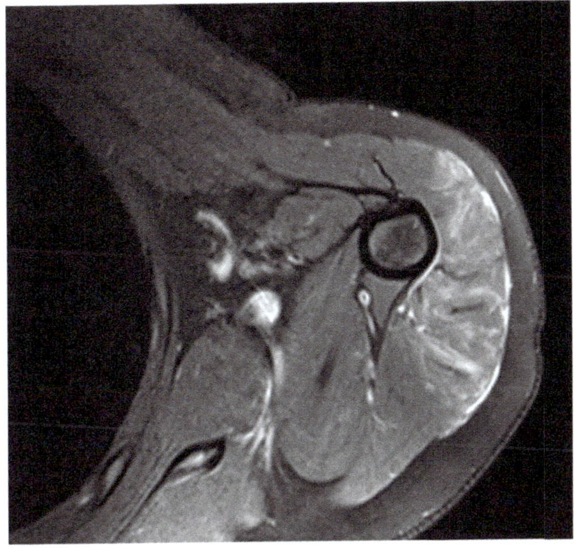

Fig. 2.10 Proton density image with fat suppression, axial section

A. Infectious myositis.
B. Muscle contusion.
C. It is sign of neuritis.
D. Myotendinous junction rupture.
E. Probable axillary nerve injury.

109. A 71-year-old patient presented with chronic shoulder pain. MRI was performed (Fig. 2.11a–e). Choose the correct statement(s) regarding this patient:

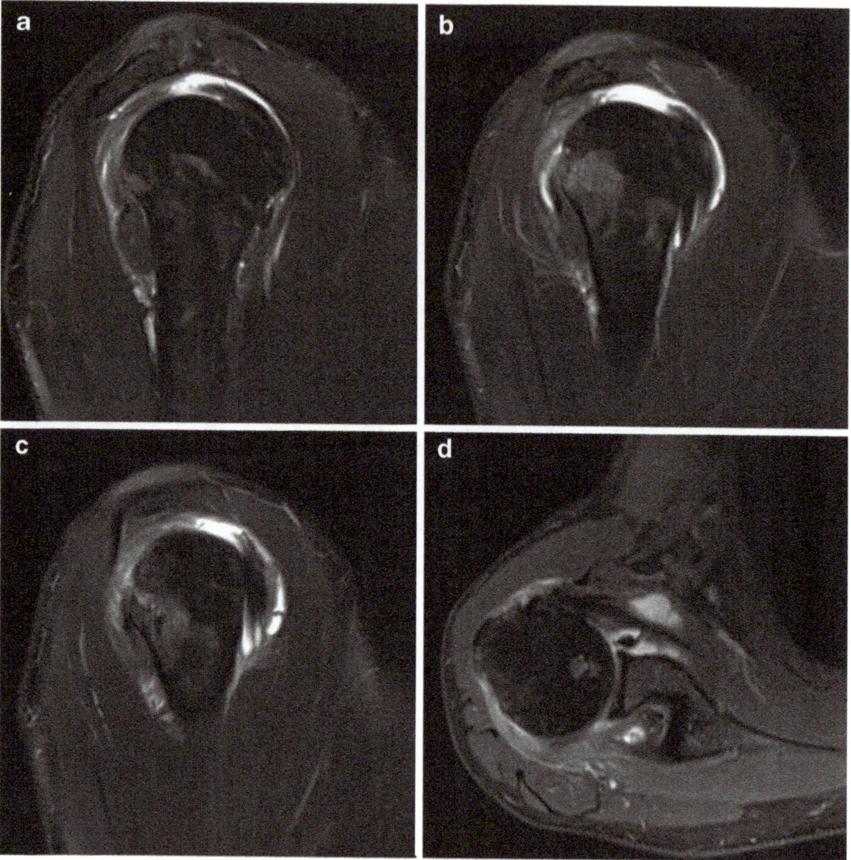

Fig. 2.11 (**a–c**) Proton density-weighted images with fat suppression, sagittal section; (**d**) axial section proton density-weighted image

A. supraspinatus total rupture
B. infraspinatus total rupture
C. subscapularis total rupture
D. teres minor total rupture
E. massive rotator cuff tear

110. The MRI of the patient from the previous question showed a lesion in the infraspinatus (Fig. 2.12a–d). Choose the correct statement(s) regarding this lesion:

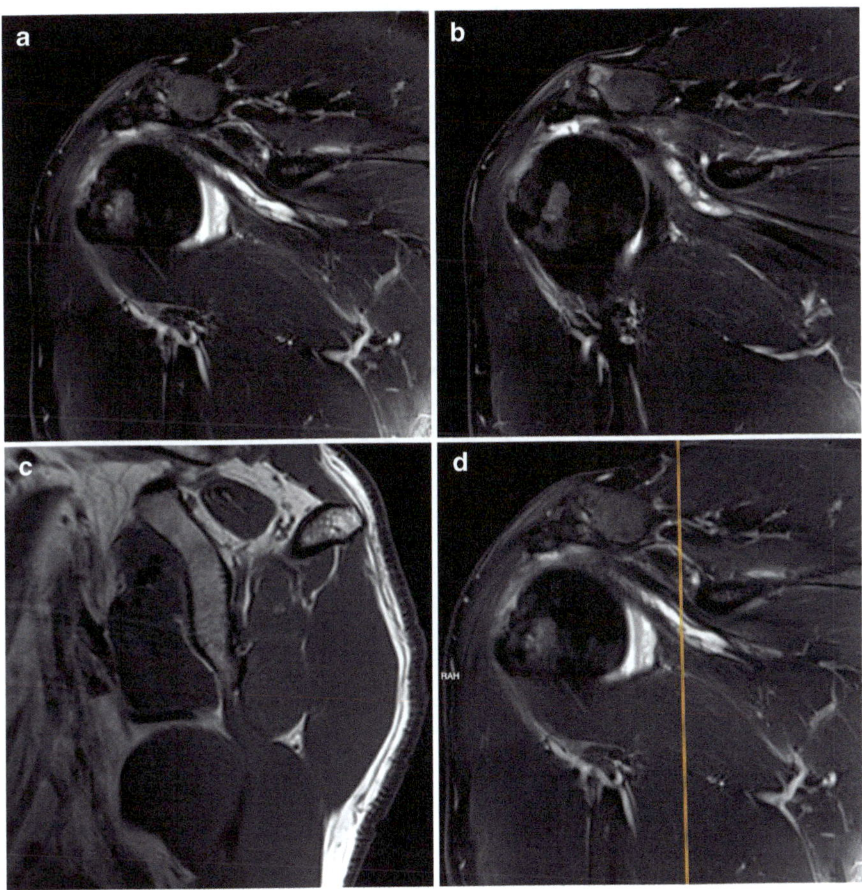

Fig. 2.12 (**a**, **b**, **d**) Proton density-weighted images with fat suppression, sagittal section; (**c**) T1-weighted image sagittal section

A. It is an unclear lesion, probably malignant.
B. It probably has a myxomatous component.
C. It is benign, no further diagnostic testing is needed.
D. It may be sign of chronic myotendinous trauma.
E. It is haematoma, which is related to acute trauma.

111. Considering the same patient from the previous question (Fig. 2.13a–e), choose the correct statement(s) regarding the long head of the biceps brachii:

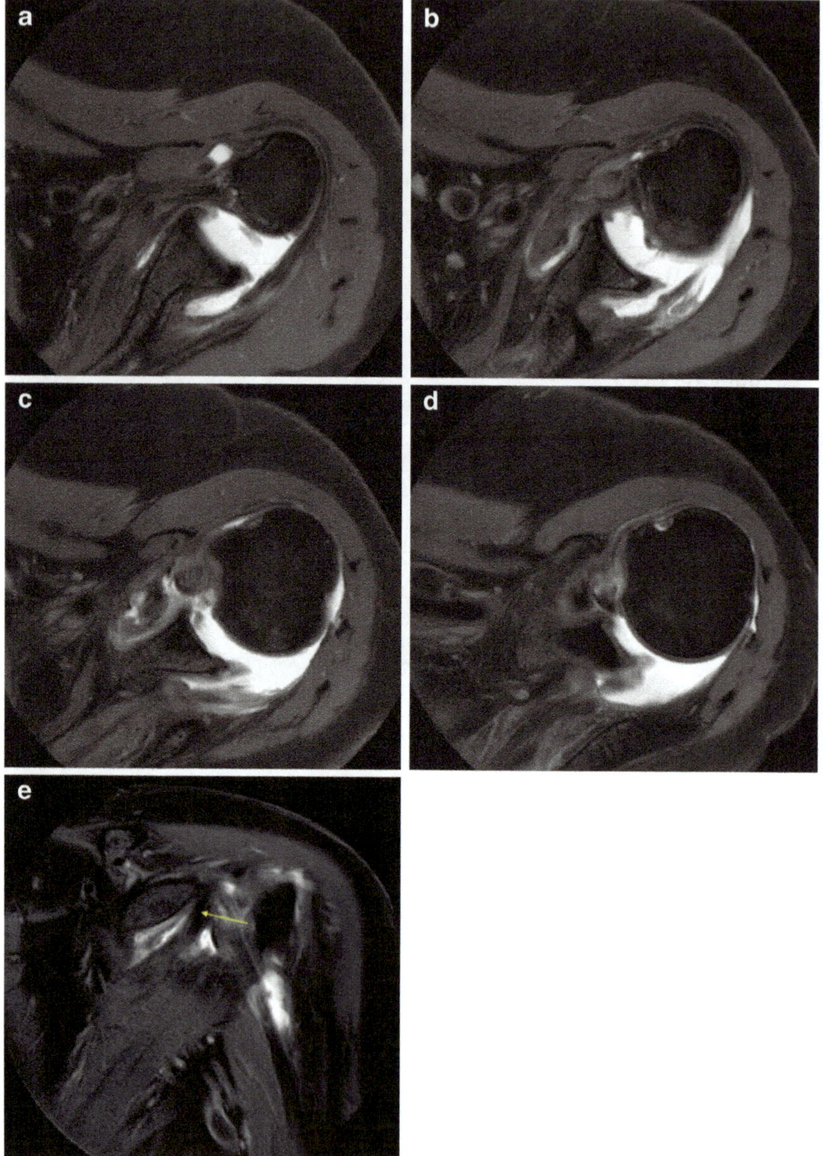

Fig. 2.13 (**a–d**) Proton density-weighted images with fat suppression, axial sections. (**e**) T2-weighted image with fat suppression, coronal section

A. Total rupture is visible.
B. Medial luxation is seen.
C. Tendinopathy is present.
D. Split rupture is visible.
E. Accessory biceps tendon is present.

112. What structure is shown by the arrow in Fig. 2.13e?
    A. the coracohumeral ligament
    B. the long head of biceps tendon
    C. the middle glenohumeral ligament
    D. the superior glenohumeral ligament
    E. the superior part of the subscapularis tendon
113. A 56-year-old patient who works on a construction site presented with shoulder pain for 3 months. MRI was performed (Fig. 2.14a–e). Choose the correct statement(s) regarding this patient:

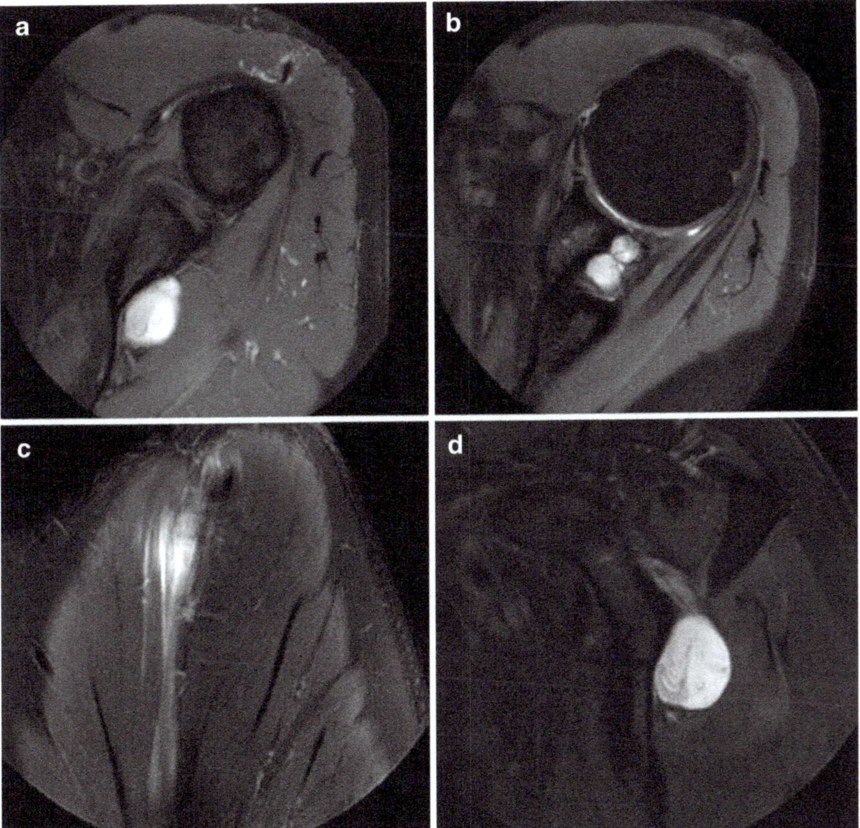

Fig. 2.14 (**a**, **b**) Proton density-weighted image with fat suppression, axial sections. (**c**, **d**) T2-weighted image with fat suppression, sagittal sections

A. A spinoglenoid notch ganglion is probably compressing the suprascapular nerve.
B. A spinoglenoid notch ganglion is present; however, there is no sign that it is compressing the suprascapular nerve.
C. There is abnormal signal in the deltoid muscle, which is related to nerve compression by a spinoglenoid notch ganglion.
D. The lesion in the infraspinatus tendon is related to a spinoglenoid notch ganglion, while the lesion in the deltoid muscle is probably related to chronic trauma.
E. The lesion in the deltoid tendon is related to a spinoglenoid notch ganglion, while the lesion in the infraspinatus muscle is probably related to chronic trauma.

114. What is the most likely diagnosis based on MRI in a patient with shoulder pain without trauma (Fig. 2.15)?

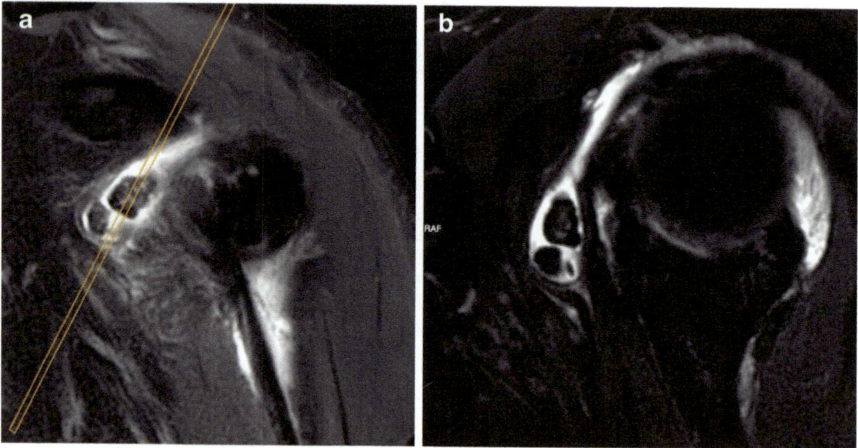

Fig. 2.15 (**a** and **b**) T2-weighted image with fat suppression, oblique sagittal section

A. scarring
B. siderotic synovitis
C. synovial chondromatosis
D. pigmented villonodular synovitis
E. frozen shoulder (capsulitis adhesiva)

115. What structure is labelled with the arrow in Fig. 2.16? What is a part of the MRI from the patient in the previous question?

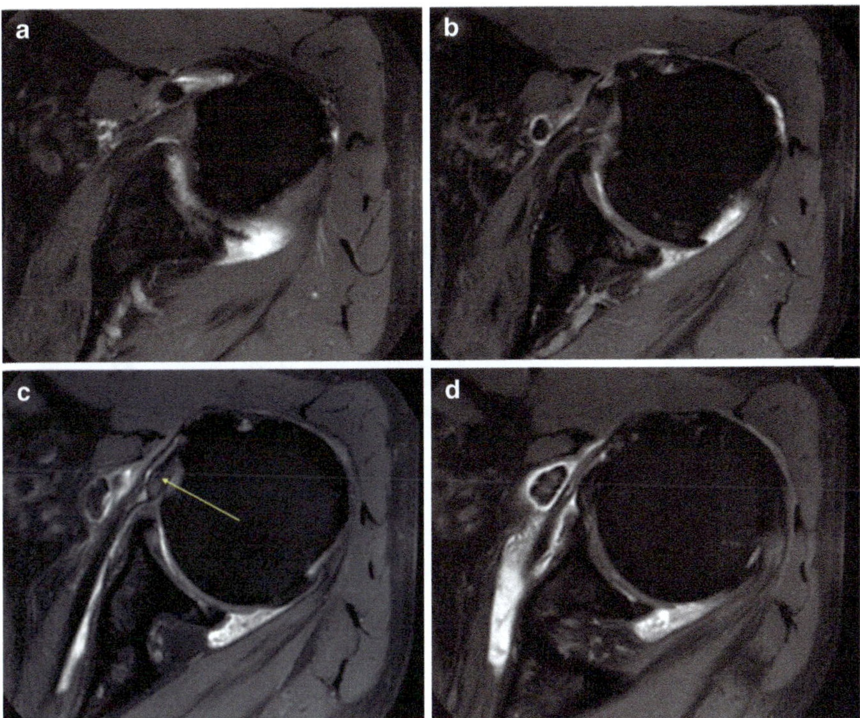

Fig. 2.16 (**a**–**d**) Proton density-weighted image with fat suppression, axial sections

A. synovial chondromatosis
B. the subscapularis tendon
C. the middle glenohumeral ligament
D. the superior glenohumeral ligament
E. the long head of the biceps brachii tendon

116. A 31-year-old patient who had several anterior shoulder dislocations presented with shoulder pain. Choose the correct statement(s) regarding this patient (Fig. 2.17):

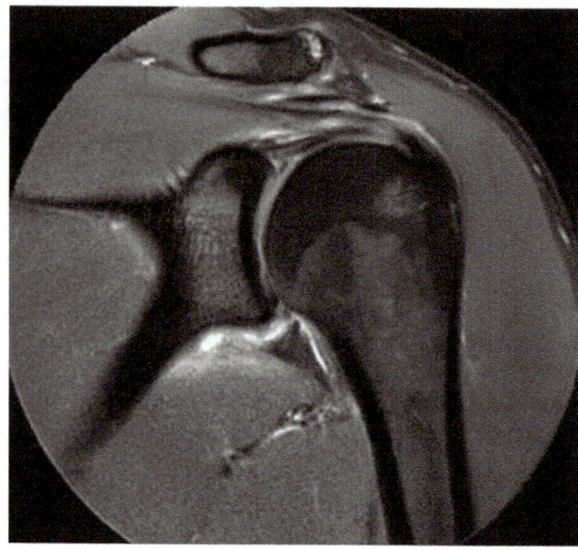

Fig. 2.17 T2-weighted image with fat suppression, coronal section

A. HAGL is seen.
B. GAGL is seen.
C. J sign is seen.
D. Supraspinatus tear.
E. abnormal signal of bone marrow in the proximal humerus.

117. What other lesion may be associated with this presented in the patient from the previous question?
    A. Bankart lesion
    B. subscapularis tear
    C. Hill-Sachs deformity
    D. reverse Hill-Sachs deformity
    E. anterior labroligamentous periosteal sleeve avulsion
118. What lesions are visible on the other MRI scans (Fig. 2.18a, b) of the patient from the previous question?

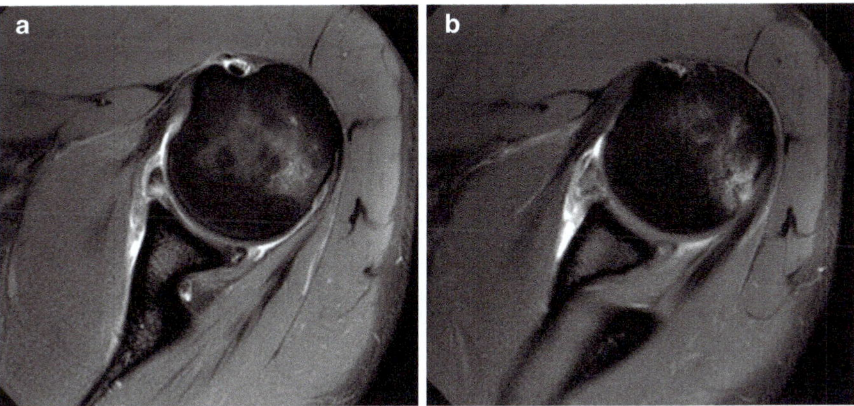

Fig. 2.18 (**a** and **b**) Proton density image with fat suppression, axial sections

A. The anterior articular capsule is abnormal.
B. Both the anterior and posterior labrum are torn.
C. Neither the anterior nor posterior labrum is torn.
D. The anterior labrum is torn, while the posterior labrum is intact.
E. The posterior labrum is torn, while the anterior labrum is intact.

119. What structure is shown by the arrow in Fig. 2.19 in this patient with chronic shoulder pain?

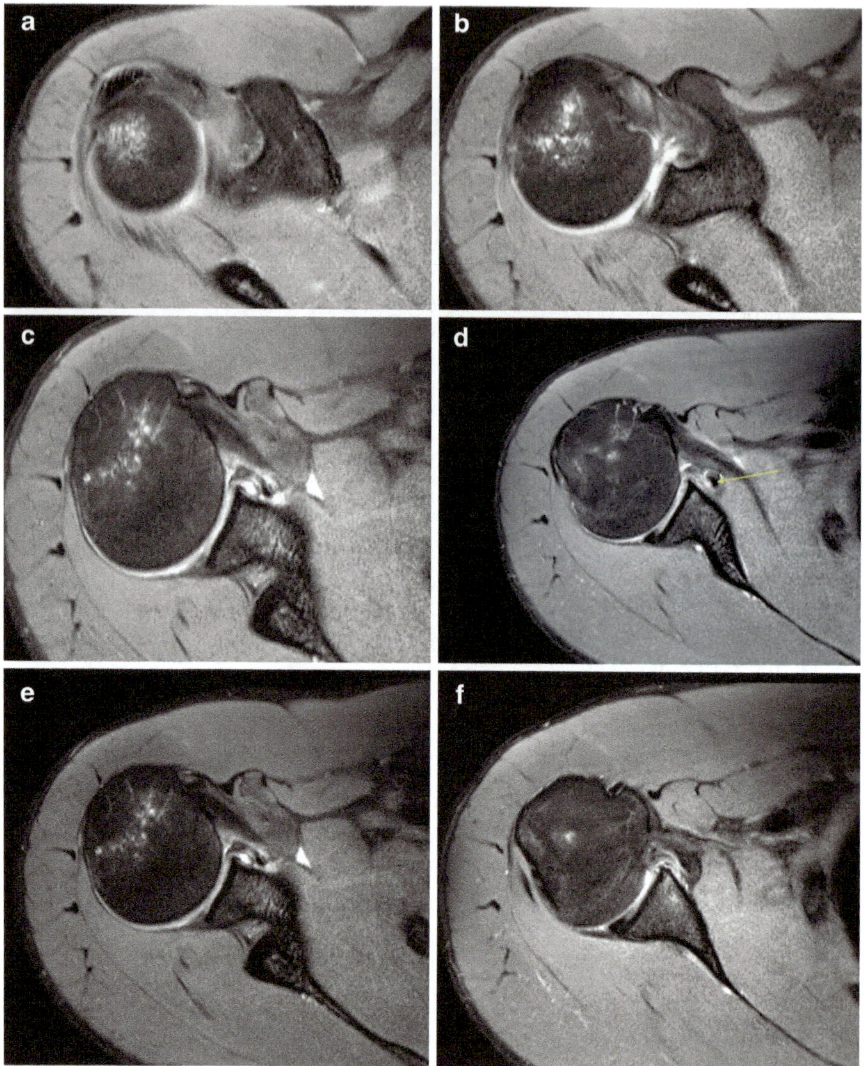

Fig. 2.19 (**a–f**) Proton density image with fat suppression, axial sections

A. free body
B. SGHL
C. MGHL
D. detached labrum
E. the long head of the biceps brachii

120. Choose the correct statement(s) regarding the patient from the previous question (Fig. 2.19):
    A. The rotator cable is intact.
    B. Both the anterior and posterior labrum are intact.
    C. Both the anterior and posterior labrum are torn.
    D. The anterior labrum is torn, while the posterior labrum is intact.
    E. The posterior labrum is torn, while the anterior labrum is intact.
121. A 45-year-old patient fell from a height of about 3 m. Now, the patient has pain and an abduction deficit. X-ray did not show any fracture or dislocation. MRI was done (Fig. 2.20a–f). Choose the correct statement(s) regarding MRI:
    A. Total rupture of the supraspinatus in the anterior part is seen.
    B. Partial bursa side rupture of the supraspinatus is seen.
    C. Articular side rupture of the supraspinatus is seen.
    D. Non-displaced fracture is seen.
    E. No fracture is seen.
122. What is the name of the structure marked with arrow 1 (Fig. 2.20)?
    A. brachialis muscle
    B. coracobrachialis muscle
    C. the short head of the biceps brachii
    D. the long head of the biceps brachii
    E. the long head of the triceps brachii
123. What is the name of the structure marked with arrow 2 (Fig. 2.20)?

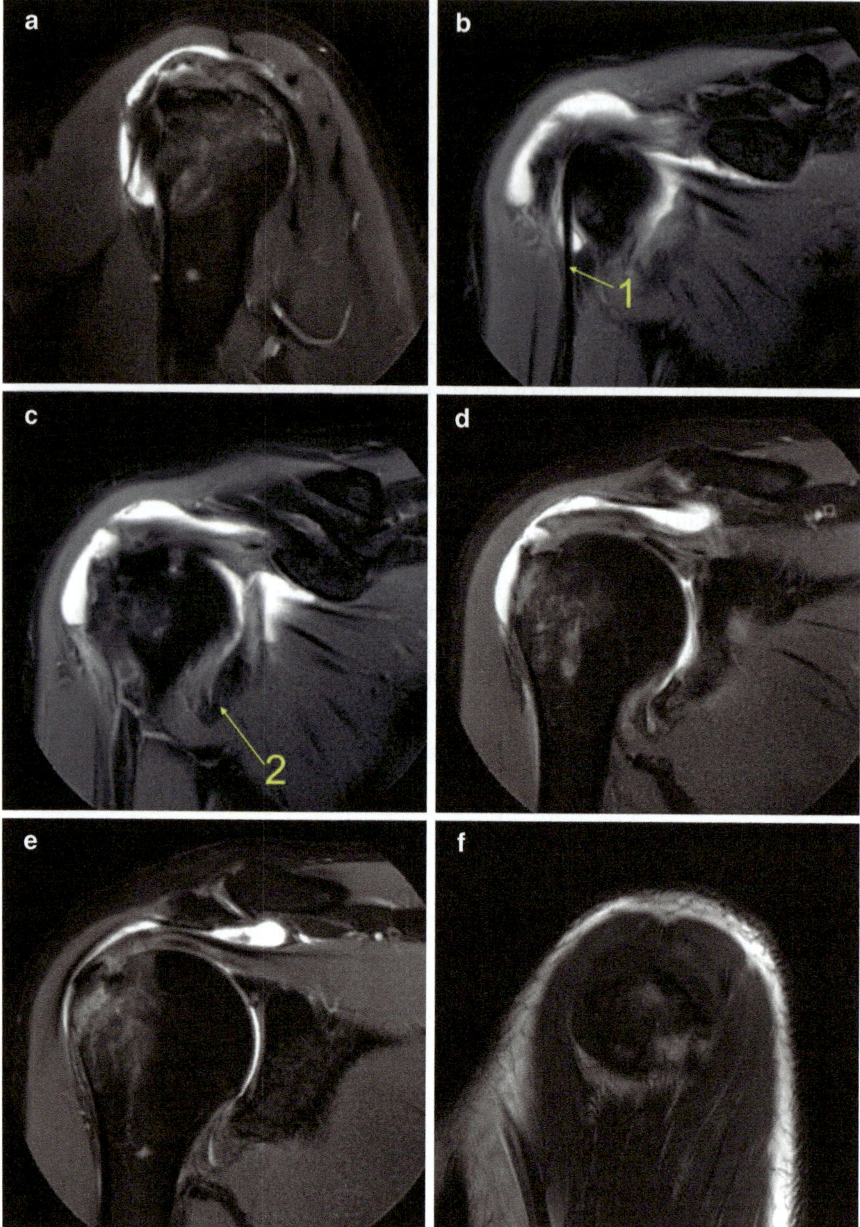

Fig. 2.20 (**a**) T2-weighted image with fat suppression, sagittal section; (**b–e**) T2-weighted images with fat suppression, coronal sections; (**f**) T1-weighted image, sagittal section

A. the long head of the biceps brachii
B. inferior glenohumeral ligament
C. middle glenohumeral ligament
D. subscapularis tendon
E. labrum

124. A 39-year-old patient fell off a bicycle and presents with arm pain and movement deficits. X-ray was done (Fig. 2.21). Choose the correct statement(s) regarding this patient:

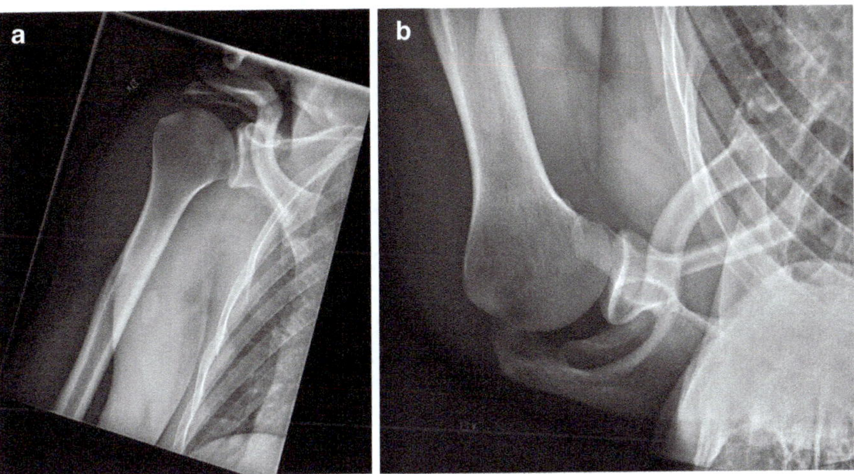

Fig. 2.21 X-ray of the shoulder, (**a**) the frontal projection, (**b**) the axial projection

A. Suspicion of non-displaced fracture of the tuberculum majus is seen.
B. Suspicion of non-displaced fracture of the surgical neck is seen.
C. Suspicion of osteonecrosis of the humeral neck is seen.
D. A Hill-Sachs deformity is seen.
E. A bony Bankart lesion is seen.

125. The patient from the previous question was referred for MRI. Choose the correct statement(s) regarding the MRI (Fig. 2.22a, b):

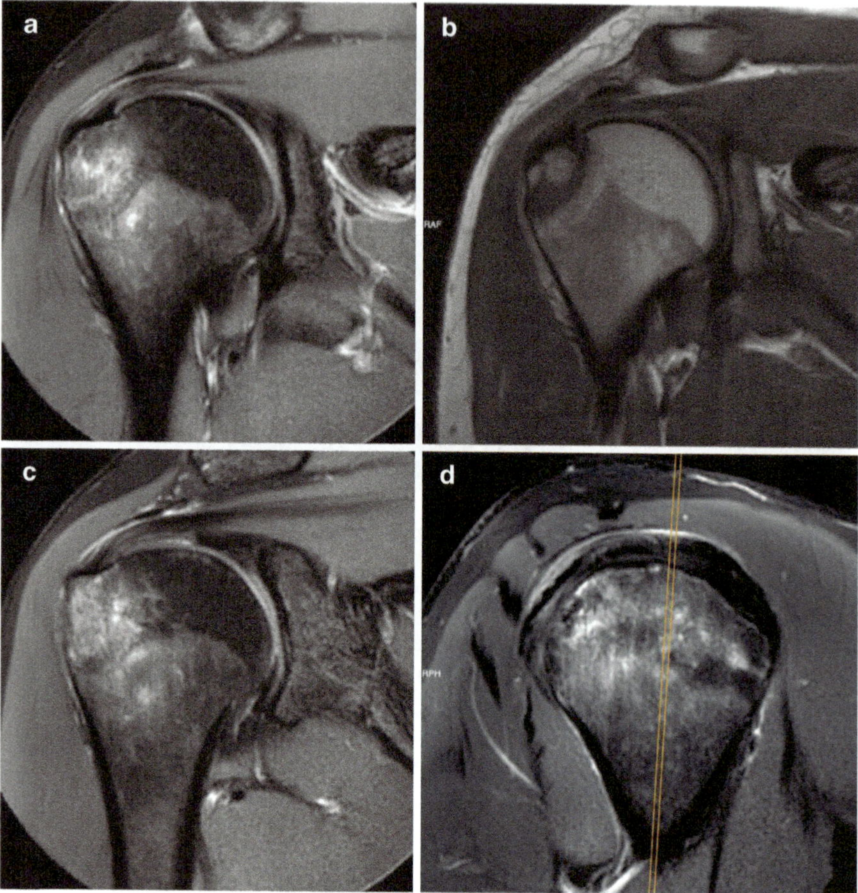

Fig. 2.22 (**a** and **c**) T2-weighted images with fat suppression, coronal sections; (**b**) T1-weighted image, coronal section; (**d**) T2-weighted image with fat suppression, sagittal section

A. MRI confirms the fracture of the tuberculum majus.
B. MRI confirms the fracture of the surgical neck.
C. MRI confirms osteonecrosis of the humeral neck.
D. MRI shows a partial tear of the supraspinatus tendon.
E. MRI shows SLAP.

126. A 52-year-old patient fell off a bicycle. Now, the patient is unable to move his arm. X-ray was done (Fig. 2.23). What is true regarding this patient?

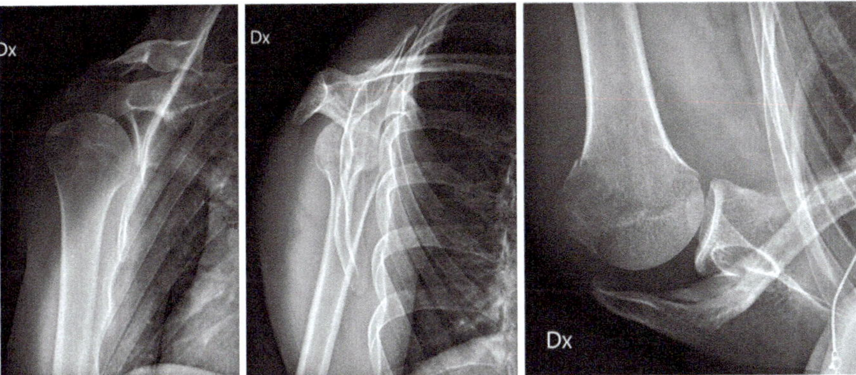

Fig. 2.23 X-ray of the shoulder

A. anatomical neck fracture
B. greater tubercle fracture
C. corpus humeri fracture
D. surgical neck fracture
E. clavicle fracture

127. A 65-year-old patient presented after trauma. X-ray was performed (Fig. 2.24). Choose the correct statement(s) regarding this patient:

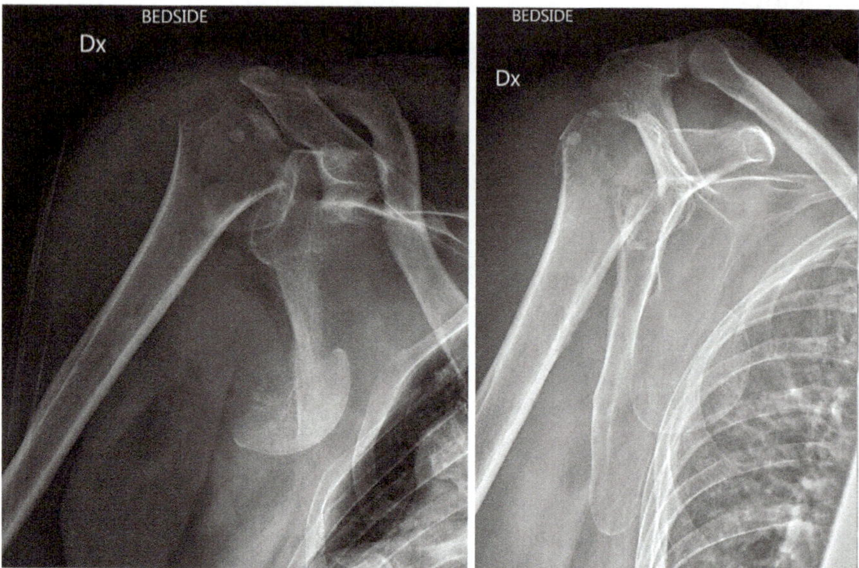

Fig. 2.24 X-ray of the shoulder

A. anatomical neck fracture
B. greater tubercle fracture
C. corpus humeri fracture
D. surgical neck fracture
E. clavicle fracture

128. The patient from the previous question got a prosthesis. Choose the correct statement(s) regarding X-ray (Fig. 2.25):

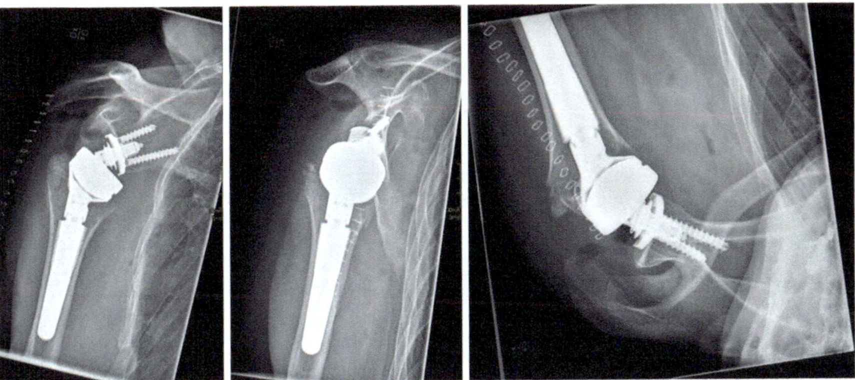

Fig. 2.25 X-ray of the shoulder

A. Irregular regions of radiolucency at the cement-bone interface.
B. Inferior scapular notching is seen.
C. Malpositioning of the prosthesis.
D. Periprosthetic fracture is seen.
E. It is normal.

129. A 32-year-old patient presented after trauma. X-ray and MRI (Fig. 2.26) were done. Choose the correct statement(s):

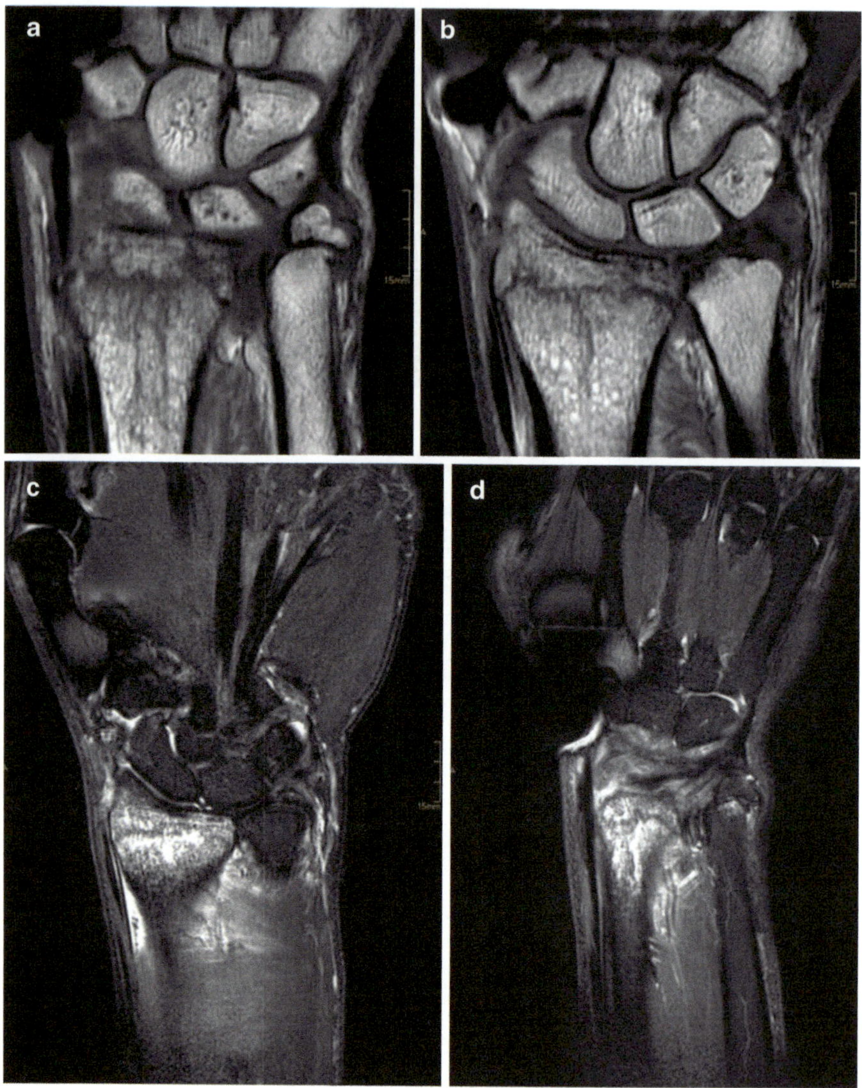

Fig. 2.26 (**a** and **b**) T1-weighted images, coronal sections; (**c** and **d**) proton density-weighted images, coronal sections

A. Distal radial fracture is acute, while ulnar styloid process fracture is chronic.
B. Ulnar styloid process fracture is acute, while the distal radial fracture is chronic.
C. Both the ulnar styloid process fracture and distal radial fracture are acute.
D. Both the ulnar styloid process fracture and distal radial fracture are chronic.
E. Intra-articular involvement of the radius is visible.

130. The patient fell on his outstretched hand about 4 weeks ago. MRI was performed (Fig. 2.27). Choose the correct statement(s) regarding MRI:

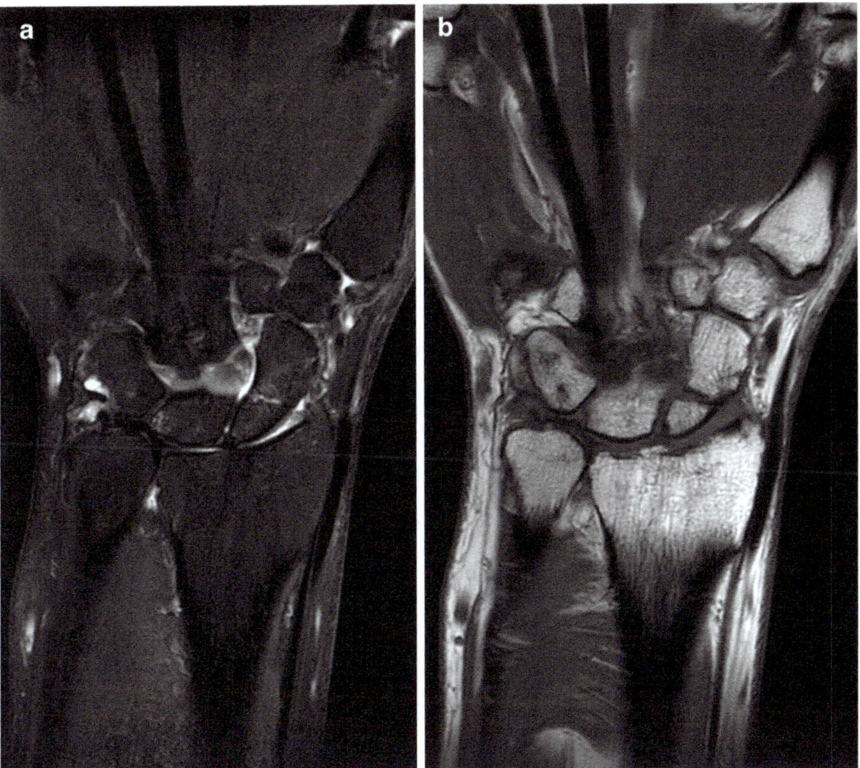

Fig. 2.27 (**a**) Proton density-weighted image with fat suppression, coronal section; (**b**) T1-weighted image, coronal section

A. It is a chronic scaphoid fracture without osteonecrosis.
B. It is a chronic scaphoid fracture with osteonecrosis.
C. It is an acute scaphoid fracture without osteonecrosis.
D. It is an acute scaphoid fracture with osteonecrosis.
E. No scaphoid fracture is seen.

131. A patient presented with wrist pain following a fall on the hand. Choose the correct statement(s) regarding X-ray (Fig. 2.28):

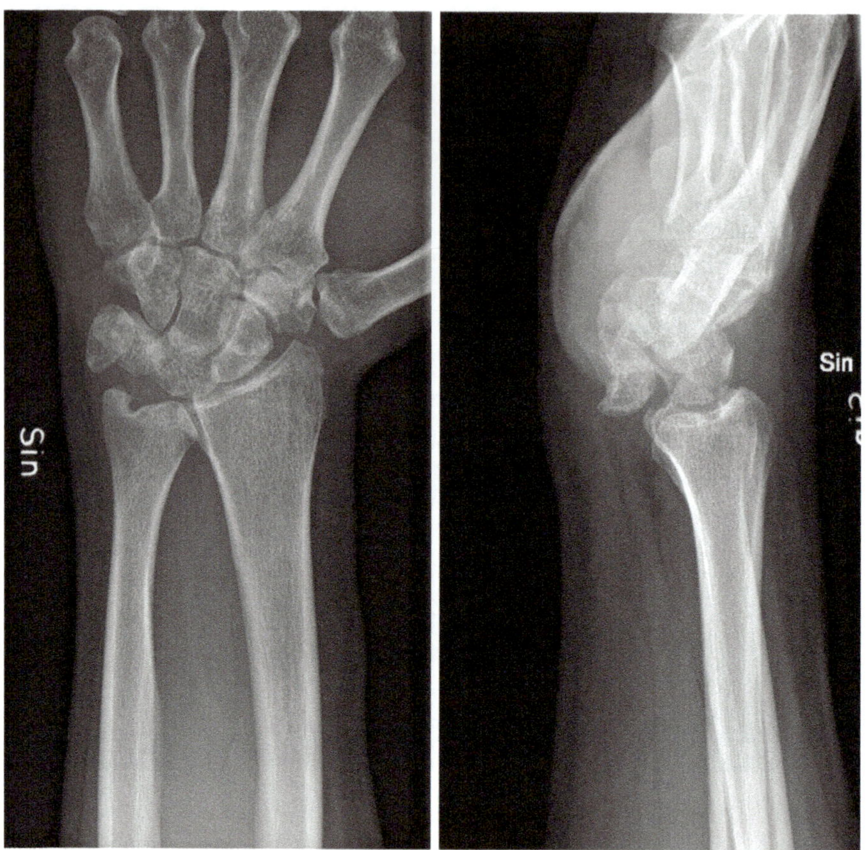

Fig. 2.28 X-ray of the wrist

A. lunate fracture
B. lunate dislocation
C. scaphoid fracture
D. triquetrum fracture
E. perilunate dislocation

132. A 39-year-old patient presented with chronic wrist pain. X-ray was done (Fig. 2.29). Choose the correct statement(s) regarding the X-ray:

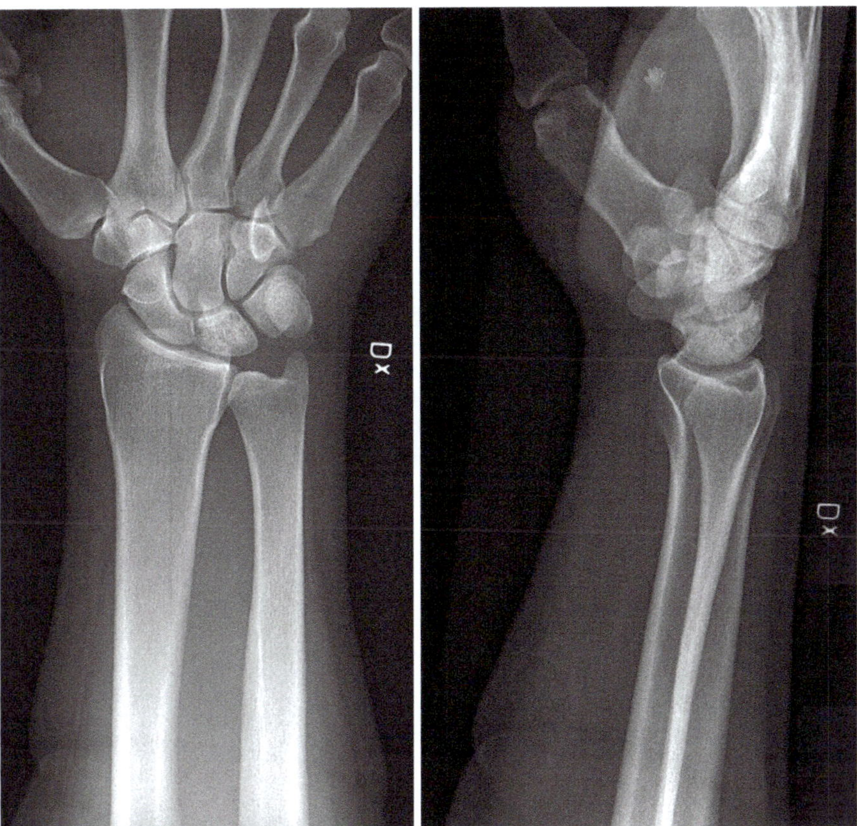

Fig. 2.29 X-ray of the wrist

A. lunatomalacia
B. scaphoid fracture
C. perilunate dislocation
D. ulnar impaction syndrome
E. scaphoid avascular necrosis

133. With regard to the patient from the previous question, MRI was done (Fig. 2.30). Choose the correct statement(s) regarding this patient:

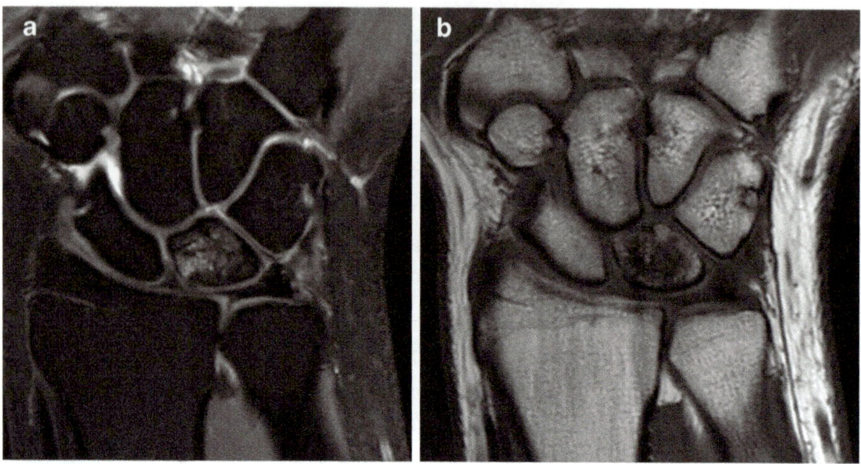

Fig. 2.30 (**a**) Proton density-weighted image with fat suppression, coronal section; (**b**) T1-weighted image coronal section

A. lunatomalacia
B. lunatum fracture
C. scapholunate dislocation
D. ulnar impaction syndrome
E. avascular necrosis of the lunate bone

134. A 43-year-old patient presented with chronic wrist pain. MRI was performed (Fig. 2.31). Choose the correct statement(s) regarding this patient:

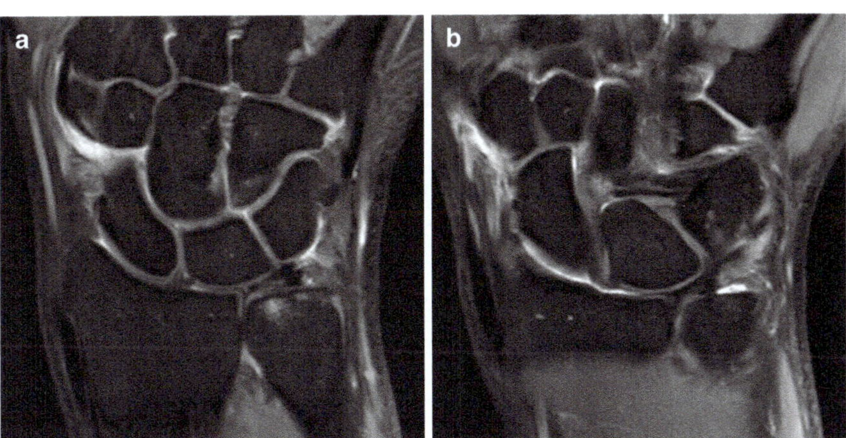

Fig. 2.31 (**a** and **b**) Proton density-weighted image with fat suppression, coronal sections

A. ulnar impaction syndrome
B. caput ulnae fracture
C. triangular fibrocartilage tear
D. avascular necrosis of the scaphoid bone
E. avascular necrosis of the lunate bone

135. A 54-year-old patient presented with chronic wrist pain. MRI was done (Fig. 2.32). Choose the correct statement(s) regarding this patient:

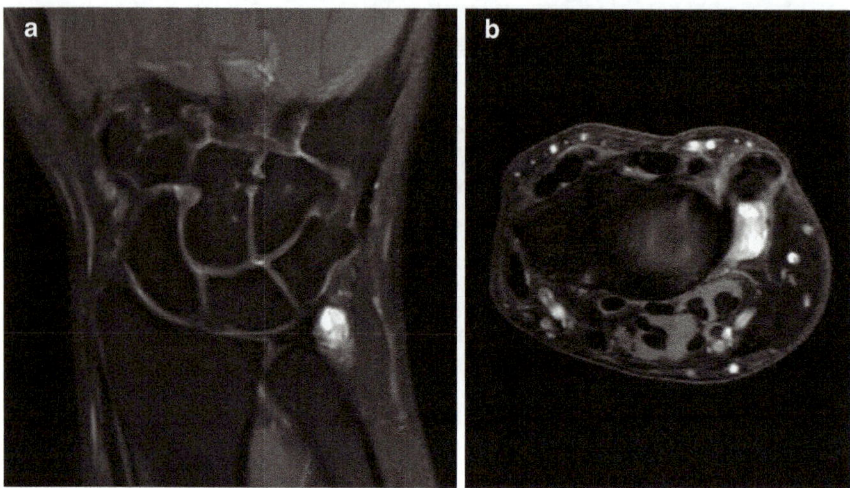

Fig. 2.32 (**a**) Proton density-weighted image with fat suppression, coronal section; (**b**) T2-weighted image with fat suppression

A. Ulnar nerve is compressed.
B. Ulnar extensor tendon is dislocated.
C. There is no sign of a complex tear of the triangular fibrocartilage complex.
D. There is an indirect sign of a complex tear of the triangular fibrocartilage complex.
E. Rupture of the radial insertion of the triangular fibrocartilage complex.

136. A 67-year-old patient presented with wrist pain. MRI was performed (Fig. 2.33). Choose in what sector or sectors can you see the abnormality?

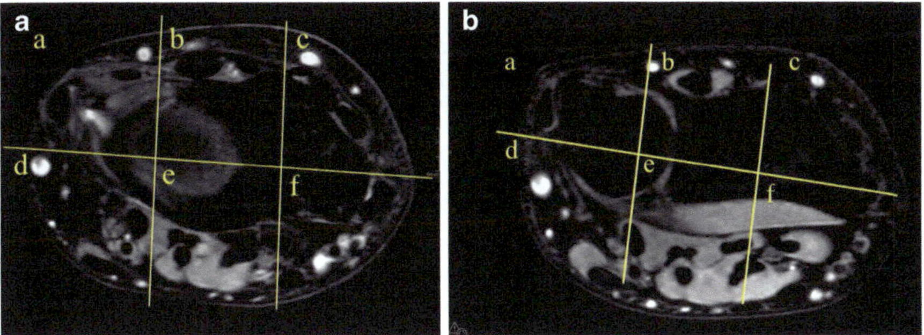

Fig. 2.33 (**a** and **b**) T2-weighted images with fat suppression, axial sections

A. a
B. b and c
C. a and c
D. d, e, and f
E. b

137. A 31-year-old patient presented with wrist pain of 5 weeks duration. MRI was performed (Fig. 2.34). Choose the correct statement(s) regarding this patient:

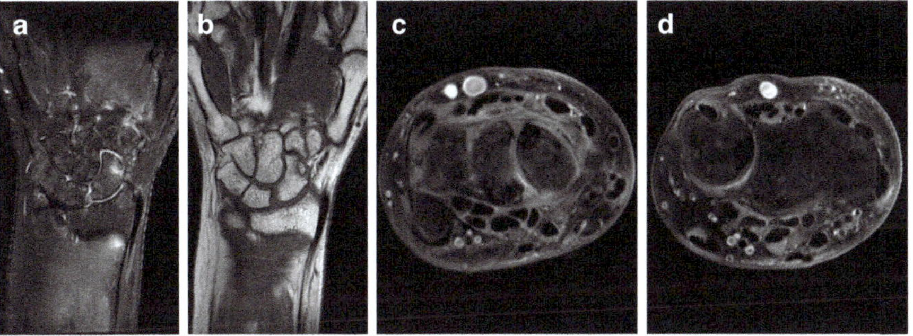

Fig. 2.34 (**a**) Proton density weighted with fat suppression, coronal section; (**b**) T1-weighted, coronal section; (**c** and **d**) T2-weighted image with fat suppression, axial sections

A. Kienböck disease
B. inactive osteopenia
C. scapholunate ligament rupture
D. fracture of the scaphoid tuberculum
E. incomplete split rupture of the extensor carpi ulnaris

138. A 49-year-old patient presented after the grand mal seizure. X-ray was performed (Fig. 2.35). Choose the correct statement(s) regarding this patient

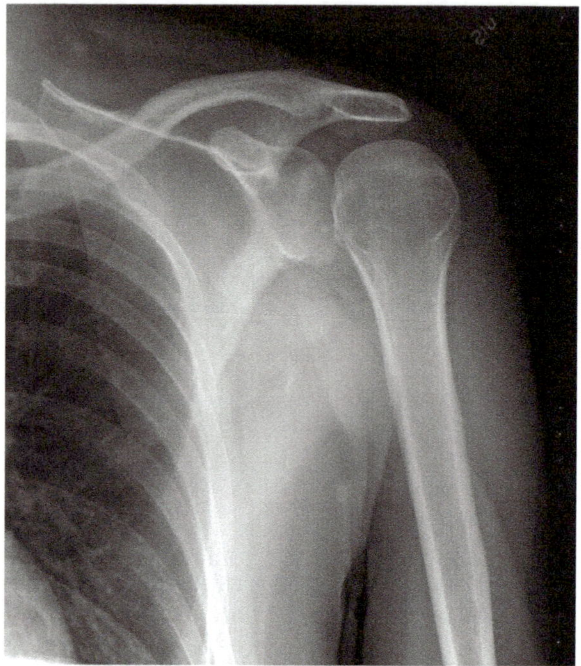

Fig. 2.35 X-ray of the shoulder

A. normal X-ray
B. anterior shoulder dislocation
C. inferior shoulder dislocation
D. posterior shoulder dislocation
E. rotator cuff tear

139. A 23-year-old patient presented after the shoulder trauma. X-ray was performed (Fig. 2.36). The patient was unable to adduct the arm. Choose the correct statement(s) regarding this patient

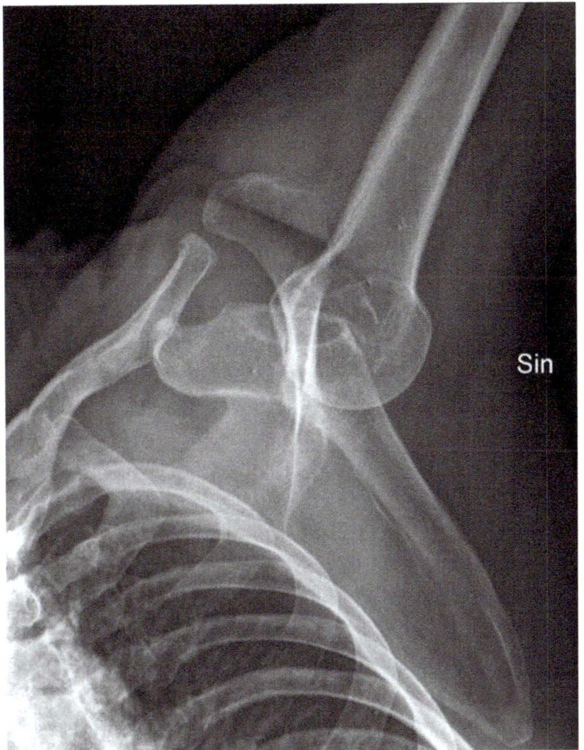

Fig. 2.36 X-ray of the shoulder

A. acromion fracture
B. anterior shoulder dislocation
C. inferior shoulder dislocation
D. posterior shoulder dislocation
E. massive rotator cuff tear

Key to Chapter 2

1. A, B, C.
2. C. MRI may show the occult fracture.
3. A, B, D. A—because no treatment is established based on the X-ray, D—X-ray is not indicated unless the pain is atypical, or the clinical presentation is unclear. CT is more appropriate.
4. B, D.
5. A, C, D.
6. A, B, C, D. It is the most common fracture of the proximal humerus (75%) after anterior dislocation.
7. A, C, E.
8. A, B, D.
9. A, D, E. Sternoclavicular dislocation is rare, the anterior dislocation is more common than posterior however the posterior is more life-threatening because of risk of vessel injury and superior mediastinum. The anterior dislocation is related more to pneumothorax. CT is the modality of choice to assess the sternoclavicular injury.
10. A, B, C. Radiologic manifestation of SAPHO (synovitis, acne, pustulosis, hyperostosis, osteitis) is located mainly in the thorax wall and sternoclavicular joints. Hallmark is an osteitis and hypertrophy of upper ribs articulations and sternal end of clavicle. Bone marrow edema and contrast enhancement may be seen in bones and thickened soft tissues [1].
11. C, D, E. Joint space more than 6 mm is considered abnormal.
12. A, C. Posttraumatic osteolysis of the clavicle is a painful condition. Reabsorption may be up to 3 cm and starts usually 1 month after trauma. Acromial lesions are minimal or are not present. MRI is an imaging tool to see subchondral fracture line which indicates fatigue of clavicle.
13. E. In rheumatoid arthritis lesions are more symmetric located. Often patient has lesion in hands and wrist.
14. B, C, D, E. Scapular fractures are located mainly in the body. Often occurs with direct trauma. Glenoid fractures indicate shoulder dislocation.
15. D. Majority of fractures are seen in children younger than 10 years of age.
16. A, C, D.
17. B, C, E.
18. A, B, D.
19. B, D.
20. B.
21. B. Monteggia fracture-dislocation is more common than Galeazzi. In Monteggia fracture is noticed the ulnar shaft fracture and dislocation of the radial head. The fracture of the distal radius and dislocation of the ulna in the distal radioulnar joint is called Galeazzi fracture-dislocation.
22. A, B, C, D, E.

23. C, E. Posterior shoulder dislocation accounts for 2–4%. Electrocution is typical but not the most common cause.
24. A, B, C, D. D is called the reverse Hill-Sachs deformity because of impaction of the humeral head on the scapula.
25. A, C, D. In the anterior shoulder dislocation Bankart lesion (or bony-Bankart), tear of the anterior limb of the inferior glenohumeral ligament and the Hill Sachs deformity are common. Tear of the anterior limb of the inferior glenohumeral ligament occurs during dislocation because of abduction and external rotation of the humerus. In this position anterior limb of the inferior glenohumeral ligament is taut.
26. B, C. Assessing the bone loss of the glenoid is an important factor which influence treatment method. Size of the glenoid defect is done by calculating the ratio between the depth and the radius of the best-fitted circle. (https://doi.org/10.12659/PJR.898566).
27. B, C, D.
28. B, C, D.
29. C, E. Little Leaguer's Shoulder is an overuse seen in teenage most commonly 11–16 years old. Widening if the lateral epiphysis on X-ray is a hallmark. Rest about 6 week is a method of treatment. No other imaging is required.
30. A, B, E. Tug lesion is a chronic avulsion injury with chronic healing. Localization in muscle insertion is a key to the right diagnosis. Surface osteosarcoma can be differential diagnosis. Other possible differential diagnosis includes fracture, osteoid osteoma, enthesophyte. Tug lesion is a do not touch lesion.
31. A, B, C, D. Floating elbow means that isolation of elbow by two fracture superior in humerus and inferior in forearm.
32. E. On the posterolateral part of capitellum is located a normal defect which should not be taken av osteochondral lesion.
33. D, E. The posterior elbow dislocation is the most common. It associates with radial head and coronoid fracture. In adult is related to Monteggia fracture while in children with chronic radial head dislocation. If a ligament is injured, it is ulnar collateral ligament.
34. B, C. Essex Lopresti fracture includes the comminute caput radii fracture, proximal dislocation of the radial shaft, tear of the interosseus membrane and disruption of the distal radioulnar joint.
35. D.
36. E.
37. A.
38. B.
39. C.
40. D.
41. B.
42. A, B, C. Humpback deformation may be seen after scaphoideum fracture when bone fragment is fused i volar angulation, this may increase risk of

arthrosis. Sclerotic fragment indicates osteonecrosis however vascularity may be recovered after some time, but sclerotic structure is going to stay.

43. B, C, E.
44. B, C, E.
45. B, C, D. Ulnar impingement syndrome is distinct from the ulnar impaction syndrome. In the ulnar impingement syndrome shorter ulnar conflicts with the radius causing bone marrow edema and thinning of the radial cortex (scalloping).
46. B, D.
47. B.
48. B, D.
49. D. PD-weighted with fat suppression used to overestimate tendinopathy. Some parts of tendinopathic tendon can be taken as rupture. T2-weighted sequences are recommend to difference tendinopathy with coexistence partial ruptures.
50. A, C, D. Non-communicate rotator cuff tear are possible but uncommon, the defect may be filled by scar, adherences or granulation tissue.
51. B, C.
52. A, C. Triad of posterosuperior glenoid impingement include humeral head deformation, undersurface tear of rotator cuff (supraspinatus and infraspinatus) and the posterior labral tear.
53. E. It is also called cartilage interface sign due to the fluid filling the defect in the rotator cuff resulting in enhancement of echo between the fluid and cartilage. Under cartilage normal cortex shows hyperechoic appearance.
54. D.
55. D. Sequences with long TE (time echo) are less susceptible because this artefact dissolve with long TE, i.e. on T2-weighted images.
56. B.
57. C.
58. A, B, D, E.
59. A, B, D.
60. A, D. Subcoracoid impingement usually affects the subscapularis tendon, middle glenohumeral ligament and long head of the biceps brachii tendon.
61. C.
62. C. Os acromiale is a slightly mobile non-fused accessory ossification centrum of the acromion. Deformation, tilt or step-off may cause impingement and rotator cuff rupture.
63. C. The most common type of rotator cuff rupture is rimrent which means that fibers from the articular side of insertion are injured.
64. B, C, E [2, 3].
65. C. The critical zone of the rotator cuff is a watershed area in the tendon. In the past, it was believed that poor vascularization was responsible for more frequent tears in this area. New research proved that there are other factors like chronic degeneration or impingement that make tears more frequent.

66. C, D, E. Geyser sign indicates communication through full-thickness rotator cuff rupture via degenerated acromio-clavicular joint which result in synovial cyst.
67. A, B, C, D, E. Long TR and short TE is PD-weighted while long TR and long TE are T2-weighted. Fluid signal or synovial proliferation in the defect may be seen in the total rupture. Synovium may obscure the defect making it more challenging to delineate.
68. A, B, D, E. Delamination of the tendon means that the horizontal intratendinous cleft is present [4]. Rupture of the superior or inferior fibers may occur with diverse combination of retraction.
69. A, B, C, D. Retraction of the tendon is an important feature of the tear. One of the most common classification is Patte classification. Grade 1 tendon retracted but is located near to the insertion, lateral to the superior outline of the humeral head. Grade 2 tendon retracted at the level of humeral head. grade 3 tendon retracted at the level of the joint space or more proximal. Goutallier classification is used to grade a muscle atrophy. Grade 1 only some fatty streaks. Grade 2 less then 50% of fatty atrophy. Grade 3 about 50% of fatty atrophy. Grade 4 more then 50% fatty atrophy.
70. C. Grade 1 less then 25%, grade 2 25–50% and grade 3 more then 50% [5].
71. C, E. Rim rent is an articular side cuff tear. PASTA (partial articular supraspinatus tendon avulsion) is a partial tear when bony insertion and articular side of the tendon are involved. All PASTA tears are rim rent because they are articular side tears. Not all rim rent tears are PASTA, because not all include bony insertion. PAINT (partial articular sided with interstitial extension) is a rim rent tear with intrasubstance involvement. CID (concealed interstitial delamination) is intratendinous tear with extension to bursal or articular side, most commonly seen in the posterior part od supraspinatus.
72. B. The rotator interval contains long head of the biceps brachii and the superior glenohumeral ligament.
73. A, B, C.
74. A.
75. A, B, C. The anterior labral lesions: Bankart and bony-Bankart, GLAD, ALPSA, Perthes lesion, HAGL.
76. A, C, E. Bankart lesion is the most common cause of anterior instability which is the commonest shoulder instability. If Bankart is present lesion is located between 6 and 9 o'clock. Often Bankart coexists with the Hill-Sachs deformity when humeral head hits the antero-lateral labrum.
77. A, C, E. There are some congenital conditions which may cause instability like mentioned in the question and medial insertion of the articular capsule.
78. B, C. MGHL is the most variable ligament absent in about 1/3 cases, however presence of shoulder instability is not directly related to absence of this ligament.
79. D.
80. C.
81. B.

82. C. Abduction and external rotation (ABER) causes stretching of the anterior limb of IGHL (inferior glenohumeral ligament).
83. C, E. Sublabral foramen is an anatomical variant of the labrum located at the level of insertion of LHB (long head of biceps brachii), rarely continue to 3 o'clock.
84. D. Buford complex is recognized when the labrum is absent in 1–3 o'clock position coexist with thickened MGHL (middle glenohumeral ligament).
85. A.
86. A, B, C, D, E. McLaughlin lesion is a reverse Hill-Sachs lesion seen in anteromedial part of the humeral head.
87. C. ALPSA (anterior labro-ligamentous periosteal sleeve avulsion) is avulsion of the labrum from the glenoid. Only periosteum is sleeved but not ruptured.
88. B, D. Not all labral tear associates with instability. Coexistence with instability is observed in Bankart and ALPSA.
89. A, B, C, E.
90. A, D, E. When two hyperintense lines are present in labrum it indicates that that sublabral recess and SLAP coexists which is known as Oreo sign.
91. A, B, D, E.
92. A, D.
93. E. Parsonage-Turner syndrome is known as acute idiopathic brachial neuritis. Pathology is unknown. MRI revels denervation changes and some atrophy.
94. B. Quadrilateral space syndrome is limited laterally by surgical neck, superiorly by teres minor, inferiorly by teres major and medially by the long head of the triceps brachii tendon.
95. B, D, E.
96. B, C, D, E.
97. C.
98. A, B, C, D.
99. B.
100. A, C, D.
101. B, C, D, E.
102. A, D.
103. B.
104. E.
105. B, C. Rimrent rupture is seen in direct posterior to the long head of the biceps brachii tendon.
106. B, C.
107. B.
108. C.
109. A, B, E.
110. C, D.
111. B, C.
112. E.
113. A, D.

114. C. The loose bodies showed layered structure which means it ossified form of synovial chondromatosis.
115. E.
116. B, C.
117. A, B, C, E.
118. A, B.
119. C.
120. A, D.
121. B, D.
122. D.
123. B.
124. A, D.
125. A.
126. B, D.
127. A, B, D.
128. E [6]
129. A, E.
130. A.
131. B.
132. A.
133. A, E.
134. C.
135. D.
136. A. Extensor carpi ulnaris dislocation is seen in the sector “a”.
137. B, D, E.
138. D.
139. C. Luxatio erecta.

References

1. Cotten A, Flipo RM, Mentre A, Delaporte E, Duquesnoy B, Chastanet P. SAPHO syndrome. Radiographics. 1995;15(5):1147–54. https://doi.org/10.1148/radiographics.15.5.7501856.
2. Taneja AK, Kattapuram SV, Chang CY, Simeone FJ, Bredella MA, Torriani M. MRI findings of rotator cuff myotendinous junction injury. AJR Am J Roentgenol. 2014;203(2):406–11. https://doi.org/10.2214/AJR.13.11474.
3. Palmer W, Bancroft L, Bonar F, Choi JA, Cotten A, Griffith JF, et al. Glossary of terms for musculoskeletal radiology. Skeletal Radiol. 2020;49(Suppl 1):1–33. https://doi.org/10.1007/s00256-020-03465-1.
4. Choo HJ, Lee SJ, Kim JH, Kim DW, Park YM, Kim OH, et al. Delaminated tears of the rotator cuff: prevalence, characteristics, and diagnostic accuracy using indirect MR arthrography. AJR Am J Roentgenol. 2015;204(2):360–6. https://doi.org/10.2214/AJR.14.12555.
5. Matthewson G, Beach CJ, Nelson AA, Woodmass JM, Ono Y, Boorman RS, et al. Partial thickness rotator cuff tears: current concepts. Adv Orthop. 2015;2015:458786. https://doi.org/10.1155/2015/458786.
6. Roberts CC, Ekelund AL, Renfree KJ, Liu PT, Chew FS. Radiologic assessment of reverse shoulder arthroplasty. Radiographics. 2007;27(1):223–35. https://doi.org/10.1148/rg.271065076.

Lower Extremity Trauma

3

140. Fracture of the ischial body is the fracture of:
    A. the anterior wall of the acetabulum
    B. the posterior wall of the acetabulum
    C. the anterior column of the acetabulum
    D. the posterior column of the acetabulum
    E. the inferior column of the acetabulum
141. Choose the correct statement(s) regarding sacral fractures:
    A. Sacrum fractures are usually not concomitant pelvis fractures.
    B. Typical patient is a young sports active female who presents with low back pain.
    C. Stress fractures are common in elderly patients.
    D. Vertically oriented lesions in the sacral alae are typical for metastatic disease.
    E. If the transverse component joins two lesions that are vertically oriented in the sacral alae, it unequivocally indicates metastatic disease.
142. Choose the typical locations of pelvic insufficiency fractures:
    A. superior pubic ramus
    B. inferior pubic ramus
    C. anterior superior iliac spine
    D. sciatic tuber
    E. iliac bone parallel to the sacroiliac joint

Supplementary Information The online version contains supplementary material available at (https://doi.org/10.1007/978-3-030-85182-8_3).

P. Szaro, *Musculoskeletal Radiology for Residents*,
https://doi.org/10.1007/978-3-030-85182-8_3

143. In which fracture is the risk of avascular necrosis the most significant?
    A. pertrochanteric femoral fracture
    B. transphyseal femoral fracture
    C. subcapital femoral fracture
    D. basicervical femoral fracture
    E. transcervical femoral fracture
144. Choose the correct statement(s) regarding the Gardner classification:
    A. Grades 1 and 2 represent more stable fractures.
    B. Arthroplasty is often needed in grades 2, 3, and 4.
    C. Despite its widespread use, it is not possible to predict the development of avascular necrosis.
    D. A valgus position of the femoral head may be observed in grade 3.
    E. It is a classification for subcapital femoral cervical fractures.
145. What fractures are intracapsular?
    A. pertrochanteric femoral fracture
    B. grade 2 according to Gardner
    C. subtrochanteric femoral fracture
    D. trochanter major fracture
    E. basicervical femoral fracture
146. Choose the correct statement(s) regarding proximal tibial fractures:
    A. The most common fracture includes the medial and lateral condyles.
    B. The most common fracture is extra-articular.
    C. A splitting fracture is a common feature of an osteoporotic fracture.
    D. Intra-articular lateral tibial plateau fracture is associated with the rupture of the anterior cruciate ligament.
    E. Avulsion of the lateral outline of the tibial plateau is positively associated with the rupture of the anterior cruciate ligament.
147. What is a Segond fracture?
    A. It is avulsion of the anterior cruciate ligament.
    B. It is avulsion of the iliotibial band.
    C. It is avulsion of the anterolateral ligament.
    D. It is avulsion of the posterolateral ligament.
    E. It is compression of the posterior part of the lateral tibial plateau.
148. What features are included in Schatzker classification?
    A. orientation of the fracture line
    B. presence of the avulsion fracture
    C. deformation of the articular surface
    D. presence of a joint effusion
    E. discontinuity of the metaphysis and diaphysis

149. Choose the features of a syndesmotic fibular fracture:
    A. Deltoid ligament is intact.
    B. Widening of the distal tibiofibular joint.
    C. Stable fracture.
    D. Frequently spiral.
    E. Narrowing of the distal tibiofibular joint.
150. Choose the correct statement(s) regarding talus and calcaneus fractures:
    A. Böhler angle less more than 20° is abnormal.
    B. Intra-articular calcaneal fracture is more common than extra-articular fracture.
    C. A vertical linear sclerotic line parallel to the calcaneal tuber indicates a stress fracture.
    D. The most common tarsal fracture is a talar fracture.
    E. Displaced fracture of the talar body is significantly associated with avascular necrosis.
151. What indicates a Lisfranc fracture?
    A. Böhler angle is 30°.
    B. Increased distance between the first and second metatarsal bones.
    C. Medial border of the second metatarsal bone lines up with the medial border of the second cuneiform.
    D. Base of the second metatarsal bone is more proximal than the other metatarsal bones.
    E. Medial longitudinal arch is fallen.
152. Choose the correct statement(s) regarding stress fractures:
    A. Female athlete triad is a condition that increases the risk.
    B. CT is the most sensitive method of diagnosing a stress fracture.
    C. Lower cortical density may be a first radiological sign.
    D. Periosteal reaction and soft tissue oedema may be revealed on MRI.
    E. Differential diagnosis is osteosarcoma and osteomyelitis.
153. What features are included in the Fredericson classification of stress fractures?
    A. presence of periosteal oedema
    B. presence of bone marrow oedema on T2-weighted without fat suppression
    C. presence of bone marrow oedema on T2-weighted with fat suppression
    D. direction of a fracture line
    E. presence of soft tissue oedema
154. Choose the correct statement(s) regarding hip dislocation:
    A. It may be associated with the posterior wall of the acetabulum.
    B. It is often related to joint capsule degeneration.
    C. Caput femoris impaction is visible.
    D. Anterior dislocation is related to anterior column fracture.
    E. There is a risk of caput necrosis.

155. Bone marrow oedema is visible in:
    A. transient osteoporosis
    B. rapidly progressive osteoarthritis
    C. stress fractures
    D. subchondral fractures
    E. the early stages of avascular necrosis
156. A football player presented with hip pain. X-ray was normal, but MRI revealed bone marrow oedema and, on sagittal T1-weighted images, the subchondral vertical orientated bowl-shaped low signal line in the anterior part of the caput femoris. What is the most likely diagnosis?
    A. stress fracture
    B. chondral contusion
    C. osteochondral fracture
    D. subcapital fracture
    E. femoral neck fracture
157. X-ray shows a complete, non-displaced femoral neck fracture with minimal angulation between the femoral neck and head. What grade is this fracture according to the Garden classification?
    A. 1
    B. 2
    C. 3
    D. 4
    E. 3 or 4
158. A 79-year-old patient with dementia presented with hip pain. The patient does not remember what happened, but he cannot go as before. No clear medical history is available. X-rays show a sclerotic line in the lateral part of the femoral neck without disruption of the cortical bone. What is your differential diagnosis?
    A. pathologic fracture
    B. femoral neck fracture, grade 1 according to Gardner
    C. transient osteoporosis of the hip
    D. healed fracture
    E. insufficiency fracture
159. Choose the correct statement(s) regarding proximal femoral fractures:
    A. Isolated lesser trochanter fracture is a pathologic fracture.
    B. Basicervical fracture is perpendicular to the intertrochanteric fracture.
    C. The population being diagnosed with intertrochanteric fractures is often older than that being diagnosed with femoral neck fractures.
    D. More significantly displaced fractures have a higher risk of avascular necrosis.
    E. Hamstring rupture should be included in the differential diagnosis.

160. A 68-year-old patient presented with chronic thigh pain. CT showed symmetric bilateral lateral cortex thickening in the femoral shaft. What is your differential diagnosis?
    A. subtrochanteric fracture
    B. shaft fracture
    C. stress fracture
    D. bisphosphonate fracture
    E. steroid-related fracture
161. Avulsion of the anterior inferior iliac spine involves the following muscle:
    A. sartorius
    B. tensor fasciae latae
    C. rectus femoris
    D. hamstring
    E. biceps femoris
162. Straddle fractures involve the:
    A. acetabulum
    B. pubic rami
    C. iliac wing
    D. sacrum
    E. anterior superior iliac spine
163. Bilateral ramus superior and ramus inferior fractures:
    A. They are considered unstable.
    B. Mechanism is often a horizontal shear injury.
    C. There is a higher risk of genitourinary tract injury.
    D. Most of them result from motor vehicle accidents.
    E. They represent insufficiency fractures.
164. Choose where the stress fracture most commonly occurs:
    A. sacrum in elderly patients
    B. femoral neck in athletes
    C. subchondral femoral caput fracture in elderly patients
    D. acetabular fracture in athletes
    E. trochanter major in elderly patients
165. Choose the correct statement(s) regarding avascular necrosis of the femur:
    A. The earliest sign is the double line sign.
    B. X-ray shows high sensitivity in detection.
    C. The anterior femoral head is affected at the beginning.
    D. Trauma, steroids, and alcoholism are the common causes.
    E. Subchondral collapse is one of the earliest signs.

166. What differential diagnosis should be considered with suspicion of avascular necrosis?
    A. subchondral insufficiency fracture
    B. idiopathic transient osteoporosis
    C. reflex sympathetic dystrophy
    D. septic arthritis
    E. synovial herniation pit
167. What is the difference between Legg-Calvé-Perthes disease and avascular necrosis of the hip?
    A. This is the same entity, but Legg-Calvé-Perthes disease is seen in children up to 10 years old.
    B. MRI shows bone marrow oedema in avascular necrosis of the hip.
    C. MRI shows bone marrow oedema in avascular necrosis of Legg-Calvé-Perthes disease.
    D. Lateral shift of the femoral head is seen in Legg-Calvé-Perthes disease.
    E. Lateral shift of the femoral head is seen in avascular necrosis.
168. What is the differential diagnosis of collapse of the femoral head?
    A. avascular necrosis
    B. subchondral fracture
    C. transient osteoporosis
    D. Pitt pit
    E. Legg-Calvé-Perthes disease
169. Choose the correct statement(s) regarding idiopathic transient osteoporosis of the hip:
    A. Middle-aged women are the most frequent patient group.
    B. It is resolved in under a few months.
    C. Differential diagnosis includes avascular necrosis.
    D. X-ray reveals sclerosis of the femoral head on the affected side.
    E. It is usually bilateral.
170. What X-ray sign is the most pathognomonic for idiopathic transient osteoporosis of the hip?
    A. joint effusion
    B. narrow joint space
    C. erosions
    D. osteopenia
    E. subchondral bone loss
171. What is the most common fracture of the proximal tibia?
    A. medial condyle
    B. lateral condyle
    C. tibial tuberosity
    D. intercondylar eminence
    E. both medial and lateral condyles

172. In which case should a non-operative approach be considered?
   A. depression 14 mm, diastasis 10 mm
   B. depression 12 mm, diastasis 8 mm
   C. depression 10 mm, diastasis 6 mm
   D. depression 7 mm, diastasis 4 mm
   E. depression 3 mm, diastasis 3 mm
173. Tibiofemoral dislocation is associated with:
   A. ACL rupture
   B. PCL rupture
   C. popliteal artery injury
   D. common peroneal nerve injury
   E. MCL injury
174. A 23-year-old male presented after trauma. You noticed a small bony fragment located directly inferior to the patellar apex. What is your differential diagnosis?
   A. bipartite patella
   B. sleeve injury
   C. osteochondral injury
   D. marginal avulsion
   E. Sinding-Larsen-Johansson syndrome
175. What is the most common localization of patellar osteochondritis dissecans?
   A. superomedial
   B. inferomedial
   C. superolateral
   D. inferolateral
   E. central
176. What type of joint connects fragments in the bipartite patella?
   A. synostosis
   B. syndesmosis
   C. synchondrosis
   D. synovial joint
   E. planar joint
177. A 32-year-old football player presented after knee trauma. X-ray of the knee showed a fracture of the fibular apex. Choose the correct statement(s) regarding this patient:
   A. This is a Segond fracture.
   B. There is a high risk for an PCL tear.
   C. There is a high risk for a posterolateral ligament tear.
   D. It is sign of iliotibial band avulsion.
   E. It is associated with popliteal artery dissection.

178. A 34-year-old runner presented with a swollen and painful leg. MRI showed extensive bone marrow oedema and thickening of the cortex, which is surrounded by a periosteal bone reaction. The extensive soft tissue oedema is visible. What is/are the correct statement(s) regarding this patient?
    A. Administration of contrast is required to make a diagnosis.
    B. An X-ray is needed to make a diagnosis.
    C. The presence of a low intensity line represents fracture.
    D. The presence of extensive oedema of the soft tissue may indicate a tumour.
    E. This is probably spontaneous osteonecrosis.
179. Choose the signs of a stress reaction on X-ray:
    A. multi-layered periosteal reaction
    B. soft tissue oedema
    C. cortical thickening
    D. line of sclerosis
    E. cortical lucency
180. What is the most common localization of osteochondritis dissecans in the knee?
    A. medial aspect of the medial femoral condyle
    B. lateral aspect of the medial femoral condyle
    C. medial aspect of the lateral femoral condyle
    D. lateral aspect of the lateral femoral condyle
    E. articular surface in the patellofemoral joint
181. Choose the signs of osteochondral fragment instability?
    A. fluid rim around fragment
    B. cyst formation under fragment
    C. shape of the osteochondral fragment
    D. localization of non-weight bearing surface
    E. localization of weight bearing surface
182. Choose the correct statement(s) regarding subchondral insufficiency fractures of the knee:
    A. The weight bearing part of the lateral femoral condyle is the most common site.
    B. A linear low intensity line in subchondral bone is the typical feature.
    C. Bone marrow oedema is usually more extensive than in osteochondritis dissecans.
    D. It is seen commonly in patients with osteoporosis.
    E. Meniscal tear or post-meniscectomy status is an often seen condition.
183. Deep sulcus sign:
    A. It is an impaction fracture of the medial femoral condyle.
    B. It is an impaction fracture of the lateral femoral condyle.
    C. It is an impaction fracture of the medial tibial condyle.
    D. It is an impaction fracture of the lateral tibial condyle.
    E. It is an impaction fracture of the lateral patellar surface.

184. A pilon fracture is associated with a(n):
    A. horizontal load
    B. axial load
    C. stress reaction
    D. tumour
    E. avascular necrosis
185. A die-punch fragment:
    A. It may be present in the intra-articular fracture.
    B. It is visible in the stress fracture.
    C. It is often located extra-articularly.
    D. It is not visible on CT.
    E. It is a sign of pathologic fracture.
186. Choose sign(s) of syndesmotic injury on X-ray:
    A. If the medial gutter is more than 4 mm on the mortise view.
    B. If the tibia and fibula overlap more than 2 mm on the AP view.
    C. If radiolucency is present in the talar dome, it indicates osteochondritis dissecans.
    D. If the medial gutter is less than 4 mm on the mortise view.
    E. If the tibia and fibula overlap less than 1 mm on the AP view.
187. A 45-year-old male presented after ankle trauma. X-ray showed a medial malleolus fracture. Choose the correct statement(s) regarding this patient:
    A. CT of the ankle is indicated.
    B. MRI of the ankle in 2 weeks is indicated.
    C. X-ray of the knee is indicated.
    D. X-ray of the contralateral ankle is indicated.
    E. X-ray of the foot is indicated.
188. A Tillaux fracture:
    A. It is a Salter-Harris type 3 fracture.
    B. It is considered if a bony fragment is visible in the posteromedial part of the distal tibial epiphysis.
    C. It is considered if a bony fragment is visible in the posterolateral part of the distal tibial epiphysis.
    D. It is considered if a bony fragment is visible in the anteromedial part of the distal tibial epiphysis.
    E. It is considered if a bony fragment is visible in the anterolateral part of the distal tibial epiphysis.
189. Choose the correct statement(s) regarding osteochondral lesions on the talus:
    A. Fluid under the osteochondral fragment indicates instability.
    B. Bone marrow oedema may even be seen in a chronic osteochondral lesion.
    C. Cartilage is intact in early osteonecrosis, which is different from an osteochondral lesion.
    D. MRI arthrography is superior to MRI without contrast.
    E. Lateral talar osteochondritis dissecans is often deeper than the medial type.

190. Choose the two most common localizations of osteochondral lesions of the talus:
    A. anteromedial
    B. anterolateral
    C. posteromedial
    D. posterolateral
    E. central
191. An axial load may result in a:
    A. Tillaux fracture
    B. pilon fracture
    C. talar body fracture
    D. lateral talar process fracture
    E. posterior process fracture
192. Which risk of avascular necrosis is the most significant?
    A. osteochondral fracture of the talus
    B. dorsal capsular avulsion of the talar neck
    C. lateral talar process fracture
    D. posterior talar process fracture
    E. non-displaced fracture of the talar neck
193. Choose the features of a calcaneal stress fracture:
    A. Böhler angle is less than 20°.
    B. Sustentaculum tali is often involved.
    C. Posterior part of the subtalar joint is depressed.
    D. Sclerotic line parallel to the calcaneal tuber.
    E. Bony trabeculae of the posterior processes are involved.
194. What structures may cause an avulsion fracture of the calcaneus?
    A. Lisfranc ligament
    B. bifurcate ligament
    C. calcaneofibular ligament
    D. plantar aponeurosis
    E. Achilles tendon
195. A navicular tuberosity avulsion is due to:
    A. plantar aponeurosis
    B. tibialis anterior
    C. tibialis posterior
    D. talonavicular capsule
    E. stress fracture
196. Choose the correct statement(s) regarding cuboid fractures:
    A. Cuboid fractures are more common than Lisfranc fracture-dislocations.
    B. The fracture line is often seen on AP view.
    C. Sclerosis and deformation are seen more often than a fracture line.
    D. When depression is seen on the inferior surface, impaction is suspected.
    E. They are often stress fractures.

197. Choose the signs of a Lisfranc fracture-dislocation:
    A. decreased distance between the bases of the first and second metatarsal bones
    B. chip fragment on the medial margin of the first metatarsal bone
    C. flattening of the longitudinal arches of the foot
    D. dorsal displacement of the second metatarsal bone
    E. overlapping bases of the second, third, and fourth metatarsal bones on AP view
198. Which os metatarsale is most commonly fractured?
    A. 1st
    B. 2nd
    C. 3rd
    D. 4th
    E. 5th
199. Choose the correct statement(s) regarding fractures of the fifth metatarsal bone:
    A. There is a high risk of non-union.
    B. A Jones fracture is more proximal than an avulsion fracture.
    C. A stress fracture is more common than a Jones or avulsion fracture.
    D. Fractures of the head are less common than proximal fractures.
    E. Most proximal fractures are transverse.
200. The flattening of the caput of the second metatarsal bone:
    A. is a sign of septic arthritis
    B. indicates avulsion
    C. indicates avascular necrosis
    D. indicates rupture of the medial collateral ligament
    E. indicates rupture of the lateral collateral ligament
201. Choose the correct statement(s) regarding femoroacetabular impingement:
    A. A pincer deformation is present on the acetabular ridge, while a cam deformation is present on the femoral neck.
    B. Reduced femoral head-neck offset is present in pincer deformation.
    C. A labrum tear is most often present at the posterosuperior part.
    D. A pistol grip deformity is related to the cam deformity.
    E. Acetabular retroversion may predispose to impingement.
202. Choose the correct statement(s) regarding an acetabular labrum:
    A. A higher intrasubstance signal in the labrum may indicate a tear.
    B. The labral recess may be seen anteroinferior.
    C. The labral recess may be seen posteroinferior.
    D. The contrast between the cartilage and superior labrum indicates a perilabral recess.
    E. A rounder outline of the labrum indicates an anatomical variant.

203. Choose the aetiology of femoroacetabular impingement:
   A. Legg-Calvé-Perthes disease
   B. slipped capital femoral epiphysis
   C. acetabular protrusion
   D. symphysitis
   E. developmental dysplasia of the hip
204. What conditions coexist commonly with osteochondral lesions of the hip?
   A. cam deformation
   B. pincer deformation
   C. acetabular labral tear
   D. hip dislocation
   E. avascular necrosis
205. What is the best imaging tool for evaluation of a labral tear after repair?
   A. MRI with IV contrast
   B. direct MRI arthrography
   C. indirect MRI arthrography
   D. ultrasound with intra-articular contrast
   E. CT with IV contrast
206. An internal snapping hip is due to the:
   A. rectus femoris
   B. gluteus medius
   C. adductor longus
   D. adductor magnus
   E. iliopsoas
207. What MRI sequence is most useful to evaluate rectus femoris injury in football players?
   A. T1-weighted
   B. T2-weighted without fat suppression
   C. T2-weighted with fat suppression
   D. T1-weighted with IV contrast
   E. PD-weighted
208. A sports hernia is tear of the:
   A. sartorius
   B. rectus abdominis
   C. rectus femoris
   D. adductor longus
   E. adductor magnus

209. What two structures are involved in the externally snapping hip?
   A. iliopsoas
   B. sartorius
   C. tensor fasciae latae
   D. gluteus maximus
   E. gluteus medius

210. What muscle is compressed in ischiofemoral impingement?
    A. quadriceps femoris
    B. quadratus femoris
    C. gemellus superior
    D. gemellus inferior
    E. obturator internus
211. What hamstring muscle is included in the conjoined tendon origin?
    A. biceps femoris and semimembranosus
    B. semimembranosus and semitendinosus
    C. semitendinosus and biceps femoris
    D. adductor longus and biceps femoris
    E. semitendinosus, semimembranosus, and biceps femoris
212. Delayed onset muscle soreness:
    A. It is visible on MRI as tendon thinning.
    B. It is related to intensive training.
    C. It includes apophysitis.
    D. It includes a partial fibre tear.
    E. Light muscle oedema is visible.
213. What is the imaging tool for an external oblique aponeurosis tear, which is called hockey groin?
    A. CT without contrast
    B. CT with IV contrast
    C. MRI without contrast
    D. MRI with IV contrast
    E. ultrasound
214. A 27-year-old football player presented with groin pain. T2-weighted with fat suppression images show extensive bone marrow oedema in the pubic bones. T1-weighted images revealed subchondral erosions. What is the most probable diagnosis?
    A. arthritis
    B. sports hernia
    C. osteitis pubis
    D. stress fracture
    E. osteomyelitis
215. MRI showed a well-limited structure located between the anterior part of the hip joint capsule and iliopsoas tendon. In T1-weighted images, the lesion showed a low signal with points of a slightly higher signal. In T2-weighted images, the lesion has a high signal with a few tiny areas of a lower signal. What is your differential diagnosis?
    A. myxoma
    B. iliopsoas bursitis
    C. paralabral cyst
    D. intramuscular lipoma
    E. synovial sarcoma

216. What nerve is compressed in piriformis syndrome?
    A. superior gluteal nerve
    B. obturator nerve
    C. saphenous nerve
    D. sciatic nerve
    E. pudendal nerve
217. What is the differential diagnosis in trauma to the lumbosacral plexus?
    A. hamstring tear
    B. sacroiliitis
    C. paralabral cyst
    D. piriformis syndrome
    E. femoroacetabular impingement
218. A 32-year-old male presented with athletic pubalgia. MRI revealed asymmetry of the inferior rectus abdominis muscles with scarring at the deep inguinal ring. What two nerves can be involved in this region?
    A. femoral nerve
    B. sciatic nerve
    C. obturator nerve and lateral cutaneous nerve of the thigh
    D. ilioinguinal nerve
    E. genitofemoral nerve
219. A 38-year-old sedentary male truck driver presented with a 4-month history of medial groin pain on the left. The most painful activities are sitting and pushing the gas pedal. What nerve can be involved?
    A. obturator nerve
    B. saphenous nerve
    C. lateral cutaneous nerve of the thigh
    D. ilioinguinal nerve
    E. genitofemoral nerve
220. Choose the correct statement(s) regarding an ACL tear:
    A. It is associated with an impaction fracture of the medial femoral condyle.
    B. It may be suspected when anterior tibial translation is visible.
    C. It may be suspected when a fibular apex fracture is visible.
    D. It may be suspected when a fracture of the lateral aspect of the tibial plateau is noticed.
    E. It may be suspected when a fracture of the medial aspect of the tibial plateau is noticed.
221. The most common total ACL tear in adults is located:
    A. proximal and distal
    B. avulsion of the tibial attachment
    C. proximal and in the midportion
    D. avulsion of the femoral attachment
    E. distal and in the midportion

222. Choose the correct statement(s) regarding the anatomy of the ACL bundles:
    A. The posterolateral bundle is bigger than the anteromedial bundle.
    B. The anteromedial bundle is bigger than the posterolateral bundle.
    C. Both the posterolateral and anteromedial bundles are taut in flexion.
    D. The posterolateral bundle is taut in flexion, while the anteromedial bundle is taut in extension.
    E. The posterolateral bundle is taut in extension, while the anteromedial bundle is taut in flexion.
223. What are indirect signs of an ACL tear?
    A. subluxation of the posterior horn of the lateral meniscus
    B. PCL angle more than 90°
    C. anterior tibial translation more than 10 mm
    D. arcuate sign
    E. Segond fracture
224. Choose the correct statement(s) regarding post-operative ACL evaluation:
    A. Bone marrow oedema in direct relation to bone tunnels is visible for months.
    B. The tibial tunnel on sagittal images should be located anterior to the Blumensaat line.
    C. The femoral tunnel on sagittal images should be present at the intersection of a line through the posterior femoral cortex and Blumensaat line.
    D. When the femoral tunnel is placed too anterior, graft tension increases in flexion.
    E. Anterior stabilization is decreased when the tibial tunnel is placed too posterior.
225. Choose the correct statement(s) regarding cyclops eye on MRI:
    A. It limits extension.
    B. It is often surrounded by fluid.
    C. It may be attached to the graft.
    D. It is a diffuse form of arthrofibrosis.
    E. It is a result of conflict with the intercondylar notch.
226. What is the reverse Segond sign?
    A. avulsion of the articular capsule from the lateral femoral condyle
    B. avulsion of the MCL from the medial femoral condyle
    C. avulsion of the MCL from the medial tibial condyle
    D. avulsion of the LCL from the fibular apex
    E. impaction fracture of the medial femoral condyle
227. A 34-year-old patient presented after knee trauma. MRI revealed a higher signal in the central part of the PCL on T2-weighted images. What is the differential diagnosis?
    A. focal synovitis
    B. mucinous degeneration
    C. chronic partial tear
    D. arthrofibrosis
    E. Osgood-Schlatter disease

228. Choose the typical bone marrow contusion pattern that indicates a PCL tear.
    A. lateral tibial plateau and lateral femoral condyle with medial femoral condyle
    B. anterior tibia and posterior patella
    C. inferomedial patella and anterolateral lateral femoral condyle
    D. anterior parts of the tibial plateau and femoral condyle
    E. posterolateral tibial and central part of lateral femoral condyle
229. Pellegrini-Stieda disease means calcification in the:
    A. proximal attachment of the ACL
    B. proximal attachment of the PCL
    C. proximal attachment of the MCL
    D. proximal attachment of the LCL
    E. proximal attachment of the popliteal tendon
230. After trauma, the MCL demonstrates normal signal and morphology on MRI, but the soft tissue signal is higher. What is correct regarding this patient?
    A. It is a grade 1 injury.
    B. The ACL tear may be an associated injury.
    C. It is grade 2 injury.
    D. It is consequence of a varus stress.
    E. Clinically, it is a stable ligament.
231. The reverse Segond sign is related to a:
    A. PCL tear
    B. ACL tear
    C. posterolateral ligament rupture
    D. medial patellofemoral ligament rupture
    E. medial meniscal tear
232. What structures are included in the ligamentous arcuate complex?
    A. popliteofibular ligament
    B. lateral collateral ligament
    C. oblique popliteal ligament
    D. biceps tendon
    E. fabellofibular ligament
233. What structures insert on the fibular head and form the common tendon?
    A. anterolateral ligament
    B. iliotibial band
    C. lateral collateral ligament
    D. biceps femoris tendon
    E. oblique popliteal ligament

234. Choose the one entity that is the most likely cause of synovitis in the lateral reflection of the knee:
   A. posterolateral ligament injury
   B. luxation of patella
   C. iliotibial band friction
   D. lateral ligament insufficiency
   E. biceps femoris tendinopathy
235. What structures may be a potential pitfall in meniscal evaluation?
   A. meniscofemoral ligaments
   B. coronal ligament
   C. intermeniscal ligament
   D. lateral collateral ligament
   E. oblique meniscomeniscal ligament
236. Choose the correct statement(s) regarding the discoid meniscus:
   A. More often it is seen in the medial compartment.
   B. On coronal plane, it is usually less than 14 mm.
   C. More than 50% of the tibial condyle is covered.
   D. It is less prone to degeneration.
   E. It is less prone to tear.
237. An intrasubstance higher signal in the meniscus, without changing of the meniscal outline, revealed on proton density sequence may be due to:
   A. rupture
   B. degeneration
   C. post-operative changes
   D. contusion
   E. bucket handle
238. MRI revealed an irregularity of the free edge of the meniscus without a higher intrasubstance linear signal. What is your diagnosis?
   A. radial rupture
   B. fraying
   C. vessels
   D. mucoid degeneration
   E. cleft rupture
239. What lesions give the ghost meniscus sign?
   A. clef rupture
   B. radial rupture
   C. root rupture
   D. horizontal rupture
   E. degeneration

240. Choose the vertical meniscal rupture types:
   A. cleft rupture
   B. root avulsion
   C. bucket handle
   D. flap tear
   E. flipped meniscus
241. Choose the horizontal ruptures:
   A. cleft rupture
   B. root avulsion
   C. parrot beak
   D. flap tear
   E. flipped meniscus
242. What alternative represents radial rupture?
   A. parrot beak
   B. flap
   C. flipped meniscus
   D. cleft rupture
   E. stellate rupture
243. Meniscocapsular separation occurs most often in the:
   A. anterior horn of the medial meniscus
   B. posterior horn of the medial meniscus
   C. anterior horn of the lateral meniscus
   D. posterior horn of the lateral meniscus
   E. body of the medial and lateral menisci
244. A parameniscal cyst indicates a meniscal rupture, except in the:
   A. anteromedial region
   B. posteromedial region
   C. anterolateral region
   D. posterolateral region
   E. central medial region
245. Choose conditions where the patellar ligament is affected:
   A. Osgood-Schlatter disease
   B. patellar luxation
   C. jumper's knee
   D. Sinding-Larsen-Johansson disease
   E. iliotibial band friction
246. Choose the correct statement(s) regarding patellar luxation:
   A. Bone marrow oedema in the patella is located in the inferolateral part.
   B. Intra-articular bodies are common.
   C. Bony avulsion may be seen on the medial patellar outline.
   D. During knee extension, patellar luxation reduces.
   E. Minor Q angle is a predisposing factor.

247. Choose the correct statement(s) regarding pes anserine bursitis:
    A. It is related to overuse and is often seen in football players.
    B. Parameniscal cyst is a differential diagnosis.
    C. Aspiration and steroid injection is contraindicated.
    D. The fluid is located between the superficial and deep part of the pes anserine.
    E. The fluid is located between the semimembranosus and medial gastrocnemius tendons.
248. Choose the correct statement(s) regarding a popliteal cyst:
    A. It may have connection with the articular space.
    B. Part of it may be located anterior to the gastrocnemius.
    C. If it ruptures, fluid may be seen in different muscle compartments.
    D. It is located between the medial head of the gastrocnemius and semimembranosus tendon.
    E. It is more common in patients with rheumatoid arthritis.
249. What is the differential diagnosis of a popliteal cyst?
    A. popliteal artery aneurysm
    B. haematoma
    C. popliteal lipoma
    D. parameniscal cyst
    E. schwannoma of the common peroneal nerve
250. A 45-year-old male presented with knee pain. MRI showed a cystic lesion in the intercondylar fossa medial to the ACL and superior to the PCL. What is your diagnosis?
    A. popliteal cyst
    B. parameniscal cyst
    C. haematoma
    D. rupture of popliteal cyst
    E. intercruciate cyst
251. Housemaid's knee is:
    A. prepatellar bursitis
    B. quadriceps fat pad impingement syndrome
    C. tendinopathy of the quadriceps tendon
    D. tendinopathy of the patellar tendon
    E. deep infrapatellar bursitis
252. What muscles are affected in a common peroneal nerve injury?
    A. popliteus
    B. tibialis anterior
    C. tibialis posterior
    D. flexor hallucis longus
    E. extensor hallucis longus

253. What may cause injury to the common peroneal nerve?
   A. fracture of the lateral tibial condyle
   B. total knee arthroplasty
   C. femoral tunnel placement during arthroscopy
   D. casting for fracture
   E. tibial osteotomy
254. A 23-year-old male presented after a comminuted tibial fracture with more pain than after trauma. MRI of the leg showed enhancement in the periphery of the muscles in the compartment, while the muscle showed no central enhancement. What is the next stage?
   A. acute operation
   B. CT without contrast
   C. ultrasound-guided steroid injection
   D. X-ray
   E. control MRI in 2 days
255. A meniscoid lesion in the ankle is referred to as:
   A. articular cartilage on the posterior talar process
   B. a scar after anterior talofibular rupture
   C. osteochondritis dissecans of the tibia
   D. synovitis of the tibialis anterior
   E. peroneus quartus
256. What is the typical and most common sequence of ligament tear?
   A. anterior talofibular ligament, posterior talofibular ligament, and calcaneofibular ligament
   B. anterior talofibular ligament, calcaneofibular ligament, and posterior talofibular ligament
   C. posterior talofibular ligament, anterior talofibular ligament, and calcaneofibular ligament
   D. anterior talofibular ligament, deltoid ligament, and calcaneofibular ligament
   E. deltoid ligament, spring ligament, and anterior talofibular ligament
257. A 45-year-old patient presented with chronic ankle pain. MRI revealed that the fibular tendons are displaced in the pouch between the superior peroneal retinaculum and distal fibula. What is your diagnosis?
   A. split rupture of the peroneus brevis tendon
   B. split rupture of the peroneus longus tendon
   C. superior peroneal retinaculum tear
   D. anterior talofibular ligament tear
   E. peroneal tenosynovitis

258. A 32-year-old runner presented with medial ankle swelling. MRI showed a local periosteal reaction present at the medial margin of the distal tibial metaphysis. What is the most likely cause?
    A. tibialis posterior tendinopathy
    B. osteomyelitis
    C. flexor retinaculum tear
    D. deltoid ligament tear
    E. synovitis
259. Turf toe is:
    A. tenosynovitis
    B. plantar fasciitis
    C. dorsal articular capsule rupture
    D. plantar plate rupture
    E. medial collateral ligament rupture
260. A 65-year-old patient presented with chronic Achilles tendon pain. MRI relevelled a spindle thickened Achilles tendon with a diffuse intrasubstance high signal. What is your diagnosis?
    A. partial rupture
    B. tendinosis
    C. paratendonitis
    D. Haglund syndrome
    E. partial tear
261. A 67-year-old patient presented with insertional Achilles tendon pain. MRI showed thinning of the Achilles tendon insertion and bone marrow oedema in the superoposterior calcaneus. What is the most likely diagnosis?
    A. os trigonum syndrome
    B. tendinosis
    C. paratendonitis
    D. Haglund syndrome
    E. calcaneal stress fracture
262. Choose the correct statement(s) regarding peroneal split rupture:
    A. The peroneus brevis is ruptured more often than the peroneus longus.
    B. Complete rupture is more common than splitting.
    C. Superior peroneal retinaculum tears are associated with splitting.
    D. Bone marrow oedema in the lateral malleolus may be seen.
    E. It is associated with lateral ligament rupture.
263. A 68-year-old female presented with calcaneal pain. MRI showed a higher signal in the posterior part of the plantar fascia and a plantar calcaneal spur with bone marrow oedema. What is your differential diagnosis?
    A. plantar fascia rupture
    B. plantar fasciitis
    C. plantar fibromatosis
    D. calcaneal stress fracture
    E. fibromatosis of the plantar heel pad

264. Choose ankle impingement and its cause(s):
   A. anterior osteophytes of the talar neck and anterior tibia
   B. tear of the anterior part of the deltoid ligament
   C. scarring of the anterior talofibular ligament
   D. os trigonum
   E. os naviculare accessorium
265. A 49-year-old male presented with medial ankle pain. MRI showed a low signal soft tissue on T1-weighted images filling the tarsal sinus. Bone marrow oedema in the neck of the talus and adjacent part of the calcaneus is visible. What is the differential diagnosis?
   A. talar neck stress fracture
   B. calcaneal stress fracture
   C. sinus tarsi syndrome
   D. talocalcaneal dislocation
   E. medial ankle instability
266. Choose the correct statement(s) regarding tarsal tunnel syndrome:
   A. It is a synonym of tarsal sinus syndrome.
   B. It may be caused by a ganglion.
   C. Plantar fasciitis is in the differential diagnosis.
   D. More than 75% of cases are due to bony deformation.
   E. Intramuscular oedema is not a reliable finding.

267. Choose the most likely cause of the condition seen on the X-ray (Fig. 3.1)

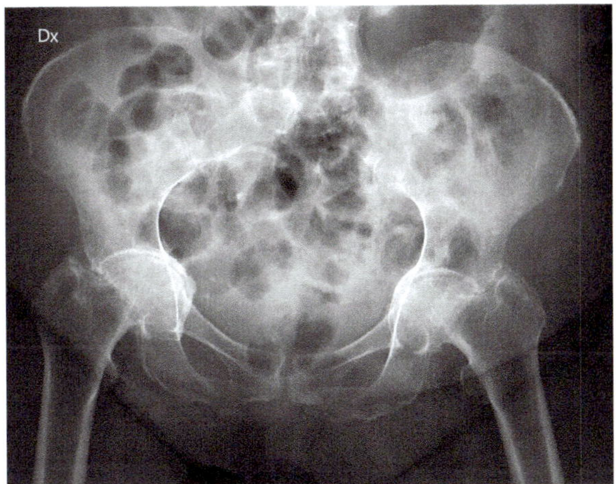

Fig. 3.1 X-ray of the pelvis

A. fracture
B. Paget disease
C. osteoarthritis
D. rheumatoid arthritis
E. ankylosing spondylitis

268. A 73-year-old patient presented after trauma. X-ray was performed (Fig. 3.2). What is your diagnosis?

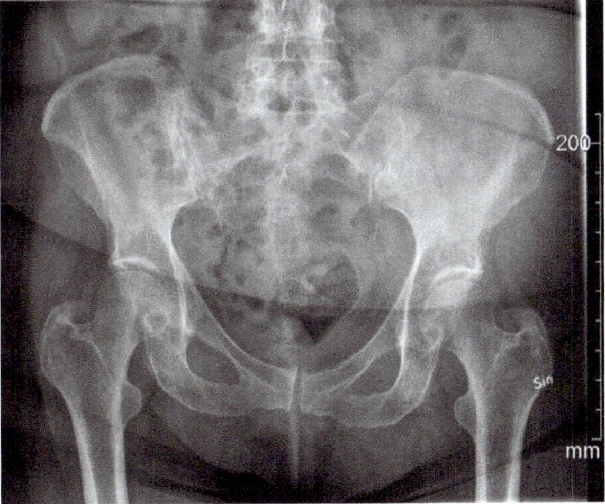

Fig. 3.2 X-ray of the pelvis

A. stress fracture of the left superior pubic ramus
B. fracture of the right superior pubic ramus
C. fracture of the left superior pubic ramus
D. fracture of the left trochanter major
E. fracture of the right acetabulum

269. What fracture is presented in Fig. 3.3?

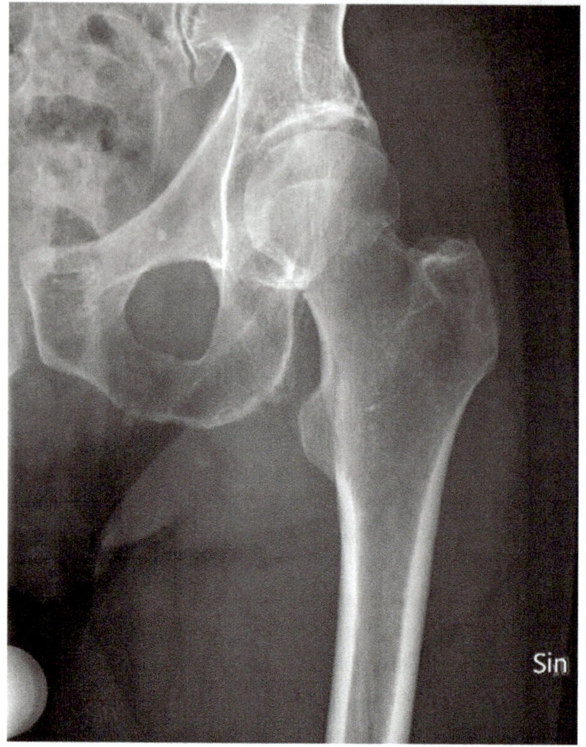

Fig. 3.3 X-ray of the left hip

A. Grade 1 according to Gardner's classification.
B. Grade 2 according to Gardner's classification.
C. Grade 3 according to Gardner's classification.
D. Grade 4 according to Gardner's classification.
E. Accessory projections are needed to answer this question.

270. Choose the correct regarding the X-ray shown in Fig. 3.4. Choose the correct statement(s) regarding this examination:
   a. stress fracture of the left ramus superior
   b. left acetabulum fracture
   c. left femoral neck fracture

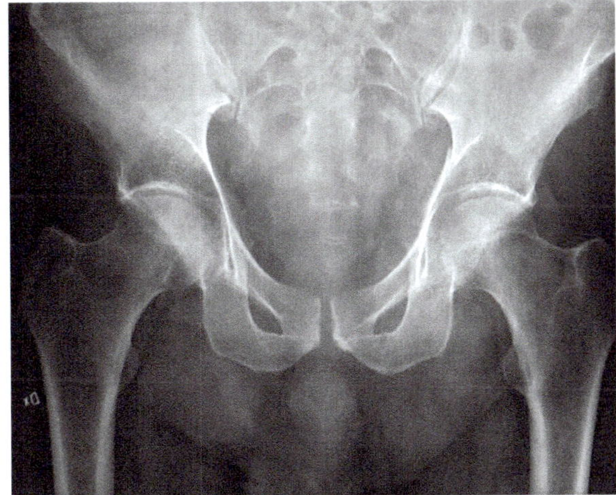

Fig. 3.4 X-ray of the pelvis

A. a, b, c
B. b, c
C. a
D. b
E. c

271. An 88-year-old patient fell off the chair. CT was done (Fig. 3.5), choose the correct statement(s) regarding this examination:
   a. osteolytic lesion in the acetabulum
   b. fracture of the trochanter minor
   c. fracture of the trochanter major

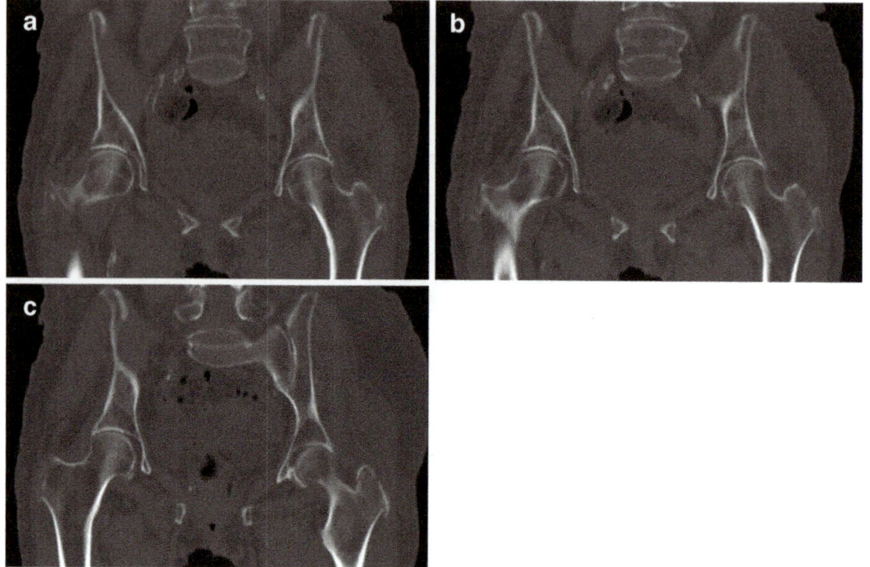

Fig. 3.5 Computed tomography (**a**–**c**) the pelvis, coronal sections

A. a, b, c
B. a, b
C. b, c
D. b
E. c

272. The patient in the previous question is unable to bear weight. MRI was done (Fig. 3.6), choose the correct statement(s) regarding this examination:
   a. The trochanter major is not fractured.
   b. Pertrochanteric femoral fracture is seen.
   c. The pathological fracture is seen.

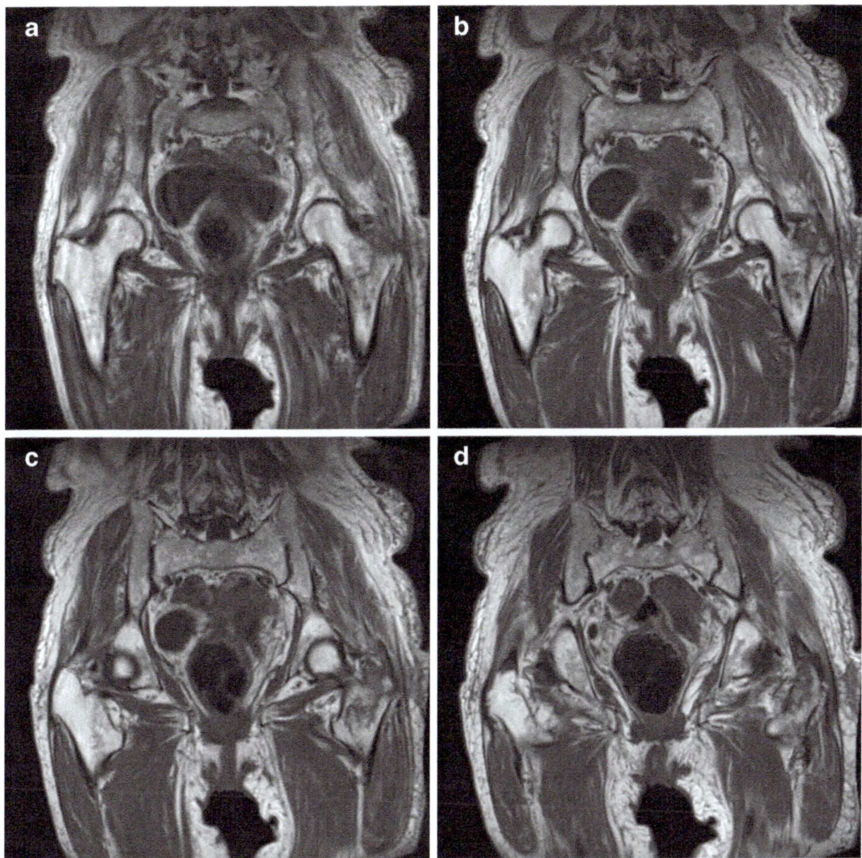

Fig. 3.6 (**a–d**) T1-weighted images, coronal sections

A. a, b, c
B. a, b
C. b, c
D. b
E. c

273. A 34-year-old patient was transported by emergency ambulance after involvement in a traffic accident. Computed tomography of the whole body was done. Choose the correct regarding fractures of the acetabulum (Fig. 3.7):
   a. the posterior wall
   b. the posterior column
   c. the anterior wall
   d. the anterior column
   e. the roof
   f. the medial wall

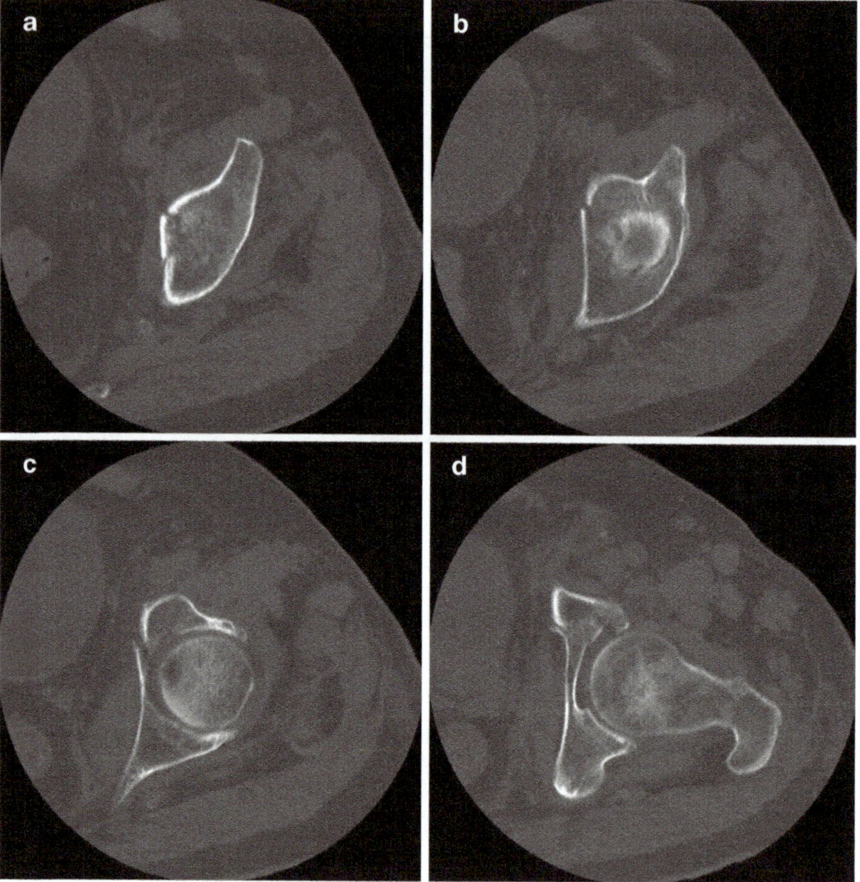

Fig. 3.7 Computed tomography of the left hip, axial sections (**a**–**d**)

A. a, c, f
B. a, c, e
C. c, e, f
D. d, e, f
E. b, e, f

274. A 42-year-old patient presented after the skiing knee injury. MRI was done (Videos 3.1, 3.2 and 3.3), choose the correct statement(s) regarding meniscus: (1) medial meniscus, (2) lateral meniscus
    a. normal
    b. radial tear
    c. vertical tear
    d. horizontal tear
    A. 1—a, 2—b
    B. 1—b, 2—a
    C. 1—c, 2—a
    D. 1—d, 2—c
    E. 1—c, 2—c
275. The patient from the previous question, choose the correct regarding the cartilage
    (1) medial femoral condyle, (2) lateral femoral condyle, (3) patella
    a. normal
    b. osteochondritis dissecans
    c. full-thickness defect
    d. focal cartilage tear
    A. 1—b, 2—a, 3—c
    B. 1—b, 2—d, 3—c, d
    C. 1—c, 2—a, 3—c, d
    D. 1—a, 2—d, 3—b
    E. 1—c, 2—c, 3—b
276. The patient from the previous question, choose the correct regarding the anterior (ACL) and posterior cruciate ligament (PCL):
    A. ACL—partial rupture, PCL—partial rupture
    B. ACL—total rupture, PCL—partial rupture
    C. ACL—partial rupture, PCL—total rupture
    D. ACL—total rupture, PCL—normal
    E. ACL and PCL normal

277. What structure is showed by the arrow (Fig. 3.8)?

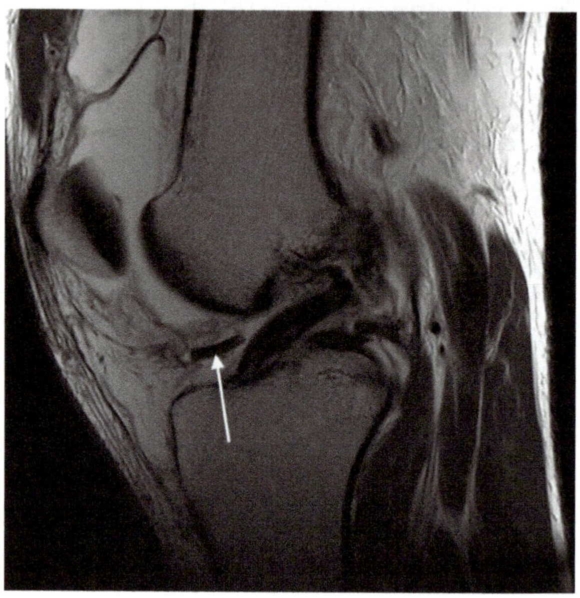

Fig. 3.8 A capture from Videos 3.1, 3.2 and 3.3. T2-weigted image, sagittal section

A. the part of the torn ligament
B. the part of the torn meniscus
C. the part of the torn cartilage
D. the free bone fragment
E. the anatomical variant

278. What indirect signs can be noticed on the MRI showed on Video 3.4.
   a. angle between lateral tibial plateau and ACL less than 45°
   b. angle between Blumensaat line and ACL is open posterior
   c. posterior displacement of the posterior horn of the lateral meniscus
   d. bone contusions in lateral compartment
   e. lateral femoral sulcus

A. a, b, c, d, e
B. a, b, c, d
C. a, b, c
D. a, b, d
E. c, d, e

279. A 34-year-old patient after sport trauma. MRI was done (Fig. 3.9); what lesion is seen in soleus muscle?

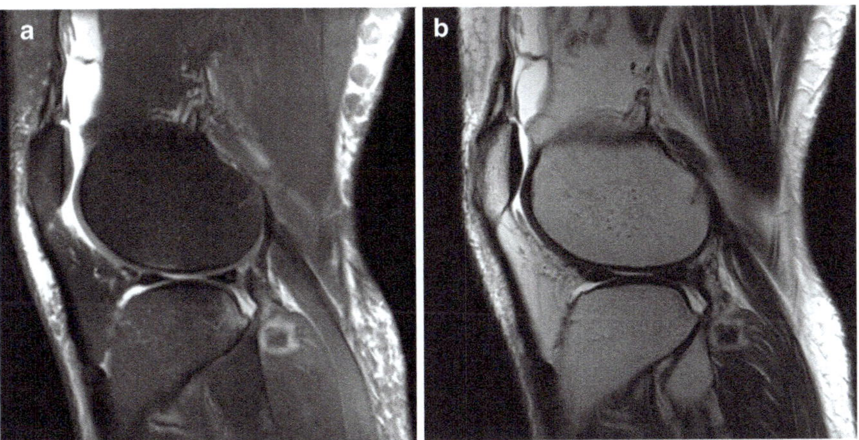

Fig. 3.9 (**a**) Proton density-weighted images with fat suppression, (**b**) T2-weighted image with fat suppression

A. sarcoma
B. ganglion
C. haematoma
D. myositis ossificans
E. it is unspecific, a further diagnostic is recommended

280. The patient from the previous question, choose the correct regarding the anterior (ACL) and posterior cruciate ligament (PCL) (Fig. 3.10):

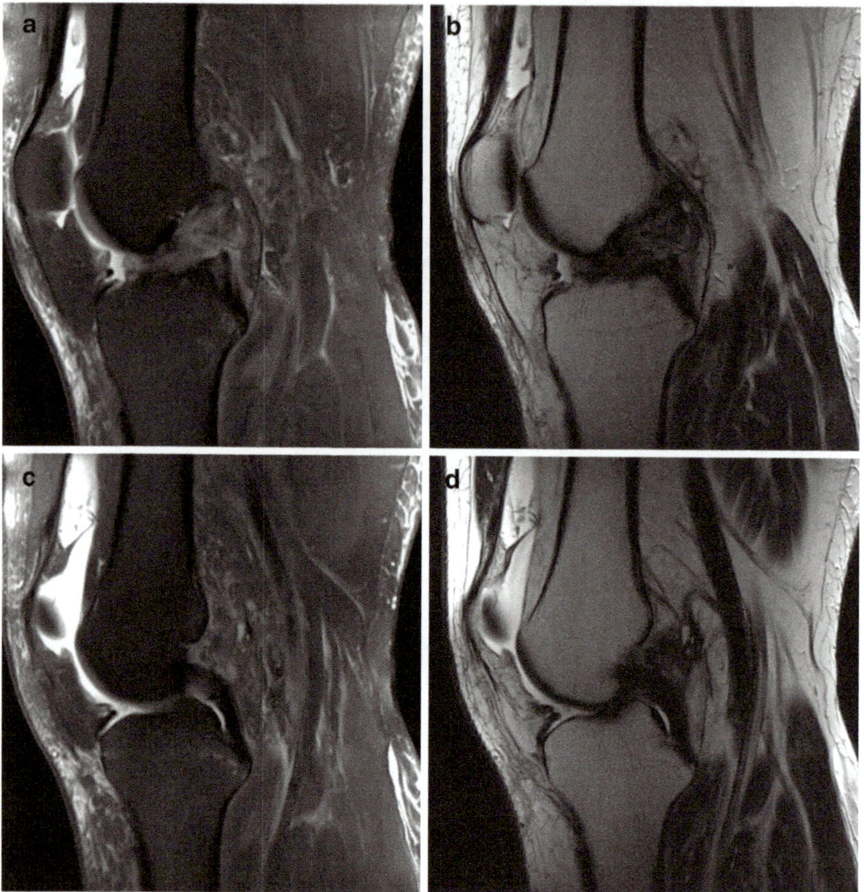

Fig. 3.10 (**a** and **c**) Proton density-weighted images with fat suppression, sagittal sections; (**b** and **d**) T2-weighted images, sagittal sections

A. ACL—partial rupture, PCL—partial rupture
B. ACL—total rupture, PCL—partial rupture
C. ACL—partial rupture, PCL—total rupture
D. ACL—total rupture, PCL—normal
E. ACL and PCL normal

281. A 22-year-old patient presented after the knee injury. MRI was done (Fig. 3.11). What structure is showed by the arrow?

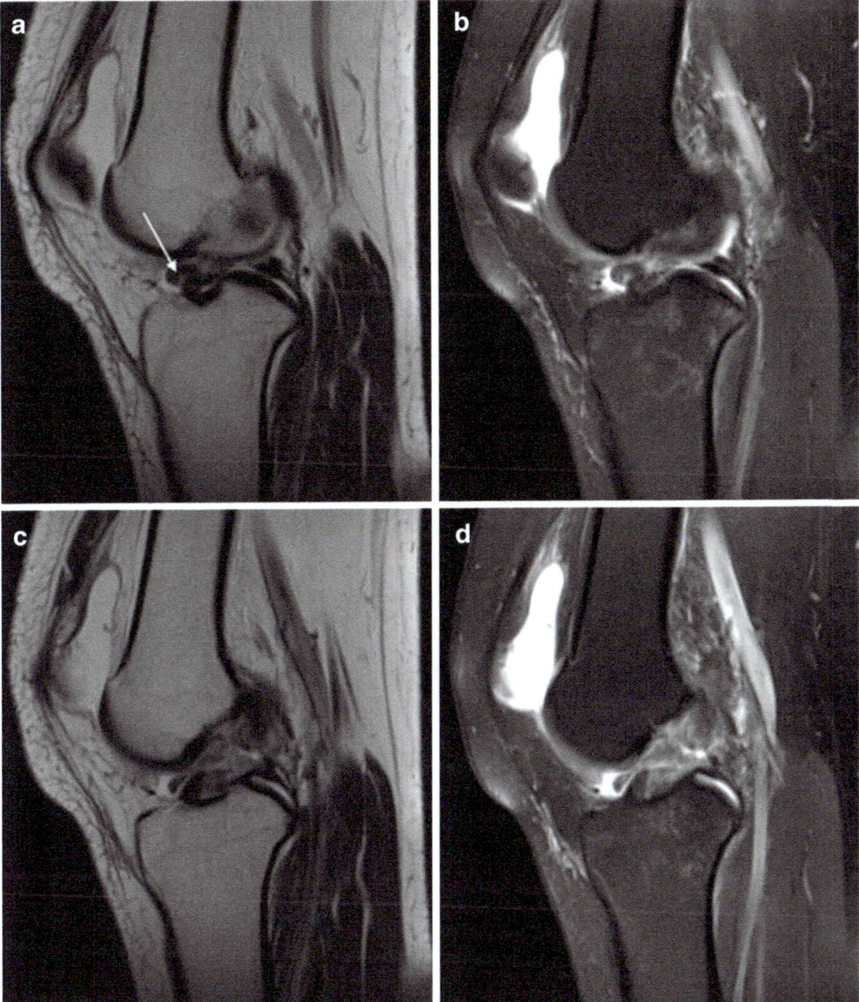

Fig. 3.11 (**a** and **c**) T2-weighted images, sagittal sections; (**b** and **d**) proton density-weighted images with fat suppression, sagittal sections

A. pigmented villonodular synovitis
B. synovial chondromatosis
C. "the cyclops eye"
D. giant cell tumour
E. no one above

282. A 42-year-old patient presenting after the skiing knee injury. MRI was done (Videos 3.5, 3.6 and 3.7), choose the correct statement(s) regarding meniscus: (1) medial meniscus, (2) lateral meniscus
    a. normal
    b. radial tear
    c. vertical tear
    d. horizontal tear
    A. 1—a, 2—b
    B. 1—b, 2—a
    C. 1—c, 2—a
    D. 1—d, 2—c
    E. 1—c, 2—c
283. The patient from the previous question, choose the correct regarding the anterior (ACL) and posterior cruciate ligament (PCL):
    A. ACL—partial rupture, PCL—partial rupture
    B. ACL—total rupture in the origin, PCL—partial rupture
    C. ACL—partial rupture, PCL—total rupture in the origin
    D. ACL—total rupture in the insertion, PCL—normal
    E. ACL—total rupture in the origin, PCL—normal
284. Choose the correct regarding the meniscus seen in Fig. 3.12:

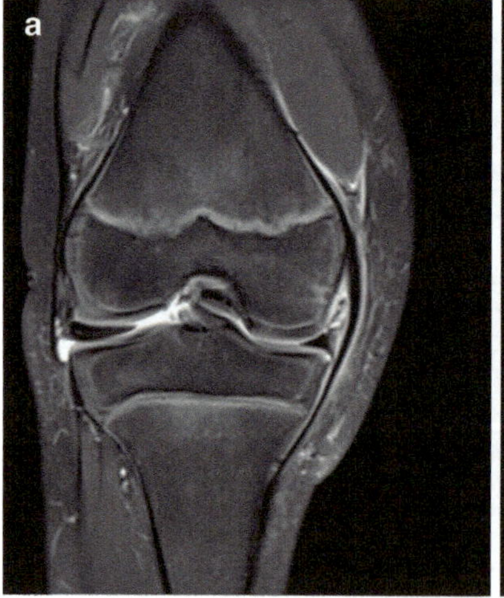

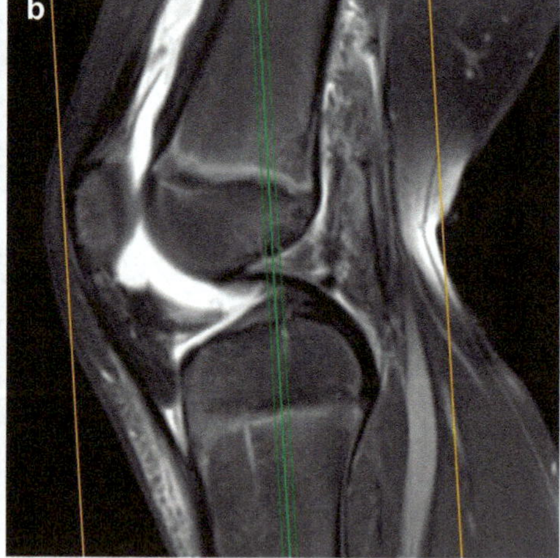

Fig. 3.12 (**a**) Proton density-weighted with fat suppression, coronal section; (**b**) proton density-weighted with fat suppression, sagittal section

    A. medial—normal, lateral—discoid
    B. medial—normal, lateral—degeneration
    C. medial—degeneration, lateral—normal
    D. medial—vertical rupture, lateral—discoid
    E. medial—horizontal rupture, lateral—discoid

285. Choose the correct regarding the medial meniscus:
    A. degeneration
    B. radial rupture
    C. vertical rupture
    D. horizontal rupture
    E. complex rupture
286. The patient from the previous question. Choose the one best description regarding the lateral meniscus:
    A. flap
    B. bucket handle
    C. meniscal fraying
    D. flipped meniscus
    E. parrot beak rupture
287. Choose the correct regarding the medial (MCL) and lateral collateral ligament (LCL) shown in Videos 3.8, 3.9 and 3.10?
    A. MCL and LCL—normal
    B. MCL—total tear, LCL—normal
    C. MCL—normal, LCL—partial tear
    D. MCL—partial tear, LCL—normal
    E. MCL—partial tear, LCL—partial tear
288. What meniscal rupture is shown in Fig. 3.13 (Video 3.11)?

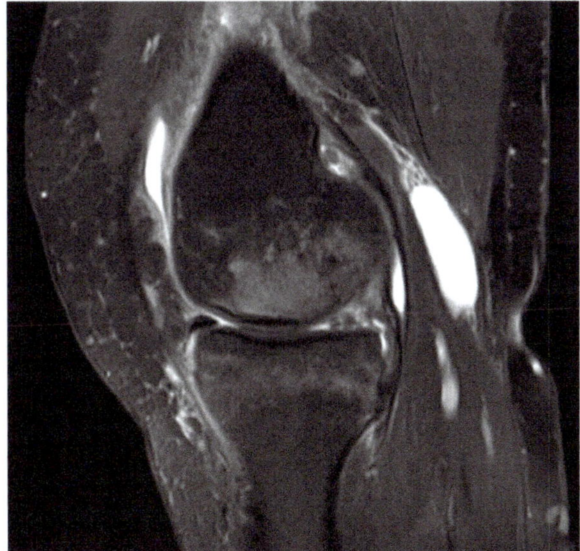

Fig. 3.13 Proton density-weighted image, sagittal section

    A. radial rupture
    B. vertical rupture
    C. flipped meniscus
    D. horizontal rupture
    E. parrot beak rupture

289. What pathology in the medial meniscus is seen in the Video 3.12?
    A. parrot beak
    B. radial rupture
    C. bucket handle
    D. vertical rupture
    E. flipped meniscus
290. Patient presented after knee trauma during a basketball match. Computed tomography was done (Fig. 3.14). Segond fracture is seen in figure(s):

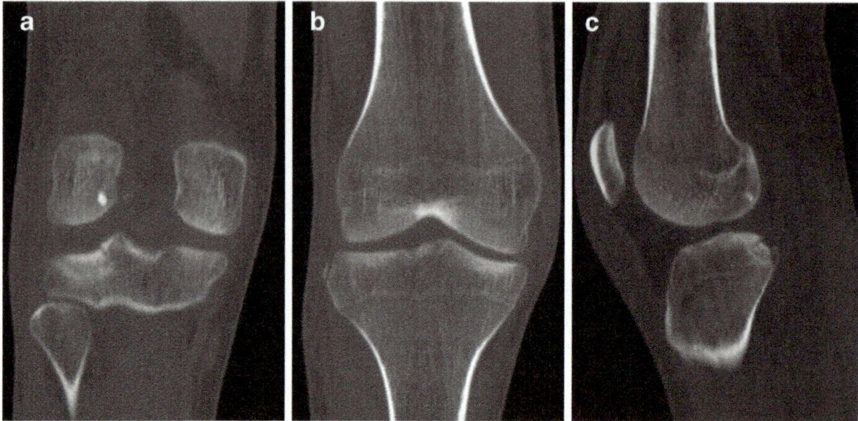

Fig. 3.14 Computed tomography of the knee. (**a** and **b**) Coronal sections, (**c**) sagittal section

    A. a, b, c
    B. a, b
    C. b, c
    D. a
    E. b

291. A 56-year-old patient presenting with acute severe knee pain without trauma. MRI was done (Fig. 3.15), what is the most likely diagnosis?

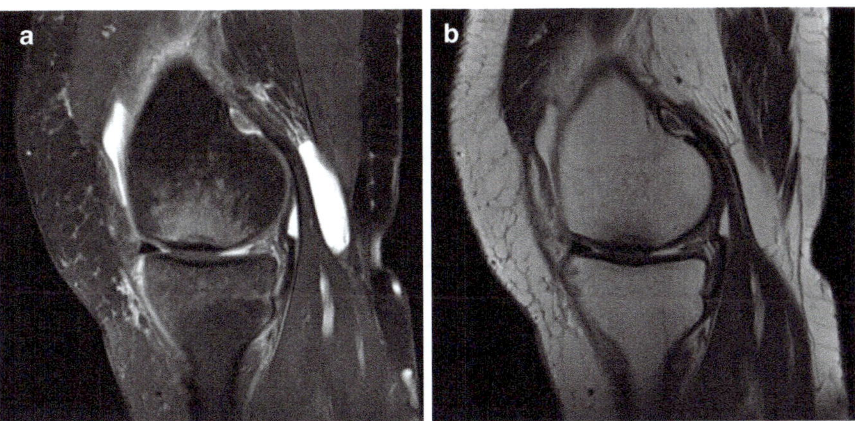

Fig. 3.15 (**a**) Proton density-weighted image, sagittal section; (**b**) T2-weighted image, sagittal section

A. bone tumour
B. osteonecrosis
C. osteochondritis dissecans
D. subchondral insufficient fracture
E. radial tear of the medial meniscus

292. A 26-year-old patient presenting with knee pain and locking. MRI was done (Fig.3.16), what is the most likely diagnosis?

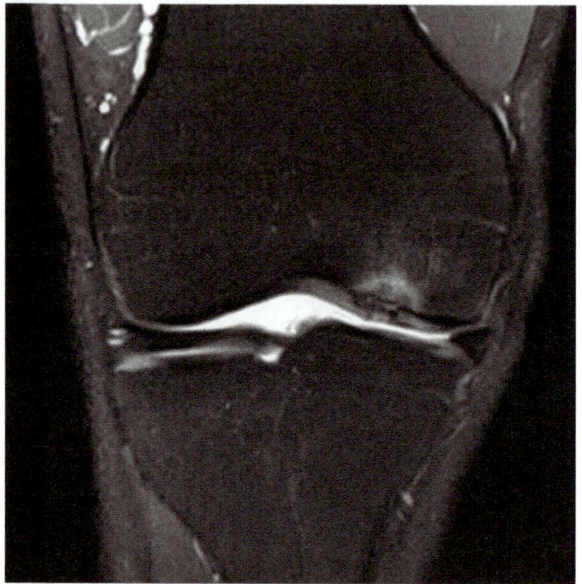

Fig. 3.16 Proton density-weighted with fat suppression, coronal section

A. cartilage tear
B. bone tumour
C. osteonecrosis
D. osteochondritis dissecans
E. subchondral insufficient fracture

293. A 34-year-old patient after ankle trauma. MRI of the ankle was done (Fig. 3.17), choose the correct regarding the anterior talofibular ligament (ATFL):

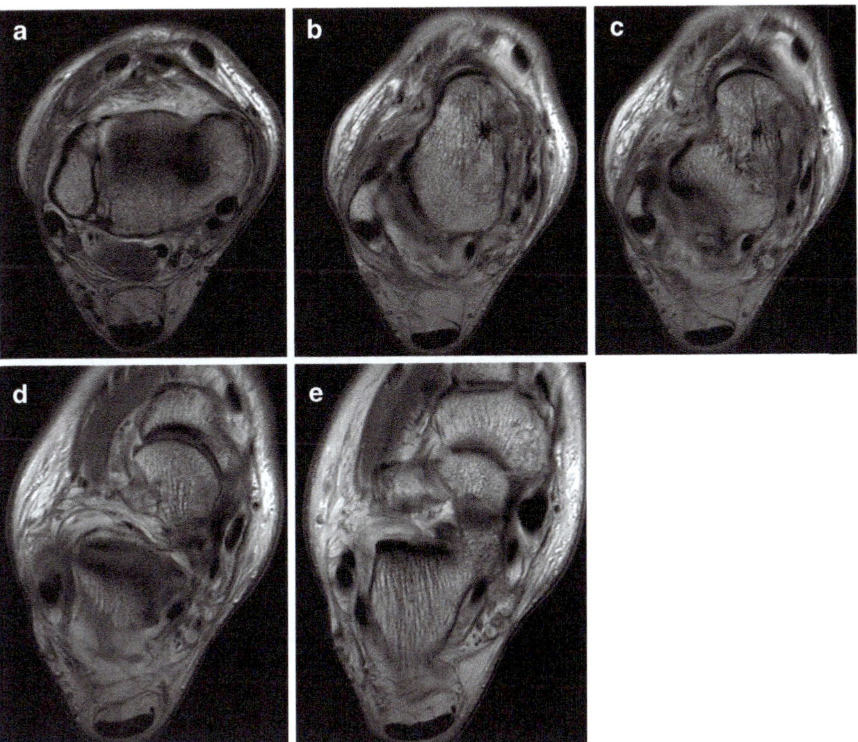

Fig. 3.17 (**a**–**e**) Proton density-weighted images, axial sections

A. ATFL is visible in Fig. 3.17b, c.
B. Acute total rupture of the ATFL is noticed.
C. Acute partial rupture of the ATFL is seen.
D. Chronic total rupture of the ATFL is noticed.
E. Chronic partial rupture of the ATFL is seen.

294. The calcaneofibular ligament is visible in the figures:
    A. 3.17a
    B. 3.17b
    C. 3.17c
    D. 3.17d
    E. 3.17e
295. Choose the structures that are normal in Fig. 3.17:
    A. Achilles tendon
    B. tibialis posterior
    C. flexor retinaculum
    D. flexor hallucis longus
    E. posterior talofibular ligament
296. Choose the correct regarding the patient after ankle injury (Fig. 3.18):

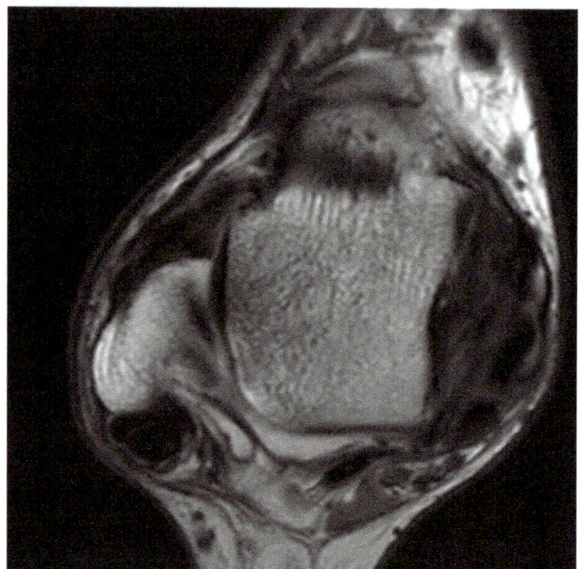

Fig. 3.18 T2-weighted image, axial section

    A. Fibrosis in the anterolateral gutter is seen.
    B. Thickened anterior talofibular ligament.
    C. Superior peroneal retinaculum is torn.
    D. Possible anterolateral conflict.
    E. Flexor retinaculum is normal.

297. A 23-year-old patient with foot pain without trauma. X-ray was done (Fig. 3.19), choose the correct regarding this patient?

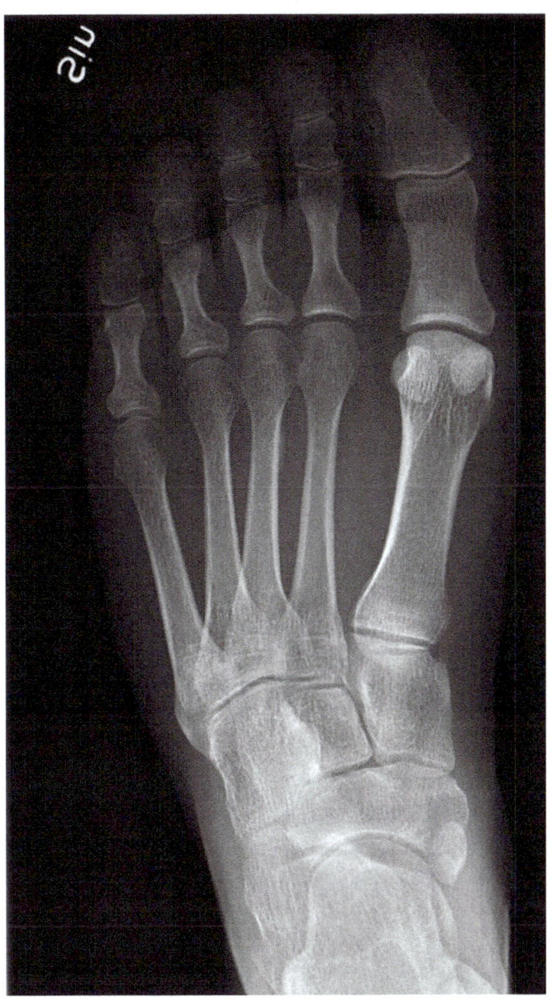

Fig. 3.19 X-ray of the foot

A. No abnormality is seen.
B. Stress fracture is seen.
C. Osteonecrosis is seen.
D. Arthritis is seen.
E. Tumour is seen.

298. A 39-year-old patient with chronic ankle pain after trauma. Choose the correct regarding radiological findings (Fig. 3.20):

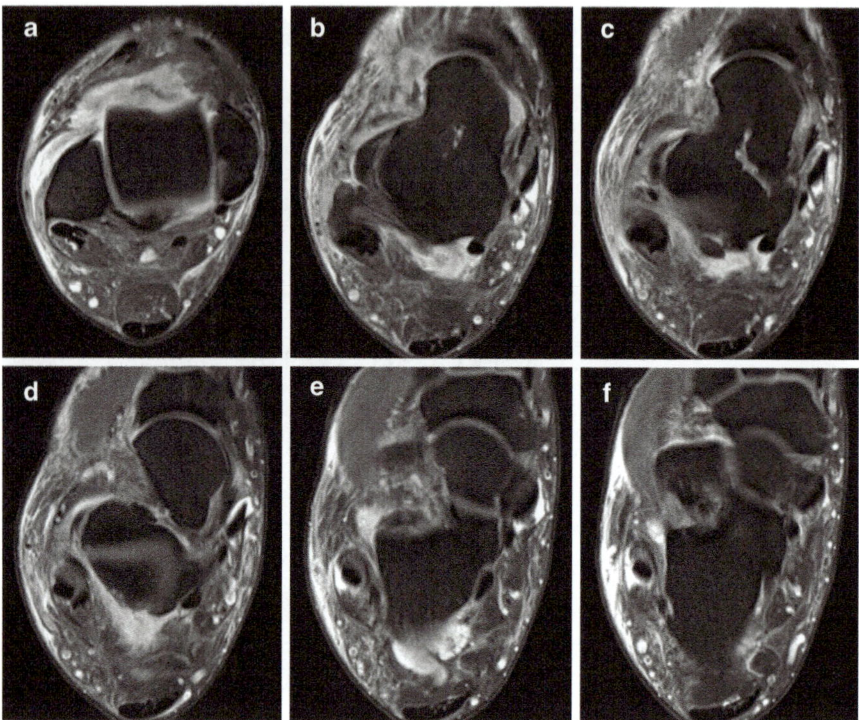

Fig. 3.20 (**a**–**f**) Proton density-weighted images with fat suppression

A. chronic avulsion of the anterior talofibular ligament
B. total rupture of the calcaneofibular ligament
C. partial rupture of the posterior talofibular ligament
D. total rupture of the posterior talofibular ligament
E. fracture of the posterior process of the talus

299. Choose the correct regarding the peroneal tendons:

A. Peroneus longus and peroneus brevis are normal.
B. Split rupture of the peroneus longus and peroneus brevis.
C. Split rupture of the peroneus longus; peroneus brevis is normal.
D. Split rupture of the peroneus brevis; peroneus longus is normal.
E. Total rupture of the peroneus longus, peroneus brevis is normal.

300. A 75-year-old patient presenting with hip pain without trauma. Choose the correct regarding the X-ray (Fig. 3.21):

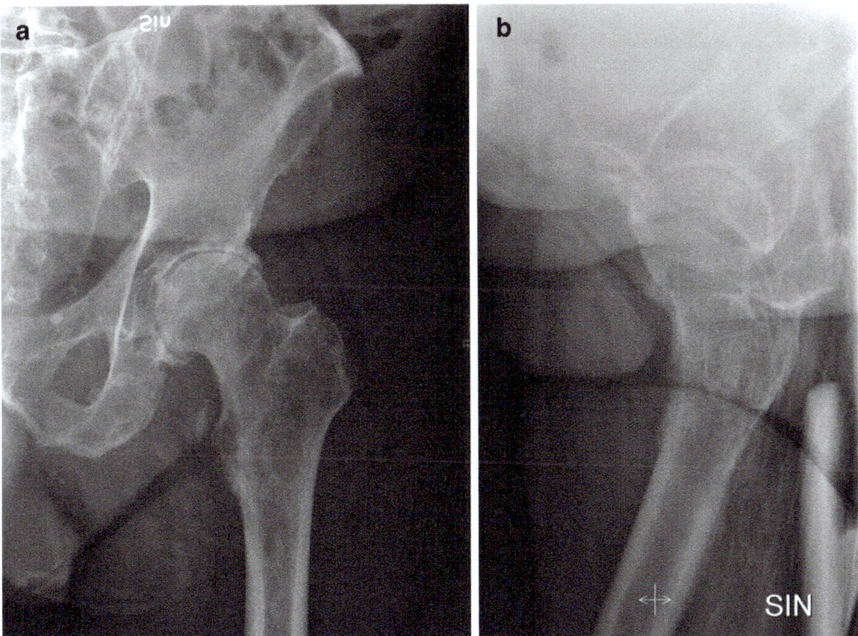

Fig. 3.21 X-ray of the left hip (**a**, **b**)

A. Hip osteoarthritis.
B. Pathologic fracture.
C. Trochanter major fracture.
D. Trochanter minor fracture.
E. Further diagnostic is indicated.

301. A 56-year-old patient presenting with right hip pain. X-ray was performed (Fig. 3.22). What is the origin of the lesion in the right hip (one answer is correct)?

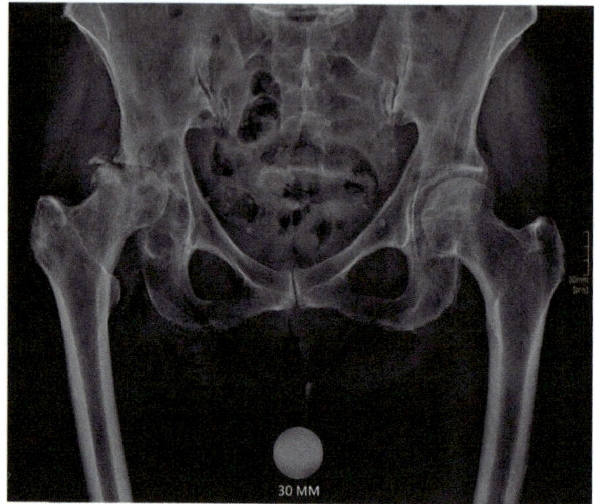

Fig. 3.22 X-ray of the pelvis

A. fracture
B. metastasis
C. osteoarthritis
D. osteonecrosis
E. septic arthritis

302. A 19-year-old patient presenting after ankle trauma, MRI was performed (Fig. 3.23). The arrow shows (one answer is correct):

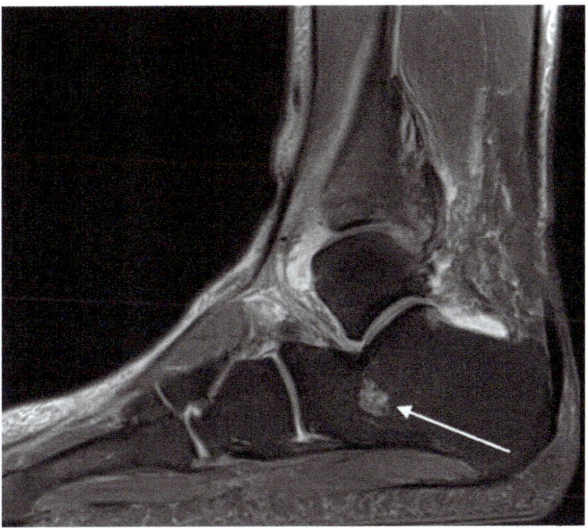

Fig. 3.23 Proton density-weighted image with fat suppression, sagittal section

A. ganglion of the talocalcaneal ligament
B. unicameral bone cyst
C. solitary bone cyst
D. vascular remnant
E. enchondroma

303. A Toddler's fracture occurs most commonly in the:
A. femur
B. tibia
C. fibula
D. talus
E. calcaneus

304. What is the name of the accessory bone present in the peroneus longus?
A. os vesalianum
B. os sustentaculi
C. os trigonum
D. os peroneum
E. os subfibulare

305. A pilon fracture:
A. It is a stress fracture of the distal tibia.
B. It is a vertical fracture of the distal tibia.
C. It is a transverse fracture of the distal tibia.
D. It is a comminuted fracture of the medial malleolus.
E. It is a stress fracture of the medial malleolus.

306. A 13-year-old boy presented with calcaneal pain aggravated by running. MRI showed a sclerotic, irregular, and fragmented calcaneal apophysis. What is the most likely diagnosis?
    A. plantar fasciitis
    B. calcaneal stress fracture
    C. juvenile idiopathic arthritis
    D. calcaneal apophysitis
    E. unicameral bone cyst
307. A 31-year-old female felt acute pain in the medial part of the leg. Choose the correct statement(s) regarding this condition:
    A. MRI is the golden standard to detect the pathology.
    B. Rupture of the plantaris tendon is a potential differential diagnosis.
    C. Medial gastrocnemius tear is a potential differential diagnosis.
    D. Rupture popliteal cyst is a potential differential diagnosis.
    E. Sprain of the gastrocnemius is a potential differential diagnosis.
308. What is the differential diagnosis of posterior ankle pain?
    A. Achilles tendinopathy
    B. calcaneal bursitis
    C. plantar fasciitis
    D. os trigonum syndrome
    E. osteochondral lesion
309. A 53-year-old patient presented with suspicion of a talar osteochondral lesion. MRI showed multiple fusiform nodules in the plantar fascia. What is the differential diagnosis?
    A. partial ruptures of the plantar fascia
    B. plantar fasciitis
    C. plantar fibromatosis
    D. neurofibromatosis
    E. schwannoma
310. A 45-year-old male presented after foot trauma. X-ray revolved dislocation of the sesamoid bone of the first toe. What is your diagnosis?
    A. flexor hallucis longus tear
    B. tears of intrinsic foot muscles
    C. plantar plate tear
    D. plantar fasciitis
    E. plantar fibromatosis

Key to Chapter 3

140. D.
141. C. A typical patient is elderly female with osteoporosis. Vertically oriented lesions with the transverse component are called Honda sign.
142. A, B, E. C and D are common localization for avulsion fractures.
143. B. Risk is about 90%.
144. A, E.
145. B, E.
146. D, E. A is not true because the lateral condyle is most commonly involved. B is not true because most fractures are intra-articular. Splitting fracture is more typical for younger individuals, while depression for patients with the osteoporosis.
147. C. It is avulsion of one of capsular ligaments which is called the anterolateral ligament. (https://doi.org/10.1111/joa.12087)
148. A, C, E.
149. B, D.
150. A, C, E.
151. B.
152. A, C, D, E. The female athlete triad is a relationship of menstrual dysfunction, low energy availability, and decreased bone mineral density. Eating disorder may associate the condition.
153. A, C [1].
154. A, C, E.
155. A, B, C, D, E.
156. C.
157. B.
158. B, D, E.
159. A, C, D, E.
160. D. Symmetric cortical thickening in elderly patient who takes bisphosphonate occurs in the lateral part of shaft. Other fractures are less possible in this context.
161. C.
162. B.
163. A, C, D. Risk of genitourinary track injury is high, about 40%.
164. A, B, C.
165. C, D.
166. A, B.
167. A, D.
168. A, B, E.
169. B, C.
170. E.
171. B.
172. E. Non-operative treatment is indicated if depression is less than 4–5 mm and diastasis less than 3–4 mm.

173. A, B, C, D, E.
174. D, E. Marginal avulsion may be seen at any outline of the patella. Sinding-Larsen-Johansson syndrome is an injury to immature osteotendinous junction, sometimes considered as jumper's knee in children.
175. B. Osteochondritis dissecans on patella accounts for about 7% of all osteochondritis dissecans seen in the knee.
176. C. Most of non-fusion ossification center is connected with synchondrosis.
177. B, C. This avulsion is called the arcuate sign demonstrating an of the arcuate ligament complex.
178. B, C, D.
179. A, B, C, D, E.
180. B.
181. A, B.
182. B, C, D, E.
183. B.
184. B.
185. A.
186. A, E.
187. C. Isolated fracture of the medial or posterior malleolus is instable and is related with syndesmotic injury and fracture of fibula (Weber C).
188. A, E.
189. A, B, C, D.
190. B, C.
191. B, C.
192. E.
193. D, E. The stress fracture usually does not involve articular surfaces. Sclerotic line involves the bony trabeculae of the posterior process or is parallel to the subtalar joint.
194. B, C, D, E.
195. C.
196. C. On the inferior surface of the cuboideum sulcus for peroneus longus tendon is present. The fracture line is seen only occasionally, and CT is recommended if sclerotic lines or deformation is seen.
197. A, C, D.
198. E.
199. A, D, E.
200. C.
201. A, D, E.
202. A, C.
203. A, B, C.
204. A, B, C, D.
205. B.
206. E.
207. C.
208. B, D.

209. C, D.
210. B.
211. C.
212. B, E.
213. C.
214. C.
215. A, B, C.
216. D.
217. A, B, D.
218. D, E.
219. C.
220. B, C, D.
221. C.
222. A, E.
223. A, C, D, E.
224. A, C, D, E.
225. A, B, C.
226. C.
227. B, C.
228. B, D. A—clip injury (MCL injury), C—patellar luxation, E—pivot shift (ACL tear).
229. C.
230. A, B, E.
231. A, E.
232. A, E.
233. C, D. Anterolateral ligament is a part of articular capsule which inserts on lateral tibial condyle. Avulsion of this ligament is called Segond sign.
234. C.
235. A, C, E. Anterior and posterior meniscofemoral ligaments unite posterior horn of the medial meniscus and insert on the medial femoral condyle. Oblique meniscomeniscal ligament unites posterior horn of the medial meniscus with the anterior horn of the lateral meniscus.
236. C.
237. B, D.
238. B. Vessels are not present in the white part of meniscus. Cleft rupture split meniscus into superior and inferior part.
239. B, C.
240. C, E.
241. A, D.
242. A. The stellate rupture is a complex meniscal rupture.
243. B.
244. C.
245. A, C, D.
246. B, C, D.
247. A, B.

248. A, B, D, E.
249. A, B, D.
250. E.
251. A. Housemaid's knee synonyms are washerwoman's knee or preacher's knee. It is superficial infrapatellar bursitis or pretibial bursitis.
252. B, E.
253. A, B, C, D, E.
254. A. This is a description of acute compartment syndrome.
255. B. Meniscoid lesion may cause anterolateral impingement.
256. B.
257. C.
258. C.
259. D.
260. B.
261. D.
262. A, C, D, E.
263. A, B.
264. A, B, C, D. Os naviculare accessorium does not cause the ankle impingement but may cause insufficiency of the tibialis posterior tendon.
265. C.
266. B, C. The tarsal tunnel syndrome is most common idiopathic condition of entrapment of the tibialis nerve or medial or lateral plantar nerve in the tarsal tunnel. Due to affecting of the nerve, muscle oedema is a reliable sign.
267. C. Causes of the acetabular protrusion are among others: Paget disease, osteoarthritis, rheumatoid arthritis (and other arthritides).
268. C.
269. A.
270. D.
271. E.
272. D.
273. D.
274. C.
275. C.
276. D.
277. C.
278. D.
279. C.
280. D.
281. E. This structure is the torn and reflected ACL fibres.
282. C.
283. D.
284. A.
285. E.
286. D.
287. D.

288. A.
289. B.
290. E.
291. D, E.
292. D.
293. A, B.
294. D, E.
295. A, B, D, E.
296. A, B, D, E.
297. B.
298. A.
299. D.
300. A, B, D, E.
301. D.
302. D.
303. B. Differential diagnosis is the trampoline fracture. It is a transverse tibial metaphyseal fracture seen in children which may occur while jumping on a trampoline.
304. D.
305. B.
306. D.
307. B, C, D, E.
308. A, B, D, E.
309. C.
310. B.

Reference

1. Fredericson M, Bergman AG, Hoffman KL, Dillingham MS. Tibial stress reaction in runners. Correlation of clinical symptoms and scintigraphy with a new magnetic resonance imaging grading system. Am J Sports Med. 1995;23(4):472–81. https://doi.org/10.1177/036354659502300418.

Part III

Spine

4 Trauma

1. Step-offs in lines in the cervical spine indicate an injury. Choose the correct statement(s) about lines:
   A. Space between the line applied to the posterior border of the airways and the line delimits the anterior wall of the vertebrae is wider superiorly.
   B. The spinolaminal line is convex posteriorly.
   C. The line which marks the anterior extent of the spinal canal is convex anteriorly.
   D. All spinal lines are convex anteriorly.
   E. All spinal lines are convex posteriorly.
2. What is the normal distance between the anterior arch of C1 and the odontoid process in adults?
   A. 2 mm
   B. 4 mm
   C. 6 mm
   D. 8 mm
   E. 9 mm
3. What is the normal distance between the anterior arch of C1 and the odontoid process in children?
   A. 2 mm
   B. 4 mm
   C. 6 mm
   D. 8 mm
   E. 9 mm

P. Szaro, *Musculoskeletal Radiology for Residents*,
https://doi.org/10.1007/978-3-030-85182-8_4

4. Choose the correct statement(s) regarding C1 fractures:
   A. Diving headfirst into shallow water may lead to a compression fracture of C1.
   B. C1 fractures are often associated with the other cervical spine fractures.
   C. Burst fractures of C1 often result in spinal cord injury.
   D. Dissection of the vertebral artery may be associated with a C1 fracture.
   E. Lateral masses of C1 extend beyond the outlines of the body of C2 in the coronal plane.
5. CT after trauma showed only that the space between the odontoid process and left of the lateral mass of C1 is wider than that corresponding to the right side. Which interpretation is correct?
   A. It is caused by the rotation of the patient's head to the left.
   B. It is caused by the rotation of the patient's head to the right.
   C. It is caused by the slight extension of the patient's head.
   D. It is caused by the slight flexion of the patient's head.
   E. It is caused by the extensive flexion of the patient's head.
6. Hyperextension of the cervical spine may result in:
   A. Jefferson fracture
   B. burst fracture
   C. clay-shoveler fracture
   D. Hangman fracture
   E. fracture of the odontoid process
7. Choose the correct statement(s) regarding teardrop fractures:
   A. Extension teardrop fractures are unstable in extension.
   B. The anteroinferior part of the vertebral body is fractured in flexion teardrop.
   C. The anterior longitudinal ligament is disrupted both in flexion and extension teardrop fractures.
   D. Flexion teardrop fracture is not as acute as extension teardrop fracture.
   E. Extension fractures more commonly occur in the lower cervical spine.
8. What are the features of the flexion teardrop fracture?
   A. anterior-superior fracture of the vertebral body
   B. anterior disc space widening
   C. injury of the posterior ligaments
   D. cervical kyphosis
   E. retropulsion of the posterior part of the vertebral body
9. The Hamburger sign is seen in:
   A. avulsion of the anterior tubercle of C1
   B. avulsion of the posterior tubercle of C1
   C. luxation of the odontoid process
   D. luxation of the intervertebral joint
   E. luxation in the atlantooccipital joint

10. Fracture of the medial occipital condyle suggests:
    A. impaction of the skull
    B. avulsion of the anterior longitudinal ligament
    C. avulsion of the alar ligament
    D. distraction
    E. hyperflexion
11. Choose the feature(s) of the most common odontoid fracture:
    A. fracture of the odontoid fracture apex
    B. high risk of non-union
    C. relatively stable
    D. superior the level of the transverse part of the cruciform ligament
    E. oblique course fracture
12. Bilateral locked facet joints are associated with:
    A. rupture of the posterior ligament complex
    B. rupture of the posterior longitudinal ligament
    C. injury to the annulus fibrosus
    D. injury of the anterior longitudinal ligament
    E. spinal cord injury
13. What structures are located in the posterior column of the spine?
    A. ligamentum flavum
    B. posterior longitudinal ligament
    C. posterior part of the annulus fibrosus
    D. supraspinal ligament
    E. facet joints
14. Choose the typical feature(s) of seatbelt fractures:
    A. Distraction occurs anteriorly during compression posteriorly.
    B. Abdominal injuries are relatively uncommon.
    C. Widening of the interpedicular distance.
    D. Increased intercostal distance.
    E. Decreased interspinal distance.
15. Choose the correct statement(s) regarding typical compression fractures:
    A. Osteoporosis is a common background.
    B. There is cortical breakage in the posterior outline of the vertebrae.
    C. Sclerosis parallel to the endplate indicates acute fracture.
    D. Most often fracture of the middle column is noticed.
    E. The most common cause is anteflexion.
16. Choose the right pair:
    A. intravertebral fluid cleft—pathological fracture
    B. multiple compression fractures—osteoporotic fractures
    C. intravertebral vacuum cleft with the collapse of the endplate—pathological fracture
    D. posterior bulging of the vertebral body—osteoporotic fracture
    E. low-signal intensity line on T1- and T2-weighted images—osteoporotic fracture

17. Choose what the known risk factor for Kümmell disease is?
    A. cement augmentation
    B. osteoporosis
    C. steroid therapy
    D. alcoholism
    E. radiation therapy
18. What is the most common level for a burst fracture?
    A. Th9
    B. Th11
    C. Th12
    D. L1
    E. L2
19. A patient fell from a 5 m height and landed on his/her feet, what do you expect in this situation?
    A. Fracture of the anterior and middle column of the vertebral column.
    B. Fracture involves the posterior outline of the vertebral body.
    C. Posterior contour of the vertebral body is concave.
    D. Widening of the interpedicular distance.
    E. Spinal canal narrowing.
20. Choose the feature that is more typical for burst fracture than compression fracture:
    A. Loss of the posterior part of the vertebral body.
    B. Spinal cord injury.
    C. Stable fracture.
    D. Interpedicular widening.
    E. Posterior vertebral body cortex is normal.
21. Choose when the distance between the pedicles of the vertebrae are widened:
    A. osteoporotic compression fracture
    B. clay-shoveler fracture
    C. Chance fracture
    D. seatbelt fracture
    E. burst fracture
22. Loss of the anterior vertebral height may be seen in:
    A. burst fracture
    B. osteoporotic fracture
    C. wedge fracture
    D. Chance fracture
    E. Hangman fracture
23. The double spine process sign may be seen in:
    A. Chance fracture
    B. clay-shoveler fracture
    C. Jefferson fracture
    D. osteoporotic fracture
    E. Hangman fracture

24. Choose the correct statement(s) regarding seatbelt fractures:
    A. Most seatbelt fractures are stable.
    B. Vertical fracture line in the vertebral body is seen.
    C. Transverse process fracture may be noticed.
    D. Increased distance between the ribs may be seen.
    E. The thoracolumbar junction is commonly involved.
25. Vertebra plana can be noticed in:
    A. skeletal metastasis
    B. multiple myeloma
    C. osteoporosis
    D. leukaemia
    E. infection
26. What features are typical for translation-rotation spine injuries?
    A. Posterior ligamentous complex is intact.
    B. Dislocated facet joints.
    C. Transverse process fractures.
    D. Vertebral body subluxation.
    E. Rib fractures.
27. What is the most common level for traumatic disc herniation?
    A. Cervical spine.
    B. Thoracic spine.
    C. Lumbar spine.
    D. There is no such prevalence.
    E. At the level of L5/S1.

Key to Chapter 4

1. C, D.
2. A. Less than 2.5 mm is normal in adults.
3. A, B. Less than 5 mm is normal in children.
4. C, D, E.
5. A.
6. D, E.
7. A, B, C.
8. C, D, E.
9. D.
10. C.
11. B.
12. A, B, C, D, E.
13. A, D, E.
14. C, D.
15. A, C, E.

16. B, E. The intravertebral fluid cleft is called fluid sign which is typical for benign fracture. The intravertebral vacuum cleft is called Kümmell disease and is a form of avascular necrosis. Posterior bulging of the vertebral body is a sign of intravertebral malign, especially if signal of pedicle is abnormal (low on T1). Whereas retropulsion of the superoposterior part of endplate with preserved concave outline of the vertebral body is seen in benign fractures.
17. B, C, D, E.
18. D [1].
19. A, B, D, E.
20. A, B, D.
21. C, D, E.
22. A, B, C, D.
23. A.
24. A, C, D, E.
25. A, B, C, D, E.
26. B, C, D, E.
27. A.

Reference

1. Lee P, Hunter TB, Taljanovic M. Musculoskeletal colloquialisms: how did we come up with these names? Radiographics. 2004;24(4):1009–27. https://doi.org/10.1148/rg.244045015.

5 Degenerative Spine

28. Choose the features of a normal intervertebral disc:
    A. Low signal in the central part on T2-weighted images.
    B. High signal in the peripheral part on T2-weighted images.
    C. Signal is similar to the muscle on T1-weighted images.
    D. Does not extend outside the outlines of the adjacent vertebral body.
    E. Somewhat lower signal than adjacent normal red marrow on T1-weighted images.
29. What is the most common level in the lumbar spine for disc abnormalities?
    A. Th12/L1 and L1/L2
    B. L1/L2 and L2/L3
    C. L2/L3 and L3/L4
    D. L3/L4 and L4/L5
    E. L4/L5 and L5/S1
30. What is the most common level in the cervical spine for disc abnormalities?
    A. C2/C3 and C3/C4
    B. C3/C4 and C4/C5
    C. C4/C5 and C5/C6
    D. C5/C6 and C6/C7
    E. C6/C7 and Th1/C7
31. Focal lumbar disc abnormalities most commonly affect:
    A. lateral recess
    B. intervertebral foramen
    C. extraforaminal region
    D. anterior longitudinal ligament
    E. spinal canal and lateral recess

P. Szaro, *Musculoskeletal Radiology for Residents*,
https://doi.org/10.1007/978-3-030-85182-8_5

32. Choose the correct statement(s) regarding small spontaneous epidural haematomas:
    A. It may be related to disc extrusion.
    B. It may cause acute back pain.
    C. It usually resolves quickly.
    D. Higher signal on T1-weighted images is a sign.
    E. It may be difficult to differentiate from a sequestered disc.
33. Gas in an intervertebral disc indicates:
    A. infection
    B. trauma
    C. distraction
    D. degeneration
    E. spondylodiscitis
34. Disc calcification may be the result of:
    A. infection
    B. ankylosing spondylitis
    C. crystal deposition disease
    D. ochronosis and haemochromatosis
    E. diffuse idiopathic skeletal hyperostosis
35. What features may help to differentiate between synovial cyst and sequestered disc fragments in the spinal canal:
    A. localization
    B. presence of calcification
    C. shape
    D. signal on T1-weighted image
    E. signal on T2-weighted image
36. Choose the features of Baastrup's disease:
    A. The interspinous ligament is fibrillated or torn.
    B. Bone marrow oedema in the spinous process.
    C. Fluid signal between the spinous processes.
    D. Spine instability.
    E. Synovial cyst.
37. Congenital lumbar spinal stenosis:
    A. It is caused mainly by facet joint degeneration.
    B. It usually occurs in patients older than 50 years of age.
    C. It occurs most commonly at the L5/S1 level.
    D. It is seen in patients with achondroplasia.
    E. It occurs in shortening of pedicles.

38. Choose the correct statement(s) regarding annular fissure:
    A. It may be associated with disc degeneration.
    B. It is a common cause of back pain.
    C. It is related to spondylodiscitis.
    D. It corresponds to a high-intensity zone on T1-weighted images.
    E. It is a sign of coexisting malignancy.
39. Extension of the intervertebral disc beyond the edges of the ring of the vertebral body is called:
    A. extrusion
    B. protrusion
    C. bulging
    D. sequestration
    E. high-intensity zone (HIZ)
40. Dislocation of disc material from the site of disc extrusion without continuity to the disc is called:
    A. bulging
    B. extrusion
    C. sequestration
    D. annular fissure
    E. asymmetric bulging
41. You noticed a disc bulge about 1.8 mm in the midsagittal plane at the L5/S1 level. Choose the correct statement(s):
    A. It is probably due to disc degeneration.
    B. It is a sign of extrusion.
    C. It is an early sign of protrusion.
    D. It is a sign of disc fissure.
    E. It is normal.
42. What can be a possible aetiology of failed back surgery syndrome?
    A. missing a sequestration
    B. spinal dura arteriovenous fistula
    C. epidural haematoma
    D. nerve root conflict with device
    E. scar formation
43. A 48-year-old patient presenting 1 year after spine surgery at the L4/L5 level. There is clinical suspicion of an L5 nerve syndrome on the left side. Axial T2-weighted MR images showed an ill-defined outline of the left L5 nerve root. The epidural space at this level was filled by an intermediate signal intensity structure, which showed some enhancement. What is the most likely diagnosis?
    A. spondylodiscitis
    B. nerve root cyst
    C. arachnoiditis
    D. post-operative scar
    E. nerve root inflammation

44. Extrusion of disc tissue to the left lateral recess L5/S1 may compress the:
    A. L5 nerve root
    B. L4 nerve root
    C. S2 nerve root
    D. S1 nerve root
    E. L5 and S1 nerve roots
45. Foraminal protrusion of the C7/Th1 disc may compress the:
    A. C7 nerve root
    B. C8 nerve root
    C. Th1 nerve root
    D. Th2 nerve root
    E. Th3 nerve root
46. A cross-sectional area of the dura sac in the lumbar spine of less than:
    A. 200 mm^2 indicated central stenosis
    B. 190 mm^2 indicated central stenosis
    C. 175 mm^2 indicated central stenosis
    D. 150 mm^2 indicated central stenosis
    E. 100 mm^2 indicated central stenosis
47. Central stenosis in the lumbar spine is considered when the anteroposterior diameter is less than:
    A. 10 mm
    B. 12 mm
    C. 15 mm
    D. 18 mm
    E. 20 mm
48. When the distance measured on the axial section between the most anterior point of the superior articular process and the posterior border of the vertebral body is less than:
    A. 2 mm is considered lateral stenosis in the lumbar spine
    B. 4 mm is considered lateral stenosis in the lumbar spine
    C. 6 mm is considered lateral stenosis in the lumbar spine
    D. 8 mm is considered lateral stenosis in the lumbar spine
    E. 10 mm is considered lateral stenosis in the lumbar spine
49. Distance between the superior articular facet and the top part of the pedicle on axial cross-section:
    A. less than 3 mm indicates lumbar stenosis
    B. less than 4 mm indicates lumbar stenosis
    C. less than 5 mm indicates lumbar stenosis
    D. less than 6 mm indicates lumbar stenosis
    E. less than 7 mm indicates lumbar stenosis

50. What values of the lateral recess angle, which is measured between the lines parallel to the superior articular process and the vertebral body at the level of pedicle, are abnormal?
    A. 40°
    B. 25°
    C. 60°
    D. 15°
    E. 50°
51. An increased risk for relative spinal canal stenosis in the cervical spine occurs when the anteroposterior diameter is less than:
    A. 10 mm
    B. 13 mm
    C. 16 mm
    D. 19 mm
    E. 22 mm
52. An increased risk for absolute spinal canal stenosis in the cervical spine occurs when the anteroposterior diameter is less than:
    A. 10 mm
    B. 13 mm
    C. 16 mm
    D. 19 mm
    E. 22 mm
53. Choose the correct statements regarding reactive changes in endplates:
    A. Sclerosis corresponds to Modic type II changes.
    B. Bone marrow oedema corresponds to Modic type I changes.
    C. Higher signal on T1- and T2-weighted images corresponds to Modic type II changes.
    D. Low signal on T1- and T2-weighted images corresponds to Modic type III changes.
    E. Low signal on T1-weighted and high signal on T2-weighted images corresponds to bone marrow oedema.
54. Choose the correct statement(s) regarding facet joint disease:
    A. It is a common cause of back pain.
    B. Synovitis is a common sign.
    C. Effusion is commonly present.
    D. Contrast enhancement is not a feature.
    E. Radiofrequency may be used in treatment.

55. Choose the correct statement(s) regarding prostate cancer metastasis and Modic type III changes:
    A. Sclerotic metastases do not enhance on MRI because only a few vessels are present.
    B. Epidural component may be seen in metastasis but is not present in Modic type III changes.
    C. Both sclerotic metastases and Modic type III changes show low signal on T1- and T2-weighted images.
    D. Non-sclerotic metastases show low signal on T1-weighted and high signal on T2-weighted images.
    E. Fat component in dense sclerotic bone is seen in Modic type III changes but not in sclerotic metastases.
56. Fibrovascular bone marrow changes correspond to:
    A. bone sclerosis
    B. bone erosion
    C. bone marrow oedema
    D. Modic type I changes
    E. Modic type II changes
57. Choose the correct statement(s) regarding post-operative changes:
    A. The most common cause of bone marrow oedema in vertebral bodies is infection.
    B. A radiolucent zone in relation to a screw is a normal finding after 6 months.
    C. Bony birding anteriorly in the disc indicates that fusion is intact.
    D. Fatty ingrowth in the fused disc indicates that fusion is intact.
    E. Distinguishing recurrent disc herniation from scar tissue is possible with contrast.
58. Which examination is the easiest method of identifying spondylolysis?
    A. MRI without contrast
    B. MRI with contrast
    C. CT without contrast
    D. oblique plain films
    E. anterior-posterior view
59. The most common cause of lateral recess stenosis is:
    A. extrusion
    B. disc bulge
    C. protrusion
    D. degenerative changes of the facet joints
    E. thickening of the ligamentum flavum

60. Choose the correct statement(s) regarding post-operative changes:
    A. Protrusion of dura through a laminar defect is always pathologic.
    B. Distinguishing a meningocele from a pseudomeningocele is possible only with MRI.
    C. Fibrosis or scarring is best demonstrated after contrast injection.
    D. Contrast enhancement of intrathecal nerve roots is common, even after 1 year.
    E. Post-operative changes in discs may continue for years.
61. Choose the correct statement(s) regarding MRI findings in failed back surgery:
    A. Diffuse contrast enhancement is seen in scarring but not in disc extrusion.
    B. Epidural fibrosis commonly has irregular margins.
    C. Epidural fibrosis may cause mass effect on the dura sac.
    D. Recurrent disc protrusions commonly have regular outlines.
    E. Epidural fibrosis and extruded disc material are the two most common causes.

Key to Chapter 5

28. C, D, E.
29. E.
30. D.
31. E.
32. A, B, C, D, E.
33. D.
34. A, B, C, D, E.
35. A, E. Synovial cyst is located near the facet joint while sequestered disk fragments are usually present anteriorly. Higher signal on T2-weighted is typical for synovial cyst. Calcifications are present in both cases.
36. A, B, C, D.
37. D, E. Congenital lumbar stenosis occurs when pedicles are shortened. However, no consensus was made regarding normal values of spinal canal. Most commonly, the pathological one is considered when AP diameter is less than 10 mm.
38. A.
39. C.
40. C.
41. E. Disc bulge at this level up to 2 mm is normal.
42. A, B, C, D, E.
43. D.
44. D.
45. B.
46. E [1].
47. A [1].
48. A [1].
49. A.

50. B, D.
51. B [2].
52. A [2].
53. B, C, D, E.
54. A, B, C, E. Facet joint syndrome may be treated with radiofrequency which causes denervation.
55. A, B, C, D, E.
56. C, D.
57. C, D, E.
58. C.
59. D.
60. C, D.
61. A, B, C, D, E.

References

1. Steurer J, Roner S, Gnannt R, Hodler J, LumbSten Research Collaboration. Quantitative radiologic criteria for the diagnosis of lumbar spinal stenosis: a systematic literature review. BMC Musculoskelet Disord. 2011;12:175. https://doi.org/10.1186/1471-2474-12-175.
2. Ulbrich EJ, Schraner C, Boesch C, Hodler J, Busato A, Anderson SE, et al. Normative MR cervical spinal canal dimensions. Radiology. 2014;271(1):172–82. https://doi.org/10.1148/radiol.13120370.

6 Infections

62. What is the most common cause of spine infection?
    A. *Streptococcus aureus*
    B. *Klebsiella pneumoniae*
    C. *Staphylococcus aureus*
    D. Tuberculosis
    E. *Pseudomonas aeruginosa*
63. Choose the correct statement(s) regarding spine infection:
    A. Endplates show the richest blood supply.
    B. Vascularization of the intervertebral disc is rich in adults.
    C. Infection in adults starts primarily in the intervertebral disc and then passes to the adjacent endplates.
    D. As in neoplasm, infection passes via the intervertebral disc.
    E. In early infection, bone marrow oedema is not visible in contrast to Modic type I changes.
64. Choose the correct statement(s) regarding spine infection:
    A. Well-capsulated liquid is very common in spine infection.
    B. Extension of the epidural phlegmon is similar to that of neoplasms.
    C. Development of bony erosions may be visible on X-ray after 4–8 weeks.
    D. Sclerotic endplates may indicate healing processes of infection.
    E. Scintigraphy may differentiate between degenerative and infectious spine disease.
65. Choose the correct statement(s) regarding spondylodiscitis:
    A. As with neoplasms, involvement of the intervertebral disc is visible.
    B. In contrast to osteoporotic fractures, usually two adjacent vertebrae are involved.
    C. Likely metastasis most visibly involves the pedicle.
    D. Signal on T1-weighted images is lower in neoplasms.
    E. Diffusion is commonly restricted, as in neoplasms.

P. Szaro, *Musculoskeletal Radiology for Residents*,
https://doi.org/10.1007/978-3-030-85182-8_6

66. Choose the correct statement(s) regarding spondylodiscitis, neoplasms, and osteoporotic fractures:
    A. As in most neoplasms and osteoporotic fractures, the disc is involved.
    B. Contrast enhancement of the disc is visible in pyogenic infection in contrast to neoplasm.
    C. Contrast enhancement of some part the vertebral body may be seen in acute fracture, neoplasm, and spondylodiscitis.
    D. An epidural component is not a classic presentation of an osteoporotic fracture but may be seen in neoplasm and spondylodiscitis.
    E. A wedge deformity of the vertebral body is seen in an osteoporotic fracture but is not typical for neoplasm and spondylodiscitis.
67. What features help in the differentiation of infectious change from Modic type 1 degenerative changes of the spine:
    A. Hyperintense disc signal on T2-weighted images is seen in infection.
    B. Hypointense endplate signals on T1-weighted images seen in degenerative changes.
    C. Erosion of at least one vertebral endplate.
    D. Presence of bone marrow oedema.
    E. Hyperintense endplate signals on T2-weighted images seen in degenerative changes.
68. What features are more typical for intervertebral osteochondrosis than infection?
    A. vacuum phenomenon
    B. T2-hyperintensity within the disc
    C. band-like subchondral oedema
    D. subchondral fat accumulation
    E. subchondral bone sclerosis
69. What features are more typical for a Schmorl's node than infection?
    A. involvement of one endplate
    B. lack of diffuse abnormal signal in the disc
    C. erosions of the vertebral body endplates
    D. paraspinal inflammatory changes
    E. squaring of the vertebral bodies
70. What abnormalities may be detected in spondylodiscitis?
    A. Increased disc height is more typical for granulomatous infections.
    B. Gas in the intervertebral disc is more typical for pyogenic infections.
    C. Destruction of the endplates is more prominent in tuberculosis.
    D. High-signal intensity of the intervertebral disc on T2-weighted images.
    E. Inflammatory phlegmon, which is detected more often than abscess.

Key to Chapter 6

62. C.
63. A, C.
64. C, D. Well-capsulated fluid collection is much less common in spine infection than phlegmon. Destruction of endplates may be seen after couple of weeks thus X-ray is not an effective method.
65. B, D. Diffusion may be restricted in infection when abscess is seen.
66. B, C, D, E [1].
67. A, C. A and C are very specific for infection show about 80% specify for infection.
68. A, C, D, E.
69. A, B. Progressive discovertebral junction destruction which is called Andersson lesion causes pseudoarthrosis it may be confused with infectious spondylitis [1].
70. C, D, E.

Reference

1. Yeom JA, Lee IS, Suh HB, Song YS, Song JW. Magnetic resonance imaging findings of early spondylodiscitis: interpretive challenges and atypical findings. Korean J Radiol. 2016;17(5):565–80. https://doi.org/10.3348/kjr.2016.17.5.565.

7 Varia

71. A flattened vertebral body may be seen in:
    A. osteoporosis
    B. Morquio syndrome
    C. osteogenesis imperfecta
    D. seatbelt fracture
    E. Jefferson fracture
72. The Genant classification is applied for:
    A. humeral fractures
    B. glenoid fractures
    C. vertebral fractures
    D. pathologic fractures
    E. pelvis fractures
73. Choose the stable fractures:
    A. most of the osteoporotic fractures
    B. fracture of the apex of the odontoid process
    C. fracture of the base of the odontoid process
    D. fracture of the middle part of the odontoid process
    E. Chance fracture
74. Horizontally orientated fractures are visible in:
    A. seatbelt fractures
    B. burst fractures
    C. Chance fractures
    D. Jefferson fractures
    E. extension teardrop fractures

P. Szaro, *Musculoskeletal Radiology for Residents*,
https://doi.org/10.1007/978-3-030-85182-8_7

75. Choose the stable fracture:
    A. flexion teardrop
    B. clay-shoveler fracture
    C. wedge fracture
    D. avulsion of the alar ligament
    E. Hangman fracture
76. Which structures include the posterior ligament complex?
    A. ligamenum flavum
    B. supraspinous ligament
    C. posterior longitudinal ligament
    D. posterior 1/3 of the intervertebral disc
    E. facet joint capsule
77. Where did joint damage range from least to the most severe?
    A. perched facet joint, subluxated facet joint, anterolisthesis
    B. subluxated facet joint, anterolisthesis, perched facet joint
    C. anterolisthesis, perched facet joint, subluxated facet joint
    D. perched facet joint, anterolisthesis, subluxated facet joint
    E. subluxated facet joint, perched facet joint, anterolisthesis
78. Choose the term and its definition:
    1. spondylosis
    2. spondylolysis
    3. spondylolisthesis
    a. degeneration of the spine
    b. displacement of one vertebra relative to the one below
    c. the neural arch defect
    A. 1—a, 2—b, 3—c
    B. 1—b, 2—c, 3—a
    C. 1—c, 2—a, 3—b
    D. 1—c, 2—b, 3—a
    E. 1—a, 2—c, 3—b
79. What is the differential diagnosis of the bony fragment directly related to the apex of the odontoid process?
    A. fracture grade 1 (according to Anderson and D'Alonzo)
    B. fracture grade 2 (according to Anderson and D'Alonzo)
    C. fracture grade 3 (according to Anderson and D'Alonzo)
    D. os odontoideum
    E. os terminale
80. What fracture(s) occur in hyperextension?
    A. lamina fracture
    B. bilateral dislocation of the facet joints
    C. Hangman fracture
    D. clay-shoveler fracture
    E. Jefferson fracture

81. What features may be associated with whiplash?
    A. increased lordosis
    B. injury to the facet joint
    C. alar ligament injury
    D. supraspinous injury
    E. loss of lordosis
82. A bony fragment located anteroinferiorly to the vertebral body of C2 indicates:
    A. Jefferson fracture
    B. burst fracture
    C. flexion teardrop fracture
    D. pathologic fracture
    E. clay-shoveler fracture
83. Pars interarticularis fractures can be seen in:
    A. Jefferson fracture
    B. Chance fracture
    C. Hangman fracture
    D. spondylolysis
    E. clay-shoveler fracture
84. A 15-year-old patient presented with low back pain. MRI showed loss of disc height, a small defect in the endplate, and a hyperintense disc on T2-weighted images. What is the differential diagnosis?
    A. disc bulge
    B. Schmorl's node
    C. apophyseal ring fracture
    D. extrusion
    E. flexion fracture of the anterior endplate corner
85. Differential diagnosis of cervical hyperflexion injury includes:
    A. burst fracture
    B. Hangman fracture
    C. flexion-rotation injury
    D. whiplash fracture
    E. distraction injury
86. Which sequence is the best to demonstrate haemorrhage in the spinal cord?
    A. T1
    B. T2
    C. T2*
    D. T1 with contrast
    E. STIR
87. The differential diagnosis of cervical hyperextension injury includes:
    A. clay-shoveler fracture
    B. whiplash injury
    C. odontoid fractures
    D. burst fracture of C2
    E. fracture of the lamina

88. Choose the correct statement(s) regarding cervical fractures:
    A. The bony fragment in an extension teardrop fracture is larger than in a flexion teardrop fracture.
    B. Distraction of the posterior column is seen in extension teardrop fractures.
    C. Facet subluxation or distraction is seen in flexion teardrop fractures.
    D. Vertebral artery dissection is more common in extension teardrop fractures.
    E. Narrowing of the spinal canal may be seen in flexion teardrop fractures.
89. Choose a feature that differs between a burst fracture and flexion teardrop fracture:
    A. Fracture of the anterior column, which is more typical for flexion teardrop fractures.
    B. Distraction of the posterior column, which is more typical for flexion teardrop fractures.
    C. Fracture of the anterior column, which is more typical for burst fractures.
    D. Distraction of the posterior column, which is more typical for burst fractures.
    E. Loss of vertebral body height, which is more typical for burst fractures.
90. Sagittal fracture through the vertebral body is a sign of:
    A. distraction
    B. compression
    C. avulsion
    D. rotatory forces
    E. compression and rotation
91. Lateral bending of the cervical spine may result in:
    A. brachial plexus injury
    B. fractures of articular processes
    C. fracture of the transverse process
    D. uncinate process fracture
    E. spinal process fracture
92. What are the typical MRI features of traumatic disc herniation?
    A. Spinal nerve compression by disc material.
    B. Most commonly associated with vertebral fracture.
    C. If compression of the spinal cord is seen, oedema is usually not visible.
    D. Disruption of the posterior longitudinal ligament may be seen.
    E. Disruption of the anterior longitudinal ligament may be seen.
93. A sclerotic line on CT in the vertebral body in the patient after trauma may indicate:
    A. callus
    B. acute fracture
    C. infarction of trabecular bone
    D. distraction
    E. compression

94. Choose the correct combination fracture and feature:
    A. compression fracture–Posterior vertebral cortex is intact.
    B. Chance fracture–Posterior elements are normal.
    C. seatbelt fracture–A horizontal fracture in the posterior elements.
    D. pathologic fracture–The destruction of the posterior vertebral cortex.
    E. burst fracture–The concave contour of the vertebral body.
95. What features are more typical for burst fractures compared to compression fractures in the thoracolumbar region?
    A. presence of kyphosis
    B. split spinous process
    C. loss of anterior body height
    D. loss of posterior body height
    E. retropulsion of the body element
96. Choose the correct statement(s) regarding thoracolumbar fractures?
    A. A haematoma between spinal processes is visible both in compression and distraction.
    B. A haematoma between spinal processes is visible only in distraction.
    C. Retropulsion of the bone fragment may be seen in both Chance and burst fractures.
    D. Horizontal fracture line is visible in both Chance and burst fractures.
    E. All spinal columns are disrupted both in compression and distraction.
97. Choose the correct statement(s) regarding the comparison between wedge fractures and burst fractures in the thoracolumbar region:
    A. Compression of more than 50% can be seen in both types of fractures.
    B. Superior endplate fracture is seen in both fractures.
    C. Posterior vertebral body involvement is seen in burst fractures.
    D. Retropulsion of the body element is more common in wedge fractures.
    E. Vertically oriented fractures are more common for burst fractures.
98. Subacute spinal subdural haematomas:
    A. They show a higher signal than cerebrospinal fluid on T1-weighted images.
    B. They show a lower signal than cerebrospinal fluid on T1-weighted images.
    C. They show a higher signal than epidural fat on STIR.
    D. They show a higher signal than cerebrospinal fluid on T2-weighted images.
    E. They show a lower signal than cerebrospinal fluid on T2-weighted images.
99. Choose the best imaging tool for imaging spinal subdural haematomas:
    A. X-ray
    B. CT with IV contrast
    C. non-enhanced CT
    D. MRI with contrast
    E. MRI without contrast

100. Choose the features of meningocele:
    A. Epidural or paravertebral localization is common.
    B. High signal on T2-weighted or STIR sequences.
    C. Absent nerve root.
    D. Pachymeningeal thinning.
    E. Contrast enhancement is seen on MRI.
101. A 72-year-old patient presented with pain in the lumbar spine for 3 days without trauma. No previous examinations of the lumbar spine are available (Fig. 7.1). What is correct regarding the X-ray?

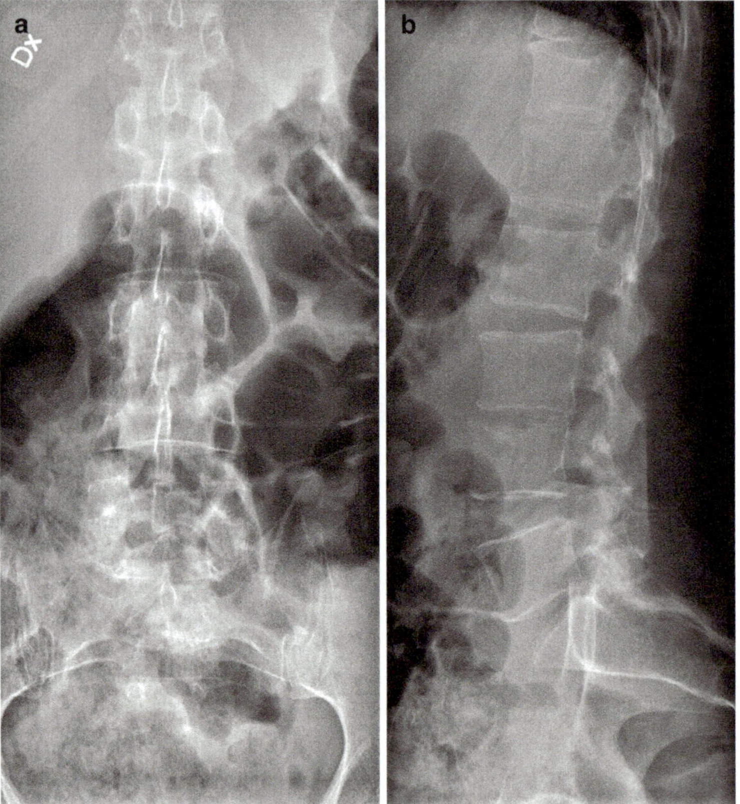

Fig. 7.1 (**a** and **b**) X-ray of the lumbar spine

A. Normal lumbar spine.
B. An unstable fracture is visible.
C. Degenerative spine mostly at the L1/L2 and L3/L4 levels.
D. Sacroiliitis.
E. Abnormality of the superior endplate of L4.

102. Regarding the patient from the previous question, what is the modality of choice?
    A. PET/CT
    B. CT (native)
    C. CECT
    D. MRI without contrast
    E. MRI with contrast
103. The patient from the previous question. CT was performed 2 weeks later because of no improvement after treatment and increasing pain. There was a fever of 38.4 °C (Fig. 7.2). What is the differential diagnosis?

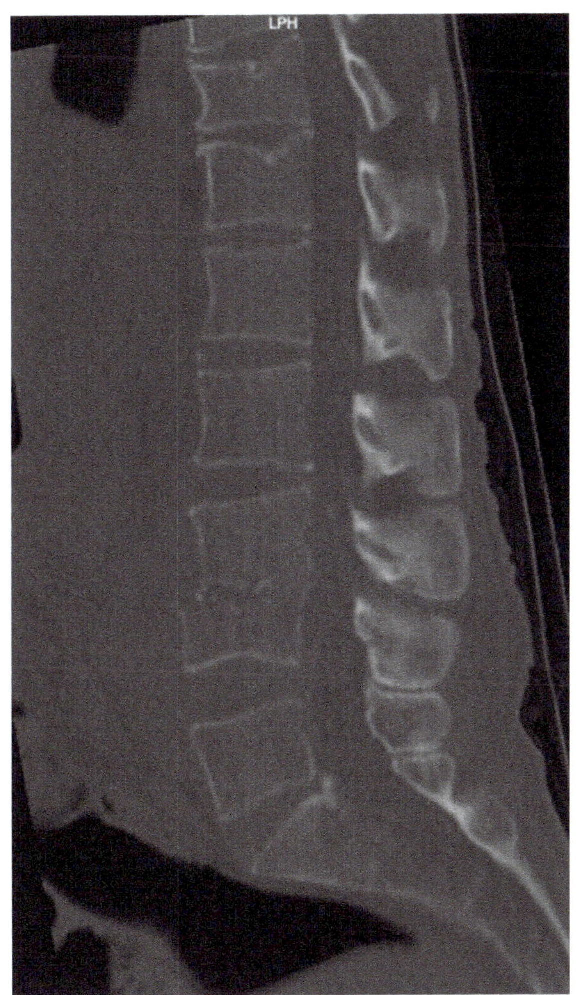

Fig. 7.2 Computed tomography of lumbar spine, sagittal section

    A. epidural metastases
    B. epidural haematomas
    C. disc extrusion
    D. spondylodiscitis
    E. pathologic fracture

104. Two days later, the patient from the previous question was referred for MRI. Choose the one best answer showing what sequence or sequences is/are most relevant to make the diagnosis?
   A. T1 sagittal without Gd
   B. T2 sagittal and axial
   C. T1 without Gd and T1 with Gd axial and sagittal
   D. STIR sagittal
   E. DWI/ADC

105. Figure 7.3 shows the MRI examination of the patient from the previous question. Which of the following findings do you recognize on these images?

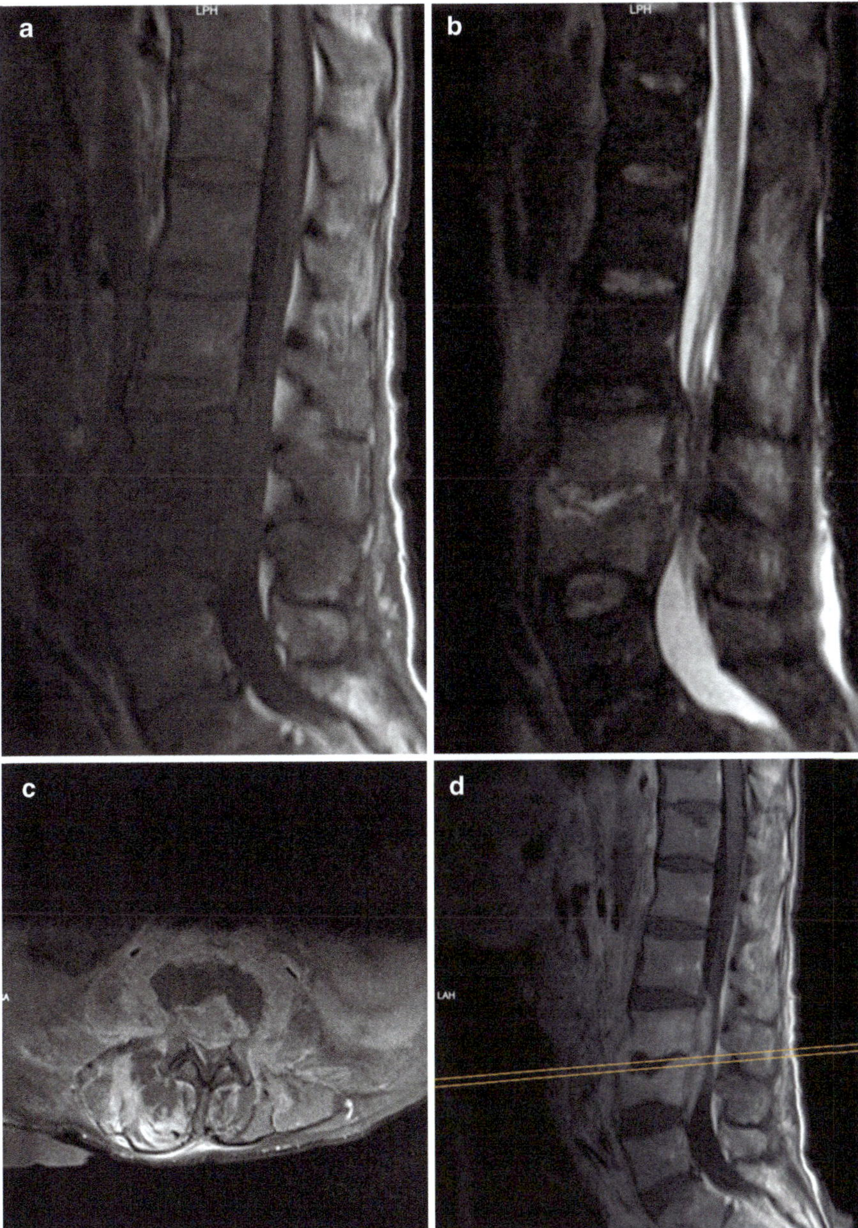

Fig. 7.3 (**a**) T1-weighted image, sagittal section; (**b**) T2-weighted with fat suppression, sagittal section; (**c**) T1-weighted with fat suppression and with contrast, axial section; (**d**) T1-weighted image with fat suppression and contrast, sagittal section

A. malignant process in the vertebral body
B. destruction of the endplate
C. subligamentous/epidural inflammatory process
D. epidural phlegmon
E. abscess in muscles

106. Choose the typical MRI features of the condition from the previous question (Fig. 7.3)?
A. low-signal intensity on T1-weighted images in marrow of the vertebral body
B. high-signal intensity on T1-weighted images in marrow of the vertebral body
C. contrast enhancement of bone marrow and endplates
D. contrast enhancement of disc if an abscess is not present
E. fluid signal in the disc on T2-weighted images

107. A 35-year-old patient presented with low back pain for 3 months. MRI of the sacroiliac joint was performed (Fig. 7.4). What abnormalities are visible?

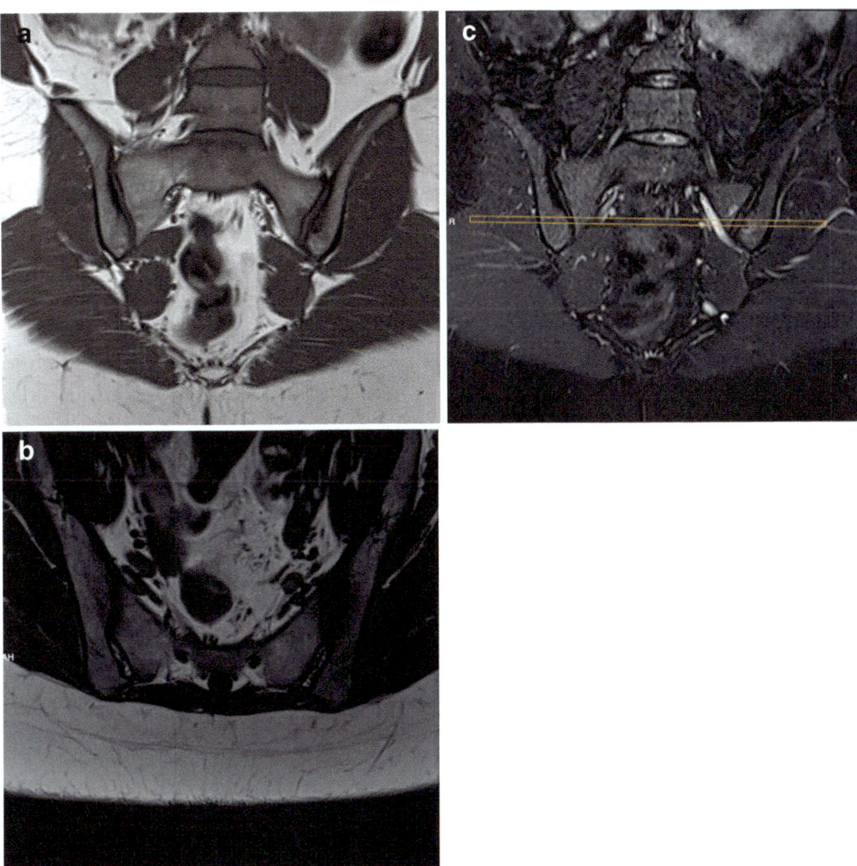

Fig. 7.4 (**a**) T1-weighted image, coronal section; (**b**) T1-weighted image, axial section; (**c**) short tau inversion recovery, coronal section

A. capsulitis
B. synovitis
C. erosion
D. subchondral sclerosis
E. osteitis condensans ilii

108. An 86-year-old patient presenting after neck trauma. CT of the cervical spine is shown in Fig. 7.5. What is the most likely diagnosis based on CT?

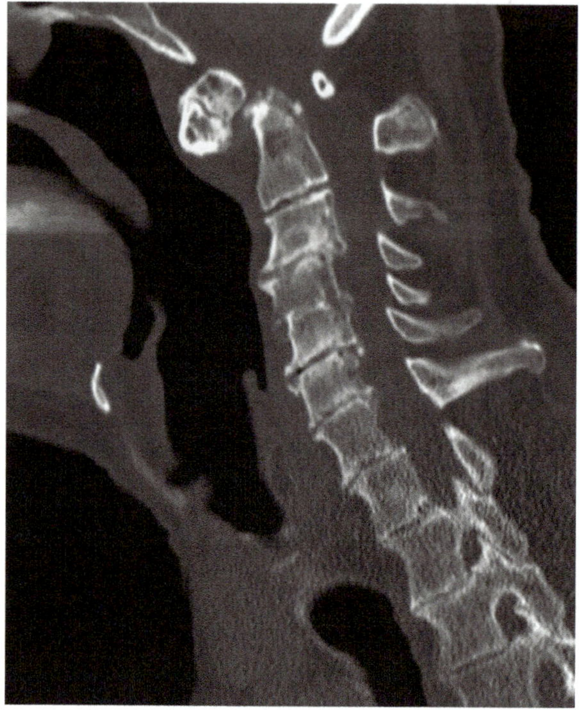

Fig. 7.5 Computed tomography of the cervical spine, sagittal section

A. acute fracture of dens, type 2
B. os odontoideum
C. os terminale
D. Chiari 1
E. pseudarthrosis

109. What is the most likely trauma mechanism regarding the MRI (Fig. 7.6)?

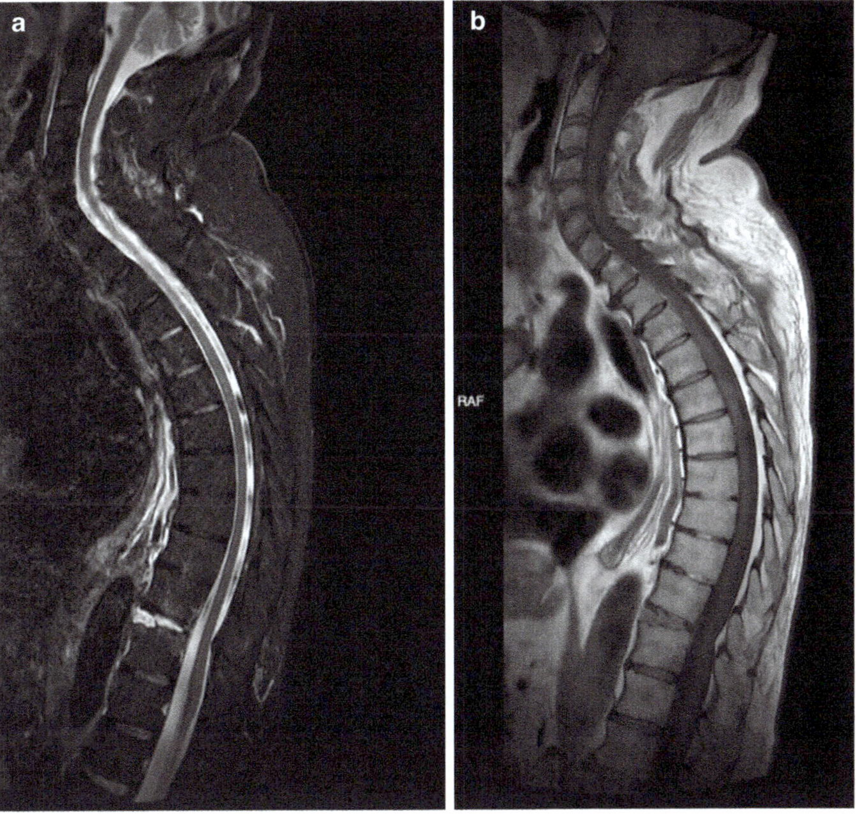

Fig. 7.6 (**a**) Short tau inversion recovery, coronal section; (**b**) T1-weighted image

A. axial compression
B. hyperextension
C. lateral flexion
D. hyperflexion
E. rotation

110. The patient after a road traffic accident. Choose the correct regarding the radiological findings (Fig. 7.7)?
   a. C2—Hangman fracture
   b. C1—Jefferson fracture
   c. C2—extension teardrop fracture
   d. C1—fracture caused by axial loading and extension

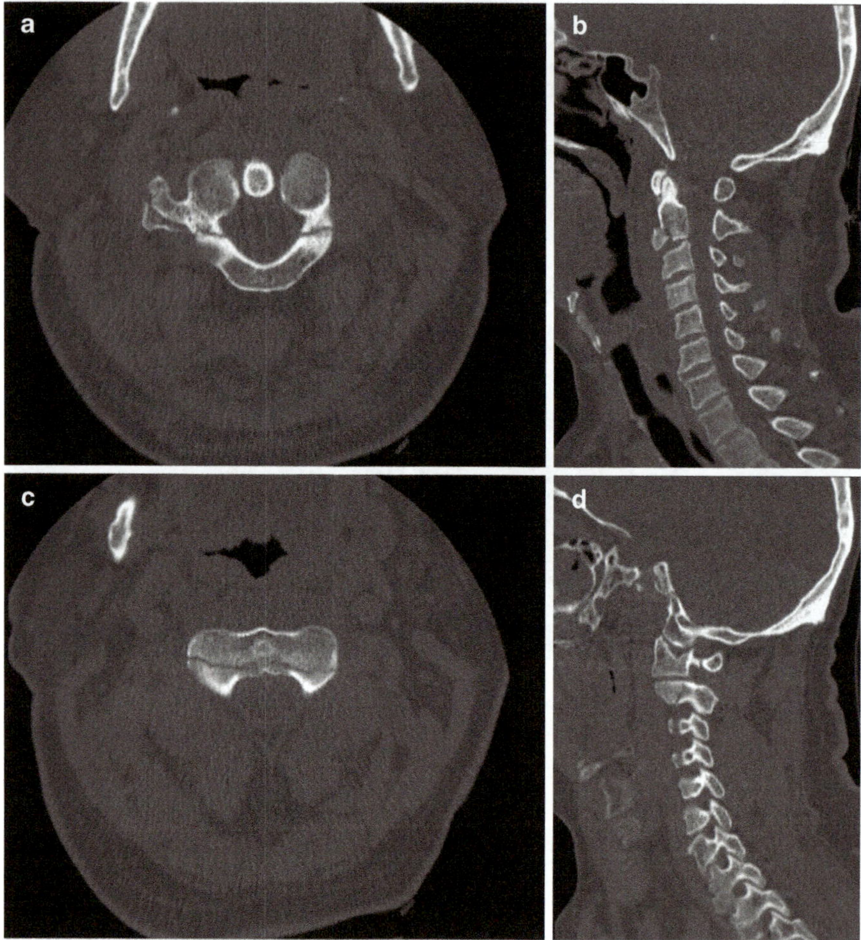

Fig. 7.7 Computed tomography of the cervical spine. (**a** and **c**) Axial sections; (**b** and **d**) sagittal sections

A. a, b, c, d
B. b, c, d
C. a, b, d
D. a, c
E. a, c, d

111. Choose the correct statement(s) regarding fractures (Fig. 7.7):
    A. There is a fracture that may cause injury of the vertebral artery.
    B. There is stenosis of the spinal canal.
    C. There is a fracture of the occipital condyle.
    D. There is a fracture of C3.
    E. There is a fracture of the skull base.
112. What is the most likely trauma mechanism regarding the CT (Fig. 7.8)?

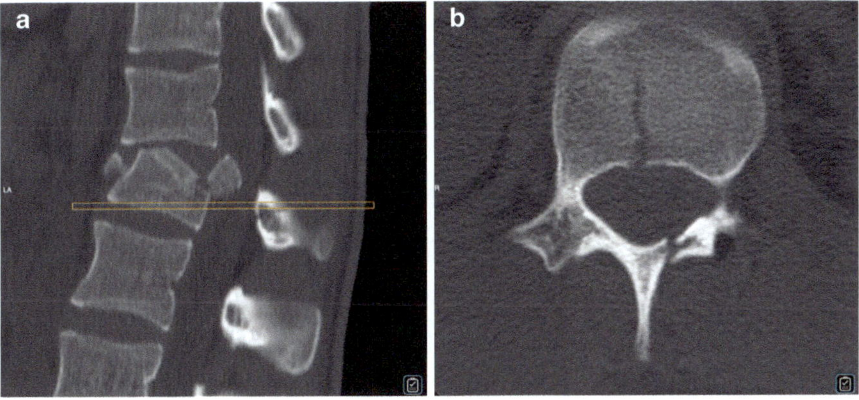

Fig. 7.8 Computed tomography of the lumbar spine. (**a**) Sagittal section; (**b**) axial section

    A. rotation
    B. extension
    C. lateral flexion
    D. Hangman fracture
    E. flexion-distraction

113. Choose the one correct answer regarding the fracture seen on CT (Fig. 7.9):
   a. It is type 2 according to Anderson and D'Alonzo classification.
   b. It is the most common fracture of the odontoid process.
   c. There is cervical spinal stenosis.

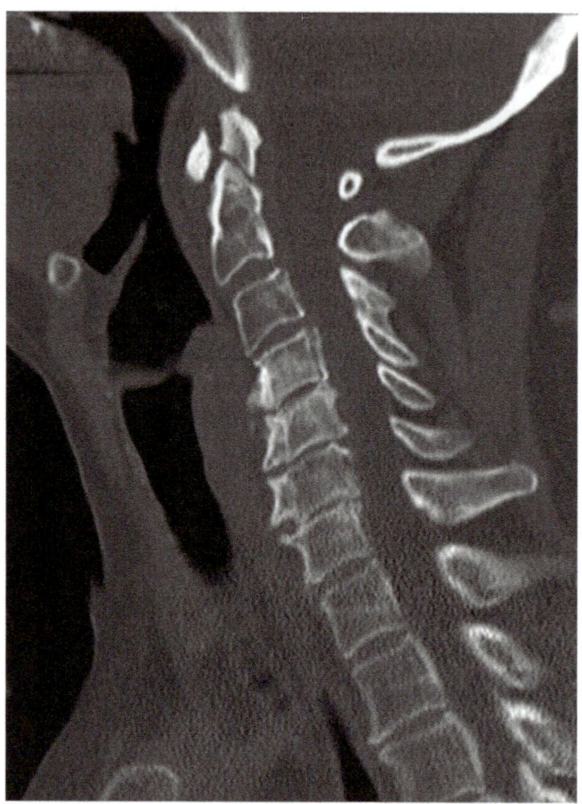

Fig. 7.9 Computed tomography of the cervical spine, sagittal section

A. a, b, c
B. a, b
C. a, c
D. b, c
E. a

114. Choose the correct regarding the radiological findings seen on MRI (Fig. 7.10)?
   a. There is no signs of instability.
   b. There is suspicion of a tumour.
   c. Acute fracture is visible.
   d. Traumatic disc herniation is seen.
   e. There is disruption of the middle vertebral column.

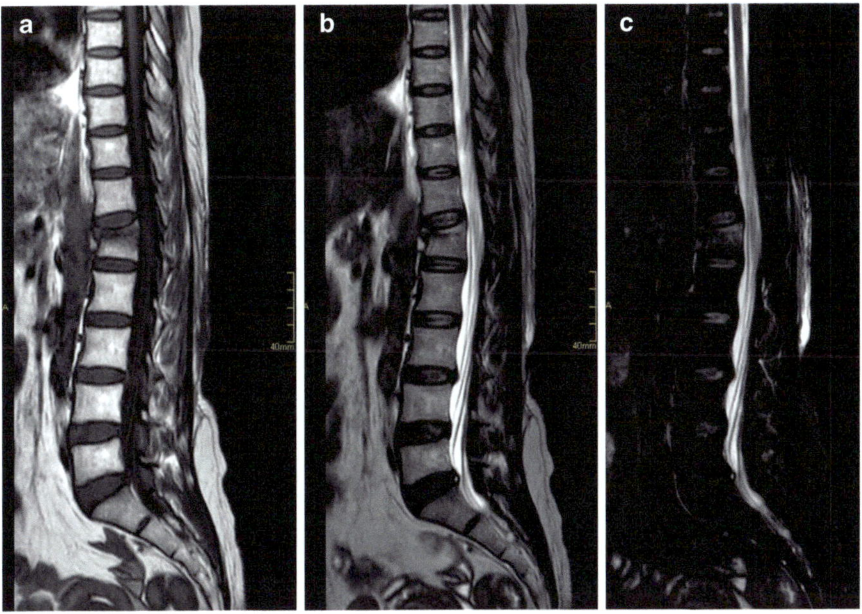

Fig. 7.10 (**a**) T1-weighted image, sagittal section; (**b**) T2-weighted image, sagittal section; (**c**) short tau inversion recovery, sagittal section

A. a, b, c, d, e
B. a, c, d, e
C. a, b, c
D. d, e
E. a, c

115. Choose one the best answer reagrding the typical radiological features of the fracture seen on CT (Fig. 7.11):
    a. It is stable.
    b. It is secondary to osteoporosis.
    c. It is related to high-energy axial loading.

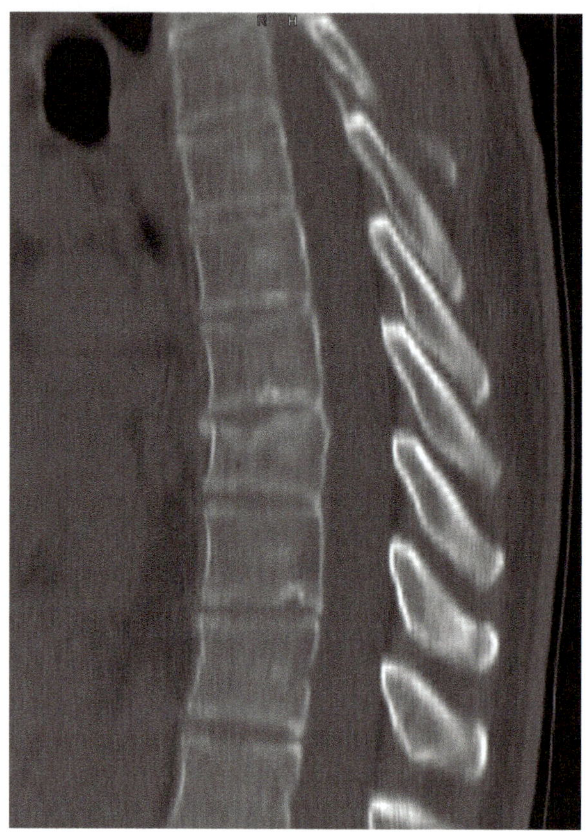

Fig. 7.11 Computed tomography of thoracic spine, sagittal section

A. a, b, c
B. a, b
C. a, c
D. b, c
E. a

116. A 68-year-old patient presenting with sacrum pain. What is the most likely diagnosis based on CT (Fig. 7.12)?

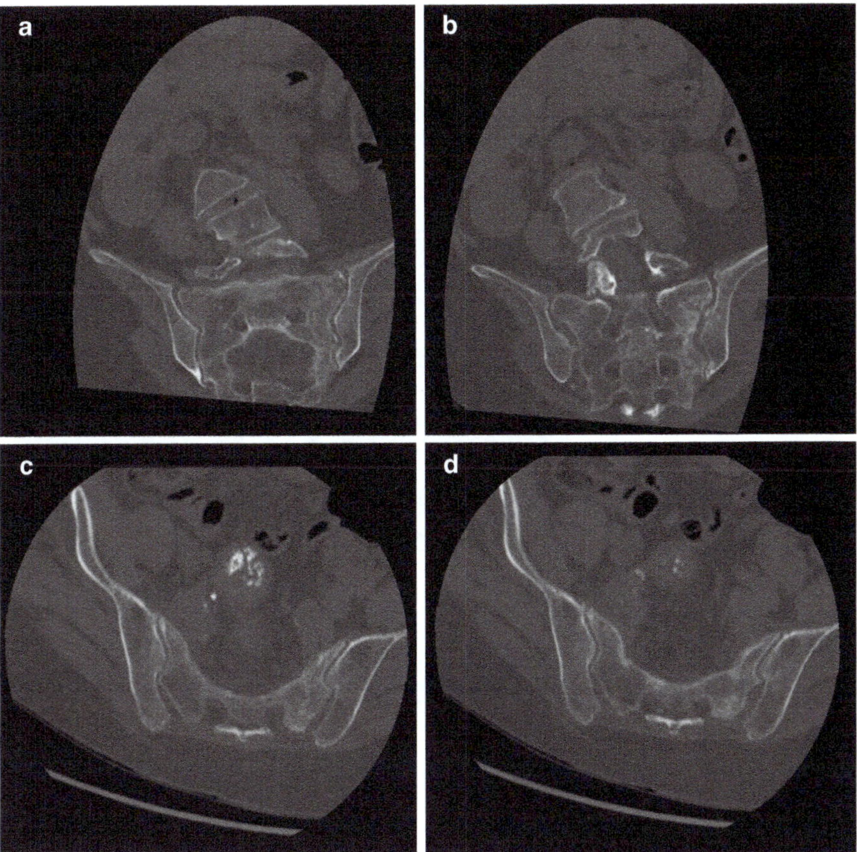

Fig. 7.12 Computed tomography of the sacrum. (**a** and **b**) Coronal sections; (**c** and **d**) axial section

A. Suspicion of a tumour, biopsy recommended.
B. Suspicion of infection, MRI is recommended.
C. Suspicion of a tumour, MRI recommended.
D. Suspected stress fracture.
E. Suspicion of sacroiliitis.

117. Choose the correct regarding radiological features seen on CT (Fig. 7.13):
   a. Extension teardrop C4.
   b. Andersson lesion is seen at the level of C5/C6.
   c. Fracture of the ossification at the level of C7/Th1.

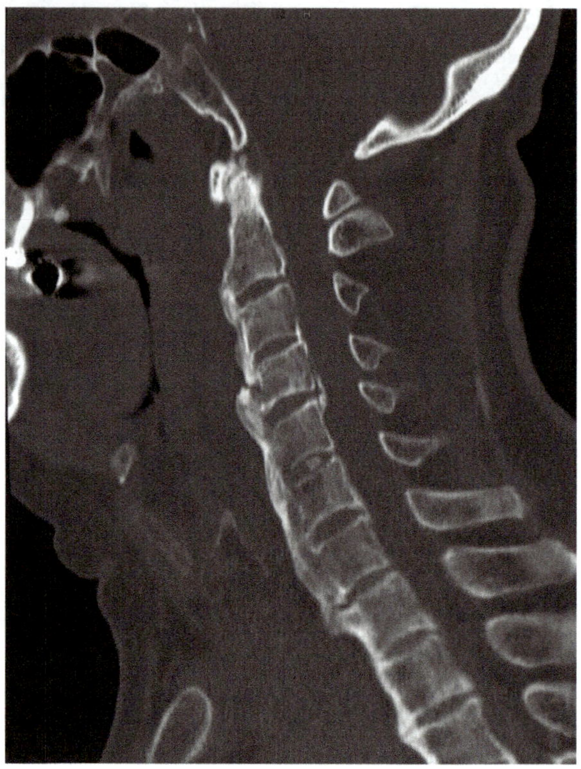

Fig. 7.13 Computed tomography of the cervical spine, sagittal section

A. a, b, c
B. a, b
C. a, c
D. b, c
E. a

118. What is the most likely trauma mechanism regarding the CT (Fig. 7.14)?

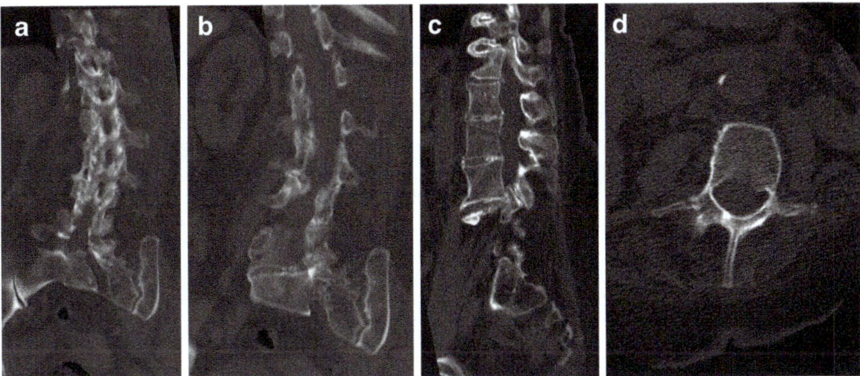

Fig. 7.14 Computed tomography of the lumbar spine. (**a** and **b**) Coronal sections; (**c**) sagittal section; (**d**) axial section

A. rotation
B. extension
C. lateral flexion
D. Hangman fracture
E. flexion-distraction

119. Choose the correct regarding stabilisation seen on X-ray (Fig. 7.15):
   a. Dynamic stabilization is seen.
   b. Markers in disc space are normal.
   c. Pedicle screws are located typically.

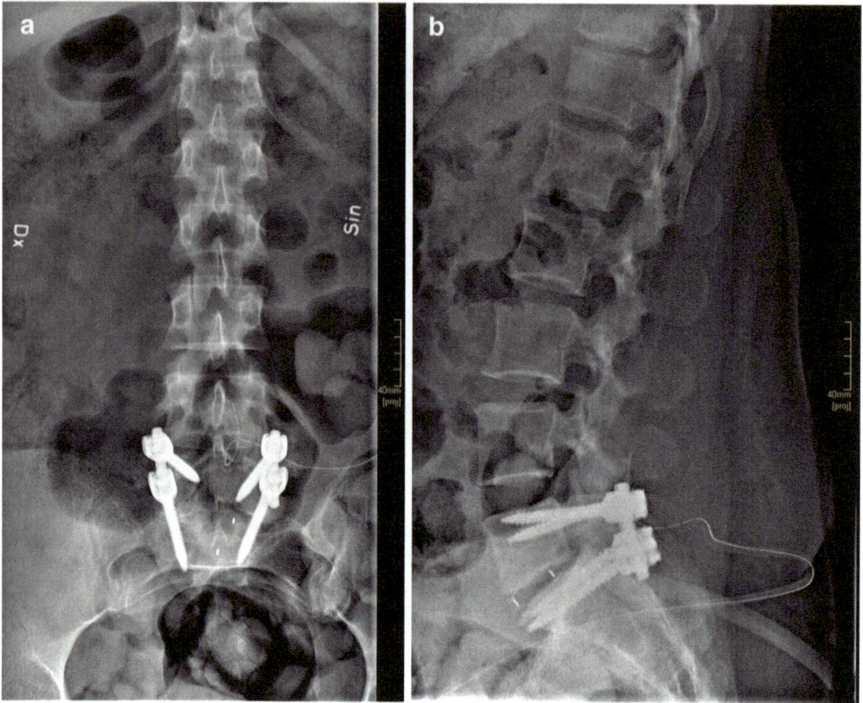

Fig. 7.15 X-ray of the lumbar spine (**a**) frontal projection, (**b**) lateral projection

A. a, b, c
B. a, b
C. a, c
D. b, c
E. a

120. A 62-year-old patient presented with a painful sacrum and fever. MRI was done (Fig. 7.16). Where is the pathology located?

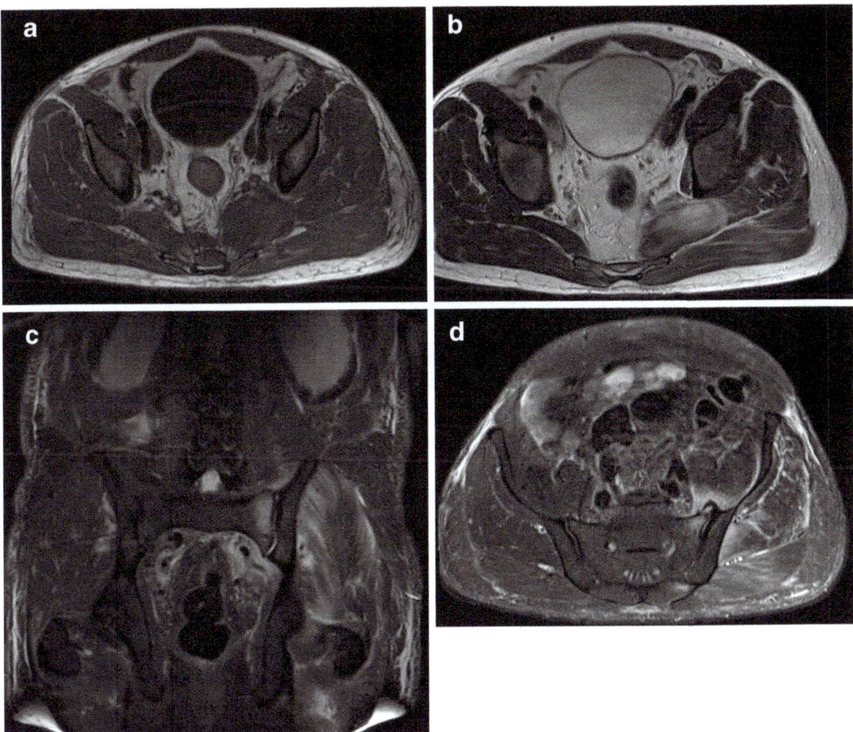

Fig. 7.16 (**a**) T1-weighted image, axial section; (**b**) T2-weighted image, axial section; (**c**) short tau inversion recovery, coronal section; (**d**) short tau inversion recovery axial section

A. sacroiliac joint
B. oedema in the gluteus medius muscle
C. oedema in the gluteus maximus muscle
D. abscess in m. obturator internus
E. abscess in m. piriformis

121. A 62-year-old patient presented with a painful sacrum and fever. MRI was done (Fig. 7.16). What is the most likely diagnosis?
A. neoplasm
B. rheumatoid arthritis
C. psoriasis
D. septic arthritis
E. ankylosis spondylitis

122. What is the name of the fracture visible on CT (Fig. 7.17)?

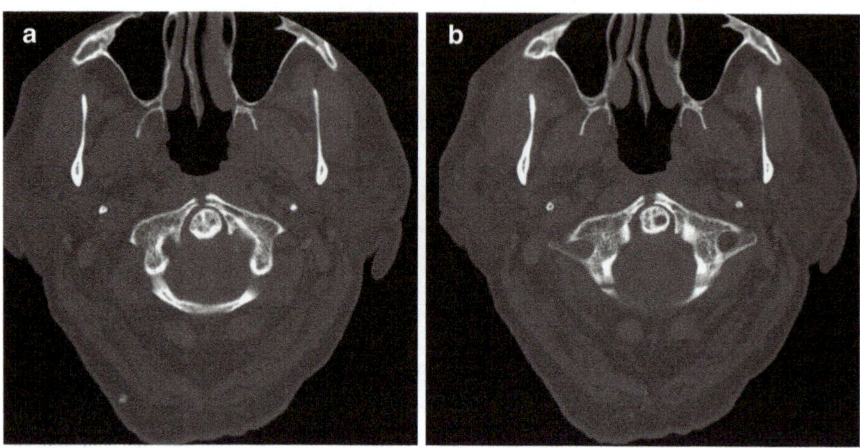

Fig. 7.17 (**a** and **b**) Computed tomography of the cervical spine at the level of the axis, axial sections

A. Chance fracture
B. Jefferson fracture
C. Hangman fracture
D. clay-shoveler fracture
E. pseudo-Jefferson fracture

123. Widespread osteophytosis without disc space narrowing is a sign of:
A. diffuse idiopathic skeletal hyperostosis
B. osteomyelitis
C. tuberculosis
D. fibrous dysplasia
E. reactive changes type 1 according to Modic

124. Horizontal fractures through the transverse process and pedicle of Th12 are the result of a:
A. seatbelt injury
B. osteoporotic fracture
C. clay-shoveler fracture
D. flexion teardrop fracture
E. extension teardrop fracture

125. Anterior wedging of the L1 vertebral body results from:
A. distraction
B. compression
C. hyperflexion
D. facet luxation
E. facet subluxation

Key to Chapter 7

71. A, B. Morquio syndrome is a mucopolysaccharidosis with musculoskeletal manifestation as deformations. The long bones became shorter and wider. In spine, platyspondyly (flatten vertebrae) and subluxation are seen.
72. C. Genant fracture of the osteoporotic vertebral fracture is one of the most commonly used. Grade 1 when loss of height is less than 25%. Grade 2 when loss of height is between 25% and 40%. Grade 3 when loss of height is more than 40%.
73. A, B, C, E. Most Chance fractures are stable because the anterior column is intact.
74. A, C.
75. B, C, D.
76. A, B, E.
77. E.
78. E.
79. A, D, E. Os odontoideum is larger than os terminale and present in direct relation to the apex of the odontoid process. Os terminale is related to the transverse atlantal ligament.
80. A, C.
81. B, C, D, E.
82. C.
83. C.
84. B, C, E. Flexion fracture of the anterior endplate corner is a common condition in adolescent. Schmorl nodule is usually present centrally not at the corner.
85. A, C, D.
86. C.
87. A, B.
88. C, E.
89. B.
90. B.
91. A, B, C, D.
92. A, B, D.
93. B, C, E.
94. A, C, D.
95. B, D, E.
96. A, C.
97. C, E.
98. A, D.
99. E.
100. A, B, C.
101. E.
102. E.
103. D.

104. C.
105. B, C, D, E.
106. A, C, D, E.
107. C, D.
108. E.
109. B.
110. E. Jefferson fracture occurs in mechanism of axial load. Posterior arch fracture occurs in axial load and extension.
111. A.
112. E.
113. C.
114. E.
115. B.
116. D.
117. E. At the level of C7/Th1, incomplete ossification is seen [1].
118. E.
119. D. It is the rigid stabilization. Dynamic stabilization is used alternative to rigid stabilization to prevent progressive degeneration by limiting the stress applied on the segment adjacent to the level of fusion [2, 3].
120. A, B, C, E.
121. D.
122. B.
123. A.
124. A.
125. B.

References

1. Shah NG, Keraliya A, Nunez DB, Schoenfeld A, Harris MB, Bono CM, et al. Injuries to the rigid spine: what the spine surgeon wants to know. Radiographics. 2019;39(2):449–66. https://doi.org/10.1148/rg.2019180125.
2. Ghodasara N, Yi PH, Clark K, Fishman EK, Farshad M, Fritz J. Postoperative spinal CT: what the radiologist needs to know. Radiographics. 2019;39(6):1840–61. https://doi.org/10.1148/rg.2019190050.
3. Murtagh RD, Quencer RM, Castellvi AE, Yue JJ. New techniques in lumbar spinal instrumentation: what the radiologist needs to know. Radiology. 2011;260(2):317–30. https://doi.org/10.1148/radiol.11101104.

Part IV

Tumors and Tumor Like Lesions

8 Bone Tumours

1. FEGNOMASHIC is a basic mnemonic that helps to identify bone lesions. What lesions are included in FEGNOMASHIC?
   A. chondromyxoid fibroma
   B. chondroblastoma
   C. osteoblastoma
   D. osteochondroma
   E. eosinophilic granuloma
2. Choose the correct features with regard to fibrosus dysplasia:
   A. Polyostotic form is more common than monostotic form.
   B. Endosteal scalloping is commonly seen.
   C. Most patients are older than 30 years.
   D. It is susceptibility to pathologic fracture.
   E. There is no periosteal reaction.
3. Choose the features of fibrous dysplasia:
   A. Femur and tibia are common localizations.
   B. It is a painful condition.
   C. Deformation of long bones is common.
   D. It may have a sclerotic appearance.
   E. It may have an osteolytic appearance.
4. Which is the most common localization of fibrous dysplasia?
   A. epiphysis
   B. metaphysis
   C. diaphysis
   D. intracortical
   E. subchondral

P. Szaro, *Musculoskeletal Radiology for Residents*,
https://doi.org/10.1007/978-3-030-85182-8_8

5. Choose one alternative indicating the less typical localization of enchondromas:
   A. pelvis
   B. phalanx
   C. humerus
   D. tibia
   E. femur
6. Enchondromas often contain calcifications, with one exception, which is:
   A. humerus
   B. fibula
   C. tibia
   D. femur
   E. phalanx
7. What are the features that may help in differentiating an enchondroma from a low-grade chondrosarcoma?
   A. Presence of calcifications.
   B. Pain, which is seen mainly in chondrosarcoma.
   C. Endosteal scalloping, which is seen in chondrosarcoma.
   D. Size, lesions larger than 6 cm are probably chondrosarcoma.
   E. It is impossible to differentiate based on imaging and a bone biopsy is indicated.
8. Choose the correct statement(s) regarding enchondroma:
   A. About half of enchondromas are located in the humerus.
   B. Metaphyseal localization is the most common.
   C. Enchondromas show less thick calcification than that in bone infarcts.
   D. It contains popcorn-like calcifications.
   E. Malignant transformation usually occurs in the hand.
9. Choose the correct statement(s) regarding multiple enchondromas:
   A. Malignant transformation is higher in Maffuci syndrome, where enchondromas are associated with haemangiomas.
   B. Malignant transformation is lower in Ollier syndrome.
   C. Malignant transformation is higher in Ollier syndrome, where enchondromas are associated with haemangiomas.
   D. Malignant transformation is lower in Maffuci syndrome.
   E. Malignant transformation is higher in both Ollier and Maffuci syndromes.
10. Choose the correct statement(s) regarding the skeletal manifestations of Langerhans histiocytoma:
    A. It can be sclerotic.
    B. It may be lytic.
    C. It may have a well-defined border.
    D. It may have an ill-defined border.
    E. Periosteal reaction may be seen.

11. What is the most common localization of eosinophilic granuloma?
    A. cranium
    B. pelvis
    C. femur
    D. ribs
    E. humerus
12. What is the differential diagnosis of eosinophilic granuloma?
    A. metastases
    B. lymphoma
    C. Ewing sarcoma
    D. osteomyelitis
    E. osteoma
13. Giant cell tumour:
    A. It may be considered in adult skeleton.
    B. It should be located about an articular surface.
    C. It showed a sclerotic margin.
    D. It is located eccentrically in the epiphysis.
    E. In solitary variant, it is located mid-diaphysis.
14. What indicates malignant giant cell tumour?
    A. presence of calcifications
    B. size of the lesion
    C. localization in the skeleton
    D. presence of sclerotic rim
    E. recurrence after operation
15. What lesion may coexist or be a part of a giant cell tumour?
    A. eosinophilic granuloma
    B. enchondroma
    C. osteochondroma
    D. fibrosus dysplasia
    E. aneurysmal bone cyst
16. Choose the most common region for the occurrence of a giant cell tumour:
    A. knee
    B. ankle
    C. hand
    D. pelvis
    E. shoulder
17. Choose the three most common diagnoses in the differential diagnosis of giant cell tumour:
    A. enchondroma
    B. fibrous dysplasia
    C. chondrosarcoma
    D. aneurysmal bone cyst
    E. chondroblastoma

18. Choose the correct statement(s) regarding non-ossifying fibroma:
    A. It is commonly located in the epiphysis.
    B. Thinning of the cortex is seen.
    C. It is usually a multiloculate osteolytic lesion.
    D. Commonly, the patient is older than 30 years.
    E. In the knee region, it may be painful.
19. Non-ossifying fibromas are commonly cortical based; however, in some rare cases, it can be seen centrally; choose the two exceptions:
    A. femur
    B. tibia
    C. fibula
    D. radius
    E. ulna
20. Choose the correct statement(s) regarding osteoblastoma:
    A. It is commonly present in the anterior elements of the vertebrae.
    B. Like osteoid, osteoma causes night pain.
    C. It may contain a secondary aneurysmal bone cyst.
    D. Sometimes cortical destruction may be seen.
    E. Osteoblastomas, unlike aneurysmal bone cysts, are not expansive.
21. What is in the differential diagnosis of osteoblastoma?
    A. giant cell tumour
    B. aneurysmal bone cyst
    C. osteoid osteoma
    D. enchondroma
    E. bone infarct
22. A 17-year-old patient was examined because of pain in the right iliac fossa. CT revealed an expansive tumour arising from the left hemisacrum. The matrix of the lesion contains some irregular sclerotic regions. No cortical break/destruction was seen. What is your differential diagnosis?
    A. enchondroma
    B. osteoblastoma
    C. myositis ossificans
    D. chordoma
    E. giant cell tumour
23. Choose the correct statement(s) regarding aneurysmal bone cysts:
    A. The most common localization is the metaphysis of long bones.
    B. In the spine, it is located in the posterior elements.
    C. It is mostly located eccentrically in long bones.
    D. A wide zone of transition is typical.
    E. It may grow rapidly.

24. What is in the differential diagnosis of a brown tumour?
    A. fibrosus dysplasia
    B. enchondroma
    C. metastatic disease
    D. multiply myeloma
    E. non-ossifying fibroma
25. Choose the correct statement(s) regarding vertebral haemangiomas:
    A. All vertebral haemangiomas show high signal on T1-weighted images.
    B. Most commonly are present in vertebral bodies.
    C. Most commonly are asymptomatic.
    D. Coarse trabeculation is a typical feature in vertebrae.
    E. Skull base is a typical localization.
26. Choose the correct statement(s) regarding vanishing bone disease:
    A. It starts usually in two or three different bones.
    B. Scintigraphy shows significant uptake of the affected bone.
    C. Shoulder region is a typical localization.
    D. Reabsorption of the bone is a hallmark.
    E. It is seen in hyperparathyroidism.
27. Choose the correct statement(s) regarding chondroblastoma:
    A. It is a diaphyseal lesion.
    B. A typical patient is younger than 20 years.
    C. A few small calcifications may be present.
    D. A wide zone of transition is typical.
    E. Occasionally, may contain fluid levels on MRI.
28. Choose the features of chondromyxoid fibroma:
    A. No periosteal reaction is seen.
    B. It is located eccentrically in the metaphysis or diaphysis.
    C. It is an osteosclerotic lesion in older patients.
    D. A wide zone of transition is usually present.
    E. Bone infarct is a common differential diagnosis.
29. Choose the most common localization of osteoma:
    A. femur
    B. pelvis
    C. femur
    D. spine
    E. skull
30. Choose the typical features of osteoid osteoma:
    A. Subchondral localization is the most common.
    B. Vertebral body is the most common spine localization.
    C. Most common age is under 25 years.
    D. Femur and tibia are the most common localizations.
    E. Nidus shows low enhancement after contrast.

31. Which intra-articular localization of the osteoid osteoma is the most common?
    A. shoulder
    B. elbow
    C. hip
    D. knee
    E. ankle
32. What is in the differential diagnosis of osteoid osteoma?
    A. stress fracture if present in the diaphysis
    B. arthritis if present intra-articularly
    C. chronic osteomyelitis if present in the diaphysis
    D. enchondroma if present in the diaphysis
    E. chondroblastoma if present intra-articularly
33. Choose possible treatment(s) of osteoid osteoma:
    A. CT-guided radiofrequency thermal ablation
    B. CT-guided cortisone injection to nidus
    C. MRI-guided laser ablation
    D. ultrasound-guided ablation
    E. surgical removal
34. Choose the correct statement(s) regarding enchondroma:
    A. Most common localization is the hand.
    B. It may cause endosteal scalloping.
    C. Expansion of the long bones is common.
    D. No contrast enhancement is present.
    E. A new region of lucency is worrisome.
35. Choose the correct statement(s) regarding osteochondroma:
    A. Femur is the most commonly affected.
    B. Calcifications in the cartilage cup are worrisome for malignant transformation.
    C. Thickening of the cartilage cup more than 1 cm is an indication for surgical treatment.
    D. A stalk that is longer than 3 cm is worrisome for malignant transformation.
    E. Osseous destruction/degeneration to chondrosarcoma can be seen.
36. Choose the correct statement(s) regarding conventional osteosarcoma:
    A. Metaphyseal localization is more common than diaphyseal localization.
    B. The most common clinical presentation is a pathological fracture.
    C. The femur, tibia, and humerus are common localizations.
    D. Most patients are younger than 25 years of age.
    E. It is present only in the appendicular skeleton.

37. What conditions are prone to sarcomatous degeneration?
    A. brown tumour
    B. giant cell tumour
    C. previous radiotherapy
    D. eosinophilic granuloma
    E. Paget disease
38. Choose the correct statement(s) regarding solitary bone plasmacytoma:
    A. Like osteoid osteoma, it is surrounded by a sclerotic reaction.
    B. It showed destruction of the cortex, unlike lymphoma.
    C. Partially calcified matrix is seen.
    D. It is present as a geographic lytic lesion in the bone marrow on X-ray.
    E. Like in lymphoma, lymphadenopathy is seen.
39. Choose the correct statement(s) regarding myeloma:
    A. Diffuse osteopenia with vertebral compression fractures are features.
    B. Endosteal scalloping may be seen.
    C. Signal on T1-weighted images is higher than the disc.
    D. If untreated, no contrast enhancement is seen.
    E. The best imaging tool is the whole-body MRI.
40. Choose the features of Ewing sarcoma:
    A. It is more common in plate bones than in long bones.
    B. A wide zone of transition.
    C. Permeative growth.
    D. Onion skin periosteal reaction.
    E. Calcified matrix.
41. Choose the correct statement(s) regarding lymphoma of the bone:
    A. Most common localization are flat bones.
    B. Endosteal thickening may be seen.
    C. Permeative growth is seen.
    D. Usually, it is present as multiple lesions.
    E. Soft tissue component is smaller than bony destruction.
42. Choose the correct statement(s) regarding bone metastases:
    A. They are more common in the axial skeleton.
    B. Sclerotic metastases should be differentiated from osteopoikilosis.
    C. Thyroid carcinoma metastases are often lytic.
    D. Lytic metastases should be differentiated from multiple myeloma.
    E. During treatment, metastases usually became more sclerotic.
43. Choose the most common localization of intraosseous lipoma:
    A. femur
    B. tibia
    C. calcaneus
    D. humerus
    E. spine

44. Choose the most common localization of chordoma:
    A. sacrum
    B. lumbar spine
    C. thoracic spine
    D. cervical spine
    E. skull
45. Choose features of chordoma:
    A. Calcifications are commonly present.
    B. Lesion is usually located in the midline.
    C. Ill-defined soft tissue mass.
    D. Matrix is similar to giant cell tumour.
    E. A narrow zone of transition.
46. Choose the correct statement(s) regarding Paget disease:
    A. Most commonly is monostotic.
    B. Thickening of bone trabeculae is a feature.
    C. Cortical thickening is common.
    D. Affected bone is enlarged.
    E. Early changes are osteolytic.
47. Choose the three most typical localizations of Paget disease:
    A. spine
    B. skull
    C. pelvis
    D. foot
    E. hand
48. Choose the right statement(s) regarding primary bone lymphoma:
    A. Moth-eaten and permeative bone destruction are typical radiological features.
    B. Most commonly involved long bones, such as the femur, humerus, and tibia.
    C. Epiphysis of the long bone is the most common localization.
    D. Most patients have a soft tissue component.
    E. Enlarged lymph nodes are commonly seen.
49. Choose most common radiological features of Hodgkin's lymphoma:
    A. Sclerotic bone lesions.
    B. Osteolytic lesions.
    C. Pathologic compression fracture.
    D. Rib involvement is uncommon.
    E. MRI signal on T1-weighted images is a typical feature.

50. Choose the correct description regarding plasmacytoma:
    A. Osteolytic lesion.
    B. Cortical thinning.
    C. Expansive character.
    D. Soap bubble appearance.
    E. Spine, pelvis, and proximal femur are typical localizations.
51. Choose the typical radiological features of multiple myeloma:
    A. diffuse osteopenia
    B. well-defined punched-out lesions
    C. multiple vertebral compression fractures
    D. endosteal scalloping with cortical thickening
    E. marginal sclerosis of primary osteolytic lesions following radiotherapy
52. Which examination shows the highest sensitivity in detection of multiple myeloma lesions?
    A. CT
    B. MRI
    C. Plain radiograph
    D. Bone scintigraphy
    E. PET scanning with the tracer 18F-fluorodeoxyglucose
53. Choose the true statement(s) regarding the radiological features of multiple myeloma:
    A. Restricted diffusion is usually seen.
    B. Low signal on T1-weighted images.
    C. Early wash-out is seen after contrast injection.
    D. Well-defined osteolytic skeletal lesions on X-ray and CT.
    E. Intervertebral disc is hypointense compared with the vertebral bodies on T1-weighted images.
54. Choose the radiological features of thalassemia major:
    A. bony expansion
    B. cortical bone thinning
    C. rib-within-a-rib appearance
    D. extramedullary erythropoiesis in the thoracic paravertebral region
    E. higher signal on T1-weigted images due to bone marrow reconversion
55. Choose the most common radiological features of sickle cell disease:
    A. asymmetrical shortening of tubular bones
    B. infarction in meta- and epiphysis
    C. infarction of the vertebral body
    D. osteomyelitis
    E. bone destruction

56. Soap bubble appearance may be seen in:
    A. plasmacytoma
    B. giant cell tumour
    C. aneurysmal bone cyst
    D. Gaucher's disease
    E. Brodie abscess
57. The fallen fragment sign is typical for a(n):
    A. aneurysmal bone cyst
    B. unicameral bone cyst
    C. solitary bone cyst
    D. giant cell tumour
    E. eosinophilic granuloma
58. CT showed irregular bone resorption and ill-defined islands of sclerosis in the diploe. Choose the differential diagnosis:
    A. haemangioma
    B. meningioma
    C. multiple myeloma
    D. metastasis
    E. hyperparathyroidism
59. A 42-year-old patient presenting with back pain. MRI of lumbar spine revealed a total compression fracture of the corpus of L1. Disc space is normal. A heterogenic soft tissue mass is visible in the paravertebral muscles. An epidural mass causes spinal stenosis. Contrast enhancement is seen in the soft tissue mass and in the epidural component. What is the differential diagnosis?
    A. haemangioma
    B. chondroblastoma
    C. osteosarcoma
    D. metastasis
    E. giant cell tumour
60. Choose the four most common osteolytic epiphyseal lesions in patients younger than 20 years:
    A. giant cell tumour
    B. chondroblastoma
    C. intraosseous ganglion
    D. eosinophilic granuloma
    E. infection
61. A 49-year-old patient is about 8 years after kidney transplantation. CT of the abdomen showed soft tissue calcifications in the soft tissue in relation to the right hip, an osteolytic somewhat bubbly appearance lesion in the acetabulum, without cortical breakthrough. What is the most likely diagnosis of the lesion in the acetabulum?
    A. brown tumour
    B. aneurysmal bone cyst
    C. low-grade chondrosarcoma
    D. giant cell tumour
    E. osteoblastoma

62. A 23-year-old patient with knee trauma. X-ray showed no fracture but in the distal femur an exocentrically located osteolytic lesion about 2 cm × 2 cm × 3 cm with a sclerotic margin was visualized. What is your diagnosis?
    A. Bone infarct, which doesn't touch the lesion.
    B. Non-ossifying fibroma, which doesn't touch the lesion.
    C. It is unspecific, CT is indicated.
    D. It is unspecific, MRI with contrast is indicated.
    E. It is unspecific, biopsy is indicated.
63. A 32-year-old patient presented after knee trauma. CT showed a pure osteolytic lesion in the metaphysis and subchondral bone with a well-defined border that is not sclerotic. Destruction of the cortex is noticed at the level of the lesion. What is the most likely diagnosis?
    A. geode
    B. chondroblastoma
    C. solitary bone cyst
    D. aneurysmal bone cyst
    E. giant cell tumour
64. A 40-year-old patient presenting with knee pain. X-ray showed an expanded osteolytic lesion of the patella. What are the two most likely diagnosis?
    A. chondroblastoma
    B. non-ossifying fibroma
    C. giant cell tumour
    D. aneurysmal bone cyst
    E. enchondroma
65. A 10-year-old child presenting after fall trauma, with pain in the right shoulder. X-ray revealed a well-defined osteolytic lesion at the level of the proximal humerus with pathologic fracture. In the inferior part of the lesion, a piece of bone can be seen. What is the most likely diagnosis?
    A. giant cell tumour
    B. aneurysmal bone cyst
    C. solitary bone cyst
    D. eosinophilic granuloma
    E. enchondroma
66. An expansile osteolytic lesion in the proximal humerus of a 60-year-old patient may represent:
    A. aneurysmal bone cyst
    B. metastasis of renal cancer
    C. osteoblastoma
    D. myeloma
    E. metastasis of colon cancer

67. Choose the lesions that may contain fluid-fluid levels:
    A. osteoblastoma
    B. giant cell tumour
    C. chondroblastoma
    D. aneurysmal bone cyst
    E. telangiectatic osteosarcoma
68. A 40-year-old patient presents with a palpable mass in relation to the medial malleolus. X-ray showed a highly expansive lesion in the distal tibia, with significant thinning of the cortex, however, without cortical breakthrough. MRI with contrast revealed fluid levels and significant enhancement of the bone marrow neighbouring the lesion. A periosteal reaction is noticed. What is the differential diagnosis?
    A. aneurysmal bone cyst
    B. telangiectatic osteosarcoma
    C. non-ossifying fibroma
    D. chondrosarcoma
    E. giant cell tumour
69. A 13-year-old child presenting after hip trauma. X-ray showed a well-defined osteolytic lesion in the intertrochanteric region, size about 3 cm × 2 cm × 2 cm. What is your differential diagnosis?
    A. giant cell tumour
    B. aneurysmal bone cyst
    C. solitary bone cyst
    D. eosinophilic granuloma
    E. enchondroma
70. X-ray of a 51-year-old patient showed subperiosteal resorption of the radial cortex of the middle phalanx. What is the differential diagnosis?
    A. enchondroma
    B. brown tumour
    C. osteomyelitis
    D. fibrous dysplasia
    E. multiple myeloma
71. A 16-year-old patient presenting after shoulder trauma. X-ray showed an eccentric osteolytic lesion in the humeral epiphysis with some punctate calcifications with a discrete expansion of the cortex. What is the most likely diagnosis?
    A. enchondroma
    B. osteoblastoma
    C. chondroblastoma
    D. osteomyelitis
    E. giant cell tumour

72. What is the most likely bony tumour of the patella in a patient who is 18 years old?
    A. aneurysmal bone cyst
    B. chondroblastoma
    C. osteoblastoma
    D. giant cell tumour
    E. unicameral bone cyst
73. What lesions do you expect in a 28-year-old patient?
    A. aneurysmal bone cyst
    B. giant cell tumour
    C. eosinophilic granuloma
    D. multiple myeloma
    E. non-ossifying fibroma
74. Periosteal reaction may be a feature of:
    A. fibrous dysplasia
    B. aneurysmal bone cyst
    C. osteomyelitis
    D. giant cell tumour
    E. eosinophilic granuloma
75. Which lesions are typically present in the epiphysis of long bones?
    A. chondroblastoma
    B. giant cell tumour
    C. osteoblastoma
    D. enchondroma
    E. bone infarct
76. Which lesions are present in the diaphysis?
    A. fibrosus dysplasia
    B. bone infarct
    C. simple bone cyst
    D. osteoblastoma
    E. aneurysmal bone cyst
77. Which lesions are not painful?
    A. non-ossifying fibroma in femur
    B. aneurysmal bone cyst in tibia
    C. enchondroma in femur
    D. spine osteoblastoma
    E. low-grade chondrosarcoma in humerus
78. What lesions may contain the fluid levels component?
    A. telangiectatic osteosarcoma
    B. giant cell tumour
    C. chondroblastoma
    D. enchondroma
    E. non-ossifying fibroma

79. Choose the lesions that may be located in the metaphysis?
    A. non-ossifying fibroma
    B. aneurysmal bone cyst
    C. giant cell tumour
    D. metastases
    E. chondrosarcoma
80. Choose the correct statement(s) regarding bony island:
    A. Both bony island and metastases may show uptake on PET/CT.
    B. Subtle extension to bone trabeculae is seen in bony island.
    C. Contrast enhancement is seen in MRI both in metastases and bony island.
    D. Eccentrically located bony islands may remain and heal as non-ossifying fibromas.
    E. Main difference with an osteoid osteoma is a lucency present in the osteoid osteoma.
81. Choose the aggressive lytic lesions in children:
    A. osteomyelitis
    B. osteosarcoma
    C. Ewing sarcoma
    D. fibrous dysplasia
    E. leukaemia
82. A 17-year-old patient presenting with left hip pain. X-ray showed a diffuse sclerotic lesion in the femoral neck with somewhat lucency in its central part and hip valgus was noticed. What is your differential diagnosis?
    A. metastasis
    B. chondroblastoma
    C. osteoma
    D. osteoid osteoma
    E. Brodie abscess
83. A 17-year-old patient presenting with back pain. X-ray showed an expanded tumour in the spinous process of L2. What is the differential diagnosis?
    A. aneurysmal bone cyst
    B. osteoblastoma
    C. chondroblastoma
    D. giant cell tumour
    E. osteoid osteoma
84. A 22-year-old patient presenting with a swollen and painful thigh. X-ray showed expansile destruction of the distal femur. Lesion is ill-defined and has permeative growth. A sizable solid soft tissue tumour is present in the popliteal fossa. What is the most likely diagnosis?
    A. osteoblastoma
    B. chondrosarcoma
    C. fracture with haematoma
    D. septic arthritis
    E. osteosarcoma

85. Choose the expansile lytic bone lesions:
    A. brown tumour
    B. aneurysmal bone cyst
    C. giant cell tumour
    D. enchondroma
    E. haemangioma
86. Sunburst periosteal reaction:
    A. It responds to aggressive periostitis.
    B. It is seen in osteosarcoma and Ewing sarcoma.
    C. It may be seen in osteoblastic metastases.
    D. It may be seen in eosinophilic granuloma.
    E. It is prominent in osteoid osteoma.
87. Choose the features of myositis ossificans:
    A. It calcifies in the centre and then continues more peripherally.
    B. A separating cleft from the cortical bone.
    C. It is seen mostly in patients older than 30 years.
    D. Usually, it is associated with trauma in anamnesis.
    E. Contrast enhancement is visible on MRI in non-calcified lesions.
88. A 25-year-old patient presenting with knee pain. X-ray showed a lytic lesion in the distal femoral meta-diaphysis with amorphous osteoid matrix, cortical breakthrough, permeative growth with some more circumscribed regions. What are three the most likely diagnosis?
    A. fibrous dysplasia
    B. osteosarcoma
    C. eosinophilic granuloma
    D. chondrosarcoma
    E. Ewing sarcoma
89. Choose the most common lesions of ribs:
    A. aneurysmal bone cyst
    B. giant cell tumour
    C. enchondroma
    D. multiple myeloma
    E. fibrous dysplasia
90. Choose multiple radiolucent bone lesions:
    A. metastasis
    B. multiple myeloma
    C. enchondroma
    D. fibrous dysplasia
    E. brown tumour

91. A 45-year-old patient presenting with lumbar back pain. MRI revealed that the bone marrow signal on T1-weighted images is lower than that of the intervertebral discs. On T2-weighted fat suppression, there is a heterogeneously low signal of the bone marrow. What is the differential diagnosis?
    A. multiple myeloma
    B. osteomyelitis
    C. lymphoma
    D. myelofibrosis
    E. leukaemia
92. Choose the ill-defined solitary bone lesions:
    A. osteosarcoma
    B. intraosseous haemangioma
    C. intraosseous ganglion
    D. unicameral bone cyst
    E. osteomyelitis
93. Choose lesions commonly located in the ilium:
    A. metastasis
    B. Ewing sarcoma
    C. Paget disease
    D. fibrous dysplasia
    E. multiple myeloma
94. Choose the one condition when the rate of degeneration to chondrosarcoma is the lowest:
    A. multiple hereditary exostosis
    B. solitary osteochondroma
    C. Ollier syndrome
    D. Maffuci syndrome
    E. Maffuci-Ollier syndrome
95. Choose the correct statement(s) regarding Ewing sarcoma:
    A. Diaphyseal and metaphyseal localization is similar to osteosarcoma.
    B. Reactive osteosclerosis is unlike osteomyelitis.
    C. Calcified matrix is similar to osteosarcoma.
    D. Aggressive periosteal reaction like in osteosarcoma.
    E. Permeative destruction like in lymphoma.
96. Choose tumours that may be commonly found in the sacrum:
    A. giant cell tumour
    B. aneurysmal bone cyst
    C. chordoma
    D. chondrosarcoma
    E. osteoblastoma

97. Choose the three most common complications caused by radiation:
    A. fracture
    B. sarcoma
    C. osteonecrosis
    D. giant cell tumour
    E. chordoma
98. Choose ill-defined osteolytic lesions:
    A. osteosarcoma
    B. giant cell tumour
    C. eosinophilic granuloma
    D. leukaemia
    E. enchondroma
99. Choose lesions which contain sclerosis:
    A. melorheostosis
    B. Paget disease
    C. stress fracture
    D. osteoma
    E. eosinophilic granuloma
100. Choose lesions that are located more often in the posterior part of the vertebrae:
    A. haemangioma
    B. osteoid osteoma
    C. osteoblastoma
    D. aneurysmal bone cyst
    E. multiple myeloma
101. Choose lesions with bony sequestrum:
    A. giant cell tumour
    B. chordoma
    C. osteoid osteoma
    D. Brodie abscess
    E. eosinophilic granuloma
102. Choose primary benign tumours found in the skull:
    A. haemangioma
    B. chordoma
    C. osteoma
    D. multiple myeloma
    E. giant cell tumour
103. What is the most common tumour of the scapula?
    A. osteochondroma
    B. chondroblastoma
    C. chondrosarcoma
    D. giant cell tumour
    E. aneurysmal bone cyst

104. What are three common calcaneal lesions?
    A. unicameral bone cyst
    B. enchondroma
    C. giant cell tumour
    D. osteoid osteoma
    E. intraosseous lipoma
105. Choose the bubbly lesions of bone:
    A. fibrous dysplasia
    B. eosinophilic granuloma
    C. non-ossifying fibroma
    D. metastases
    E. aneurysmal bone cyst
106. Choose the cortical lesions:
    A. osteoid osteoma
    B. osteomyelitis
    C. stress fracture
    D. osteomyelitis
    E. enchondroma
107. Choose three typical lesions of the distal phalanx:
    A. glomus
    B. enchondroma
    C. osteoblastoma
    D. epidermoid
    E. chondroblastoma
108. A 54-year-old male presenting with incontinence and buttock pain. X-ray revealed destruction of the sacrum and some weakly seen calcification. What is the most likely diagnosis?
    A. giant cell tumour
    B. osteosarcoma
    C. chordoma
    D. aneurysmal bone cyst
    E. osteoblastoma
109. A 17-year-old patient presenting after knee trauma during a football match. X-ray showed a well-defined radiolucent lesion in the posterior intercondylar area of the tibia. The lesion has a lobulated margin and a thin sclerotic rim. What are two most likely diagnosis?
    A. chondroblastoma
    B. giant cell tumour
    C. osteomyelitis
    D. intraosseous ganglion
    E. osteoid osteoma

110. What thickness of cartilage cap may be worrisome in osteochondroma?
    A. more than 1 mm
    B. more than 5 mm
    C. more than 10 mm
    D. more than 15 mm
    E. less than 10 mm
111. Choose signs of malignant transformation of osteochondroma:
    A. fracture
    B. bursa formation
    C. pain after puberty
    D. hyaline cartilage cap greater than 1.5 cm
    E. growth before skeletal maturity
112. A 36-year-old patient with a painful great toe. CT revealed a well-defined, peripherally calcified lesion, which arises with a broad base from the inferior outline of the cortex of the distal phalanx. No periosteal reaction is noted. What is most likely diagnosis?
    A. enostosis
    B. Nora's lesion
    C. osteoid osteoma
    D. subungual exostosis
    E. paraosteal osteosarcoma
113. Which is the most common primary malignant bone tumour?
    A. metastasis
    B. lymphoma
    C. osteosarcoma
    D. Ewing sarcoma
    E. multiple myeloma

114. A 16-year-old patient presenting with painful thigh and knee pain, as well as no trauma or fever. Choose the right option(s) regarding the lesion on X-ray (Fig. 8.1a–d):

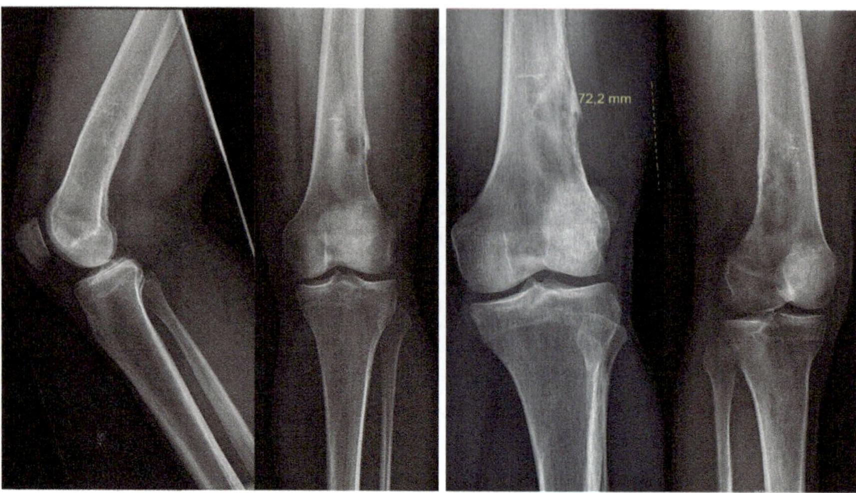

Fig. 8.1 X-ray of the knee

   A. cystic lesion
   B. sclerotic border
   C. chondroid matrix
   D. wide zone of transition
   E. aggressive periosteal reaction

115. Regarding age, localization, and morphology, which of the following is the most likely diagnosis (Fig. 8.1a–d)?
   A. cortical desmoid
   B. osteosarcoma
   C. osteomyelitis
   D. aneurysmal bone cyst
   E. giant cell tumour

116. A 38-year-old patient presenting with a tumour that was noticed 3 years ago. What is the differential diagnosis (Fig. 8.2a, b)?

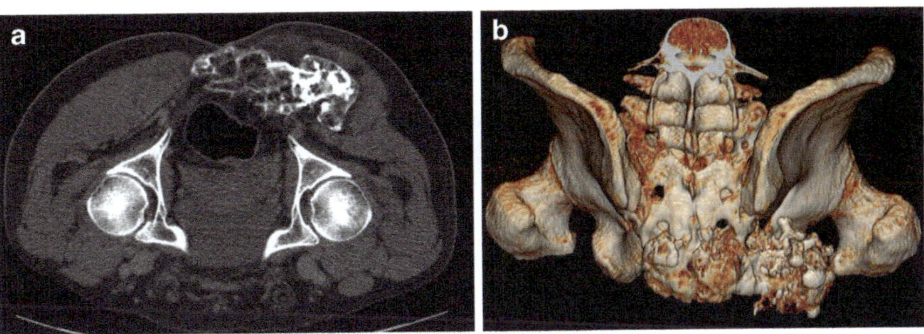

Fig. 8.2 Computed tomography of the pelvis. (**a**) Axial section, prone position; (**b**) volume rendering, posterior superior view

A. myositis ossificans
B. malunited fracture
C. osteochondroma
D. haematoma with calcifications
E. bizarre paraosteal osteochondromatous proliferation

117. Over the last 3 weeks, the patient has noticed pain. MRI was performed (Fig. 8.3a–f). Choose the correct statement(s) regarding MRI:

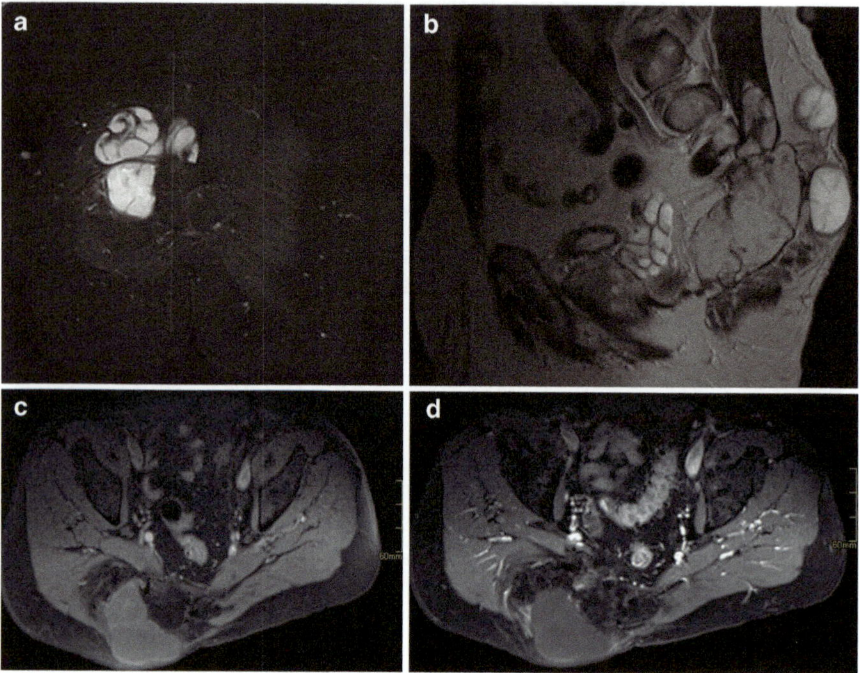

Fig. 8.3 MRI of the pelvis, supine position. (**a**) Short tau inversion recovery, coronal section; (**b**) T2-weighted image, sagittal section; (**c**) T1-weighted with fat suppression, axial section; (**d**)–T1-weighted with fat suppression and contrast, axial section

A. Soft tissue mass is visible.
B. Thick cartilage cap is noticed.
C. Aggressive periosteal reaction is visible.
D. Pathological contrast enhancement is present.
E. Osteochondroma, bursa formation is noticed.

118. A 59-year-old patient with back pain was referred for MRI (Fig. 8.4a, b). Choose the correct statement(s) regarding Th6:

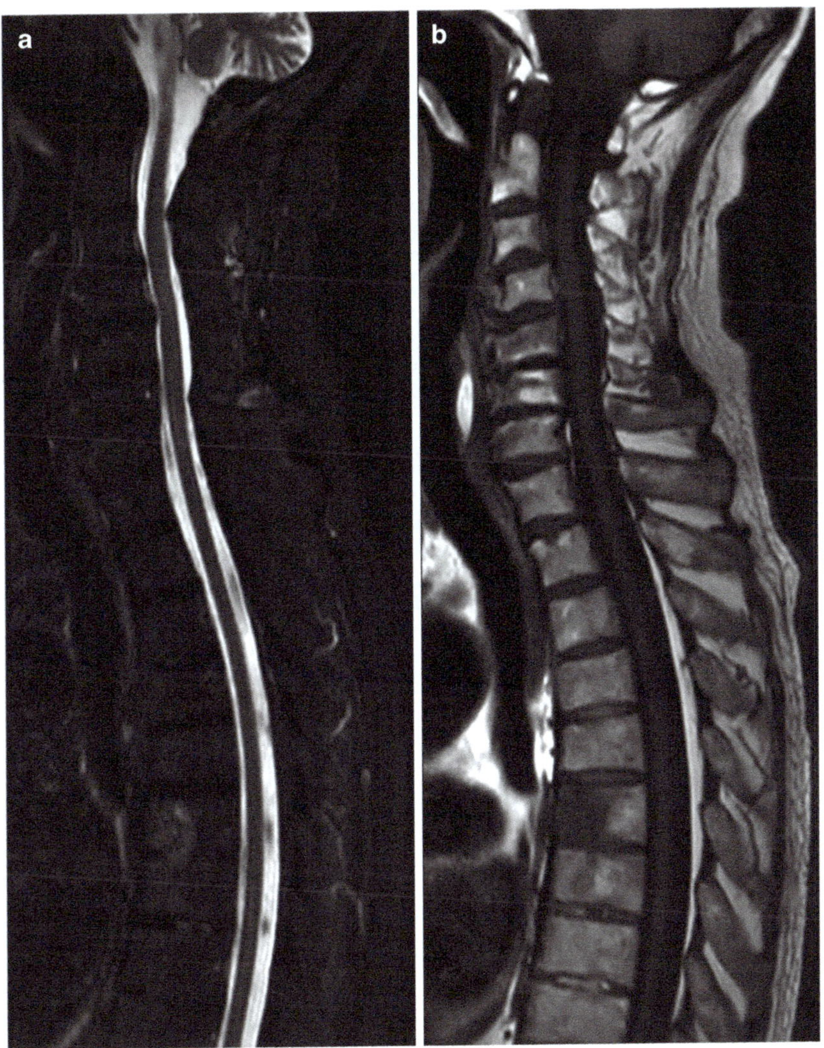

Fig. 8.4 (**a**) Short tau inversion recovery, sagittal section; (**b**) T1-weighted image, sagittal section

A. It is suspicious for metastasis.
B. It may be an atypical haemangioma.
C. It is a typical picture of Paget disease.
D. Destruction of the inferior endplate may indicate spondylodiscitis.
E. Soft tissue component is visible and is typical for primary malignant tumour.

119. An 83-year-old male with dementia presents with 4 months of pain in the pelvis, more on the left side. X-ray was performed (Fig. 8.5). What is the most likely diagnosis?

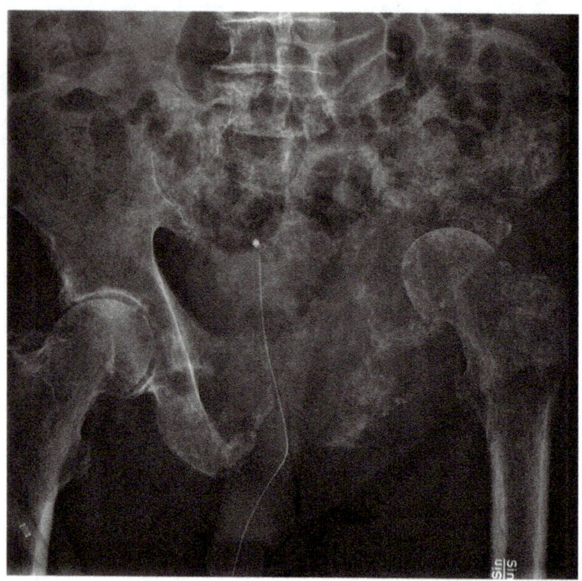

Fig. 8.5 X-ray of the pelvis

A. metastasis
B. Paget disease
C. osteomyelitis
D. osteosarcoma
E. Ewing sarcoma

120. A 56-year-old patient who had a fall from 3 m. CT of the whole body was performed (Fig. 8.6a, b). A focal lesion was noticed in the iliac bone. Choose the correct statement(s):

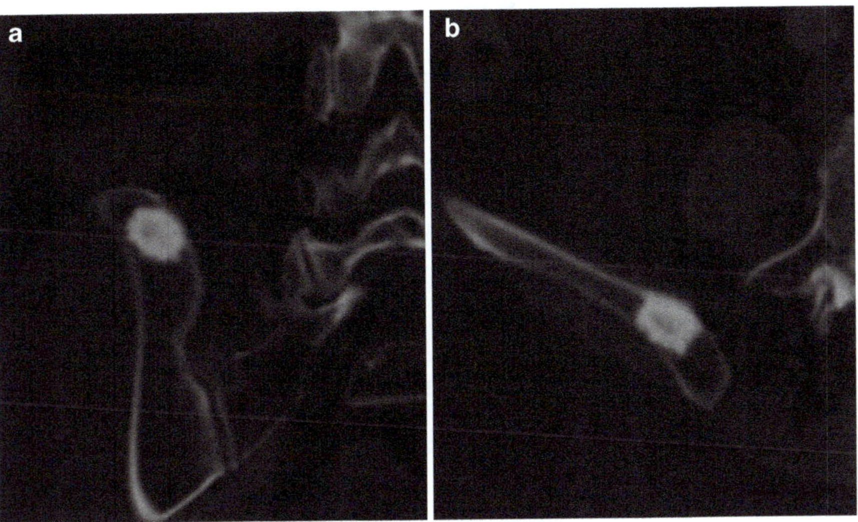

Fig. 8.6 Computed tomography of the whole body, focus on the right ilium. (**a**) Coronal section; (**b**) axial section

A. It is suspected, bone core biopsy should be done.
B. It is not suspected, biopsy is not needed.
C. MRI is recommended for better characterization.
D. CT with contrast may help for better characterization.
E. Scintigraphy is recommended.

121. What is the most likely diagnosis regarding the patient from the previous question?
A. bony island
B. chondrosarcoma
C. enchondroma
D. osseous haemangioma
E. unspecific intraosseous calcification

122. A 19-year-old patient presents with a painful arm. X-ray is provided on Fig. 8.7a, b. Choose the correct statement(s) regarding the radiological finding:

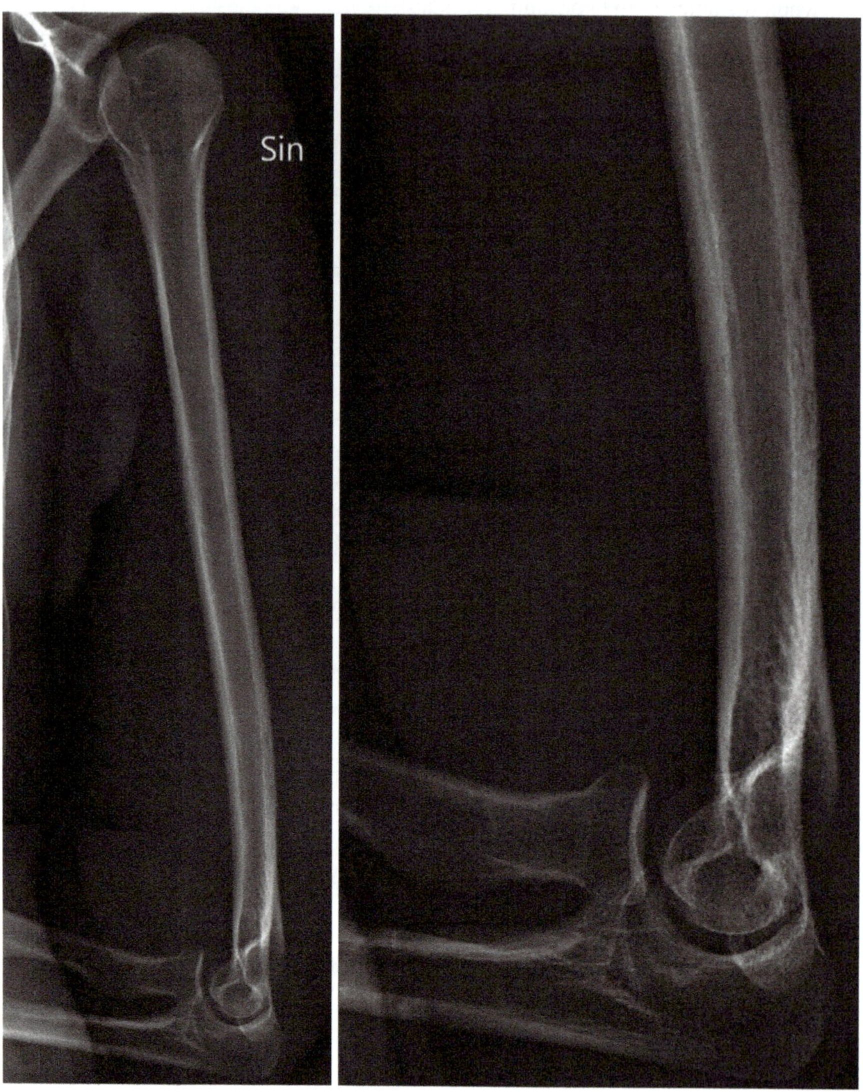

Fig. 8.7 X-ray of the elbow

A. Thinned cortex is noticed.
B. It is a visible cartilage matrix.
C. Periosteal reaction is visible.
D. There is visible permeative destruction.
E. It is normal, I recommend further diagnostic MRI.

123. Choose the correct statement regarding differential diagnosis (Fig. 8.7a, b):
   A. lymphoma because of permeative destruction
   B. Langerhans cell histiocytosis because of cortical breakthrough
   C. osteomyelitis because of permeative destruction
   D. osteosarcoma because sunburst periosteal reaction
   E. Ewing sarcoma because of no true matrix
124. MRI was performed (Fig. 8.8a–d). What is the most likely diagnosis?

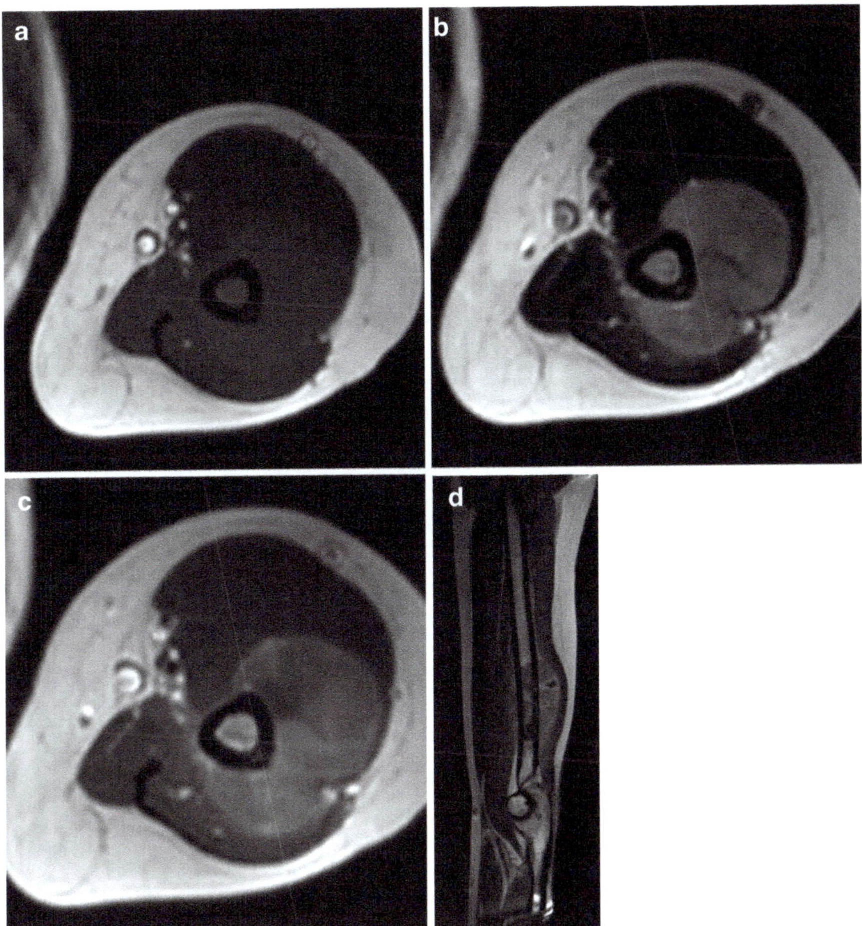

Fig. 8.8 (**a**) T1-weighted image, axial section; (**b**) T2-weighted image, axial section; (**c**) T1-weighted image with contrast, axial section; (**d**) T1-weighted image with contrast, sagittal section

   A. lymphoma
   B. Langerhans cell histiocytosis
   C. osteomyelitis
   D. osteosarcoma
   E. Ewing sarcoma

125. A 24-year-old patient presented with nocturnal pain of the forefoot. CT was performed (Fig. 8.9a–d). What is the most likely diagnosis?

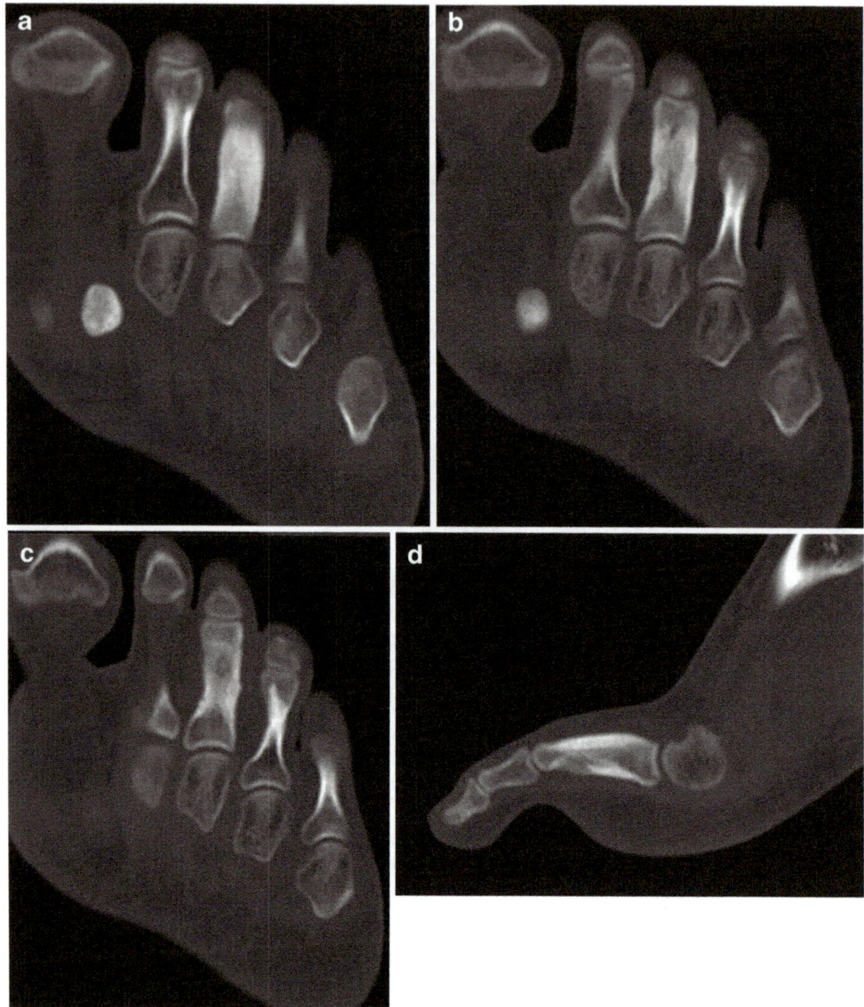

Fig. 8.9 Computed tomography of the forefoot. (**a**–**c**) Axial sections; (**d**) sagittal section

A. osteosarcoma
B. stress fracture
C. Brodie abscess
D. cortical desmoid
E. osteoid osteoma

126. In the patient from the previous question, an MRI examination without contrast was performed (Fig. 8.10a–c). Choose the most likely diagnosis:

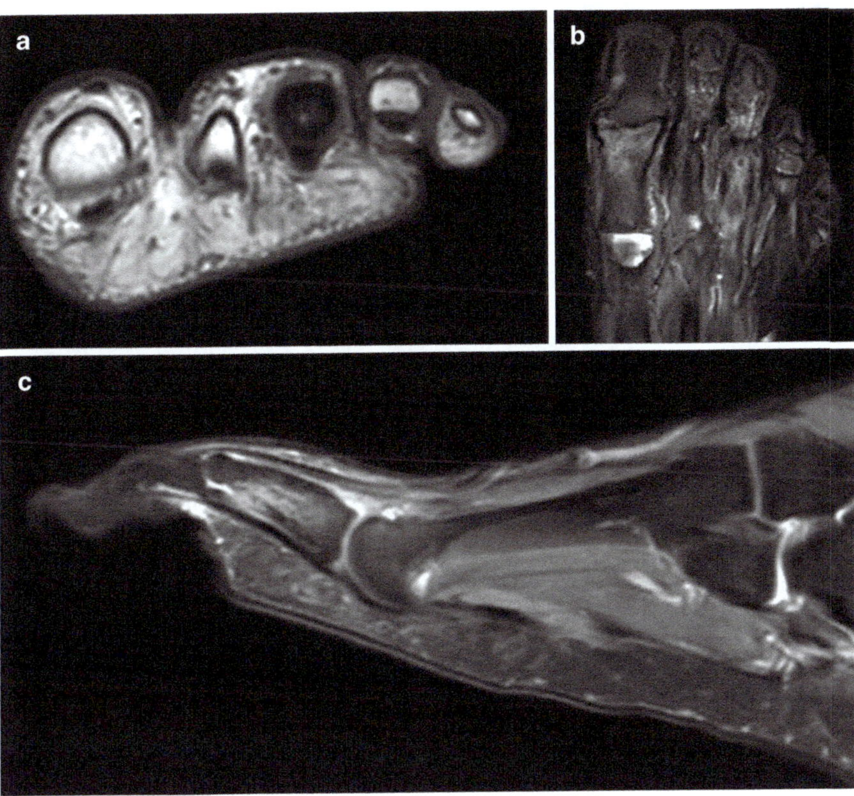

Fig. 8.10 (**a**) T1-weighted image, coronal section; (**b**) short tau inversion recovery image, axial section; (**c**) short tau inversion recovery image, sagittal section

A. osteosarcoma
B. stress fracture
C. Brodie abscess
D. cortical desmoid
E. osteoid osteoma

127. A 25-year-old patient presents with a painful and tender thigh. X-ray was performed (Fig. 8.11a, b). Choose the correct statement regarding the lesion:

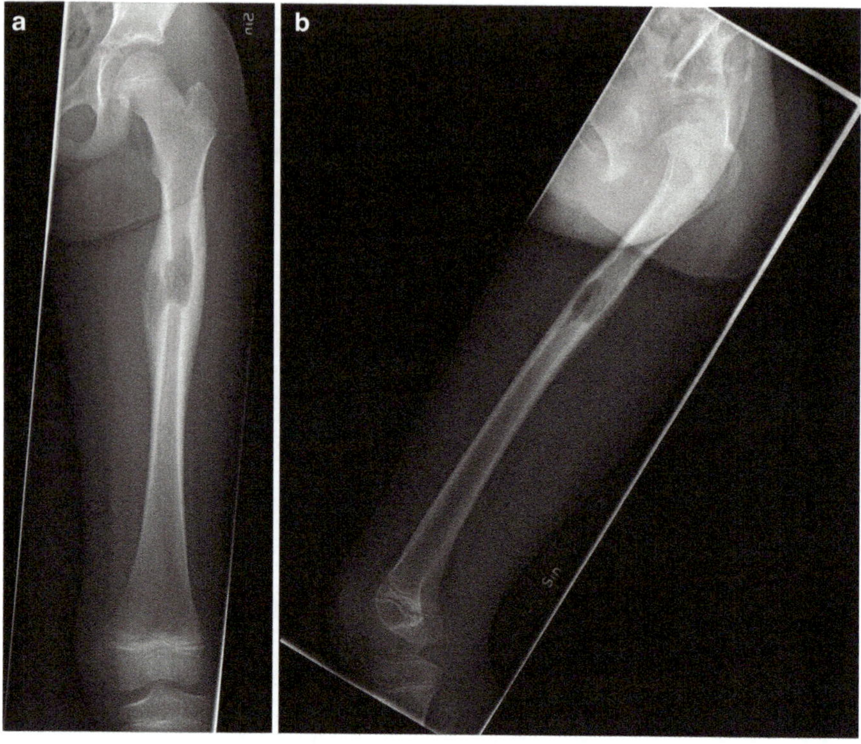

Fig. 8.11 (**a** and **b**) X-ray of the femur

A. narrow zone of transition
B. diaphyseal localizations
C. periosteal reaction
D. cortical breakthrough
E. no sclerotic margin

128. What is the most likely differential diagnosis regarding the patient from the previous question (Fig. 8.11a, b)?
A. metastasis because of diaphyseal localization
B. lymphoma because of permeative destruction
C. Ewing sarcoma because of permeative destruction
D. eosinophilic granuloma because of permeative destruction
E. osteomyelitis because of destruction and periosteal reaction

129. Ten days after the first X-ray (Fig. 8.11a, b), a control X-ray was taken (not showed). It was noticed that the lesion was more than twice bigger, while the character of the tumour remained unchanged. Regarding rapid progress, what is the most likely diagnosis?
    A. metastasis
    B. lymphoma
    C. Ewing sarcoma
    D. eosinophilic granuloma
    E. osteomyelitis
130. A 24-year-old patient presented with knee pain. X-ray was performed (Fig. 8.12a–c). What is the differential diagnosis?

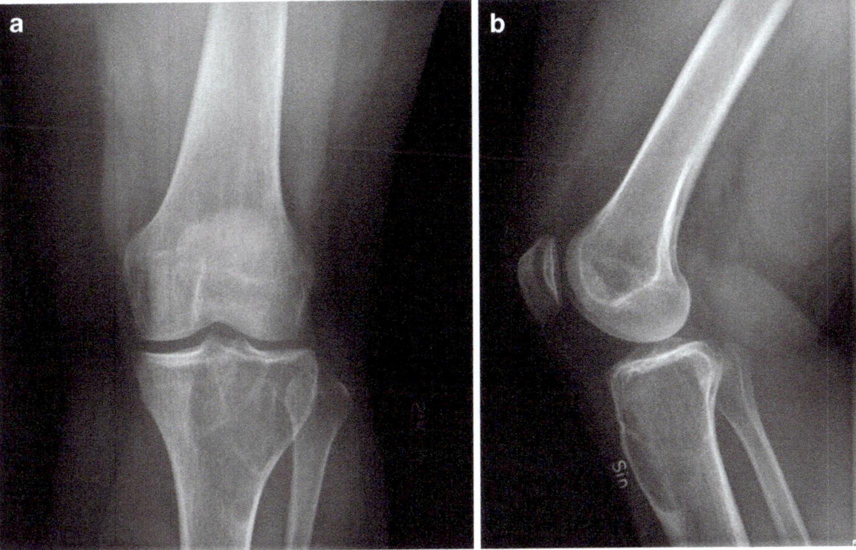

Fig. 8.12 X-ray of the knee (**a**) the fronal projection, (**b**) the lateral projection

    A. aneurysmal bone cyst
    B. fibrous dysplasia
    C. giant cell tumour
    D. chordoma
    E. metastasis

131. The patient from the previous question was referred for MRI. Choose the correct statement(s) regarding MRI (Fig. 8.13a, b):

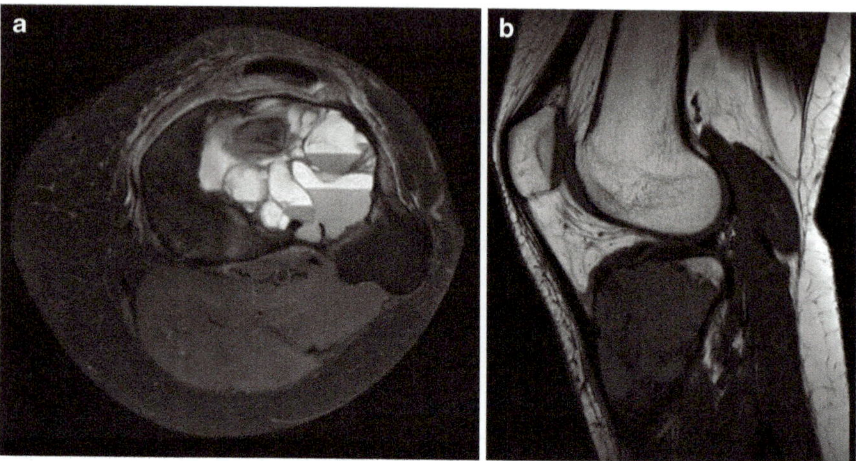

Fig. 8.13 (**a**) T2-weighted with fat suppression, axial section; (**b**) T1-weighted, sagittal section

A. Fluid levels are present.
B. Most of the lesion is solid.
C. The figure b shows cortical thinning.
D. The lesion is located in the meta-epiphysis.
E. There is direct contact with the articular surface.

132. In the patient from the previous question, what is the most likely diagnosis regarding X-ray (Fig. 8.12a–c) and MRI (Fig. 8.13a, b)?

A. aneurysmal bone cyst
B. fibrous dysplasia
C. Ewing sarcoma
D. chordoma
E. metastasis

133. A 63-year-old patient presented with bladder dysfunction. CT of the abdomen and pelvis was performed (Fig. 8.14). Choose the three most likely diagnosis?
    A. chondrosarcoma
    B. giant cell tumour
    C. plasmacytoma
    D. Tarlov cyst
    E. metastasis
134. Choose the correct statement(s) regarding the patient from the previous question (Fig. 8.14):

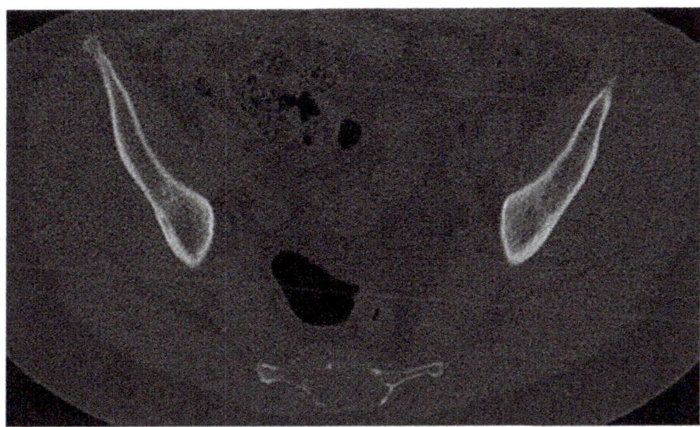

Fig. 8.14 Computed tomography, axial section

    A. The lesion causes destruction of the sacrum.
    B. Soft tissue components are present.
    C. No calcifications are present.
    D. No fat component is visible.
    E. Marginal sclerosis is visible.

135. The patient from the previous question was referred for MRI (Fig. 8.15a, b). What is the correct statement(s) regarding this patient?

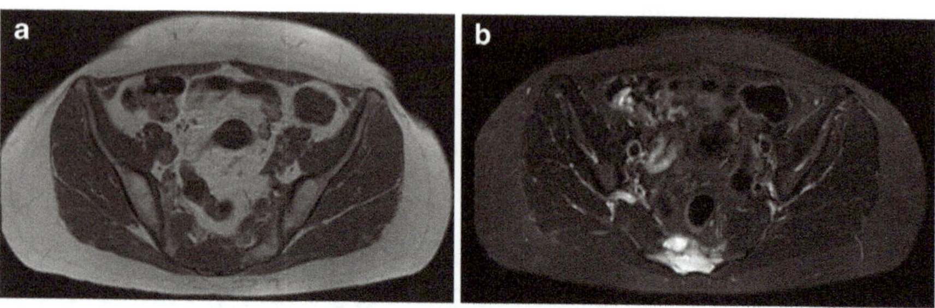

Fig. 8.15 (**a**) T1-weighted image; (**b**) T2-weighted image with fat suppression

A. Intratumoural haemorrhage is visible.
B. Cystic component is visible.
C. Well-defined lobulated mass is present.
D. Obstruction of sacral canal is noticed.
E. It bulges into the presacral space.

136. Regarding the previous question, what sequence is missing to be sure that the cystic component is visible (Fig. 8.15a, b)?

A. T1-weighted with fat suppression
B. T2-weighted with fat suppression
C. T1-weighted with contrast
D. PD-weighted with suppression
E. PD-weighted without fat suppression

137. A 58-year-old patient presented with shoulder pain. X-ray was performed (Fig. 8.16a–c). a- the frontal projection, b- the lateral projection, c- the axial projection. Choose the best answer:

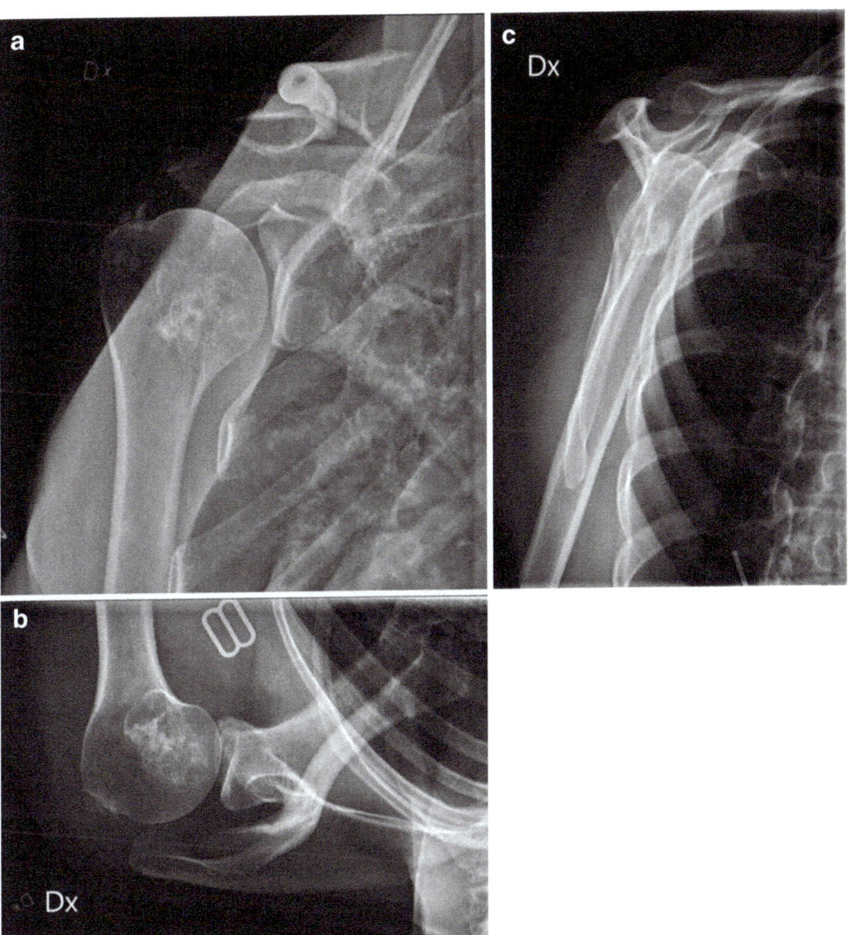

Fig. 8.16 X-ray of the shoulder

A. It is probably benign, no further diagnostic testing is required.
B. Cartilage matrix is visible, which means that further diagnostic testing is needed.
C. Periosteal reaction is visible, which means that city without contrast is compulsory.
D. No clear breakthrough is visible, which means that it is benign, and no further diagnostic testing is needed.
E. It is somewhat regular distribution of cartilage classifications further diagnostic testing is recommended.

138. The patient from the previous question is reporting much more pain, what should be done next?
   A. X-ray accessory projections
   B. CT without contrast
   C. CT with contrast
   D. MRI without contrast
   E. MRI with contrast
139. MRI was performed (Fig. 8.17a–d). Choose the correct statement regarding MRI:

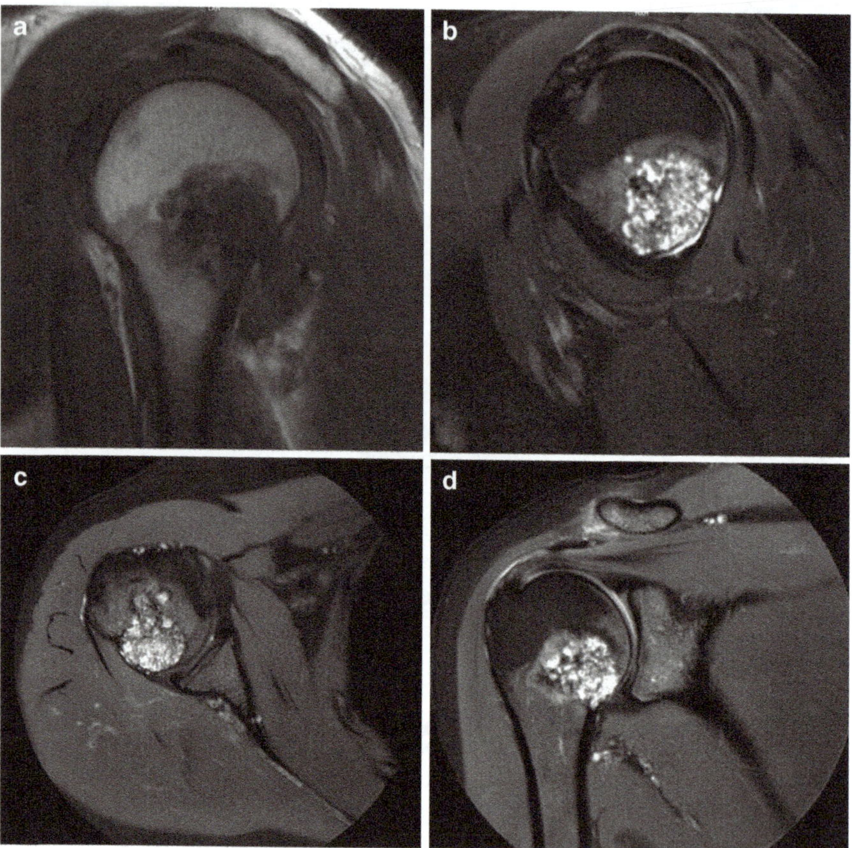

Fig. 8.17 (**a**) T1-weighted image, sagittal section; (**b**) T2-weighted spectral adiabatic inversion recovery, sagittal section; (**c**) proton density spectral adiabatic inversion recovery, axial section; (**d**) T2-weighted spectral adiabatic inversion recovery, coronal section

   A. Cortical breach is seen.
   B. Blooming artefact is visible.
   C. Calcifications are visible.
   D. Endosteal scalloping is present.
   E. The lesion is present in the epi-metaphysis.

140. Which of the following findings do you recognize on X-ray (Fig. 8.16a–c) and MRI (Fig. 8.17a–d)?
    A. metaphyseal lesion
    B. bone destruction
    C. bone production
    D. periosteal reaction
    E. pathologic fracture
141. A patient presents with knee pain. X-ray (Fig. 8.18) and MRI (Fig. 8.19) were performed. Choose the correct option regarding this patient:
    a. Permeative growth.
    b. Fluid-fluid levels are seen.
    c. Lesion is poorly marginated.
    d. Cortical destruction and soft tissue extension are seen.

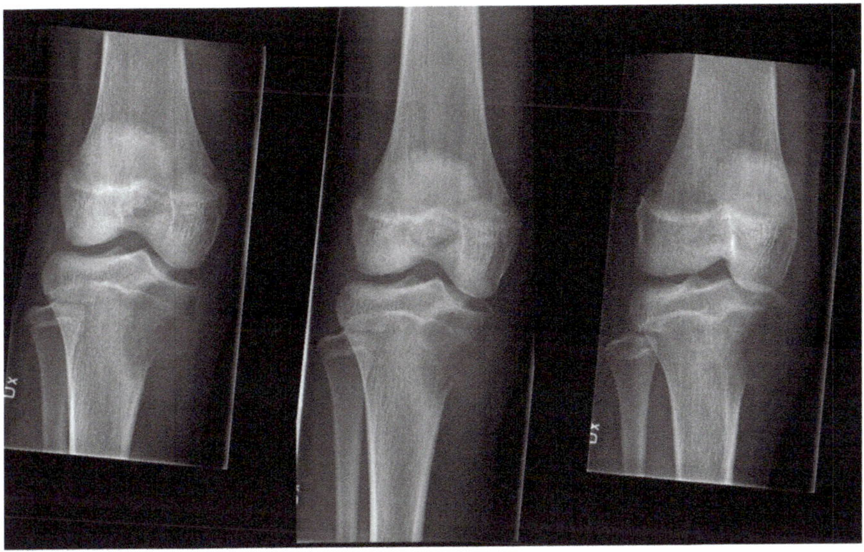

Fig. 8.18 X-ray of the knee

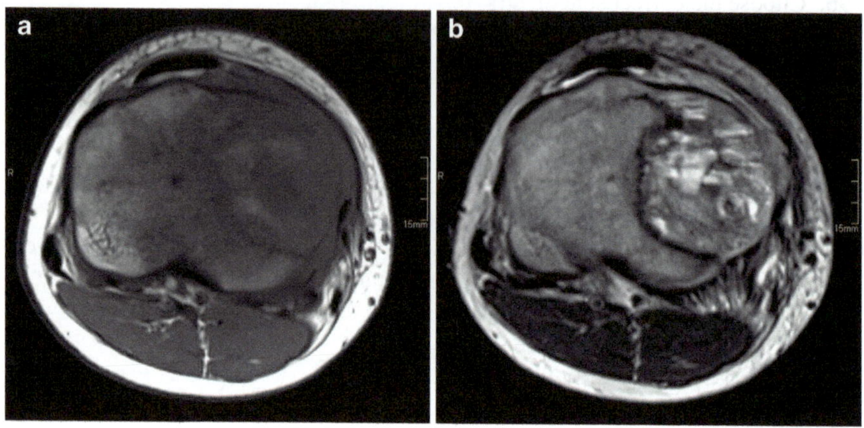

Fig. 8.19 MRI of the knee. (**a**) T1-weighted image, axial section; (**b**) T2-weighted image, axial section

A. a, b, c, d
B. a, b, c
C. a, b
D. c, d
E. b, c, d

142. What is the most likely diagnosis regarding the patient from the previous question?
A. chondrosarcoma
B. classic osteosarcoma
C. aneurysmal bone cyst
D. paraosteal osteosarcoma
E. telangiectatic osteosarcoma

143. Choose the correct option regarding the lesion seen in Fig. 8.20:
   a. Lesion in the metaphysis.
   b. A juxtacortical lesion is seen.
   c. Permeative bone destruction.
   d. Periosteal reaction is present.

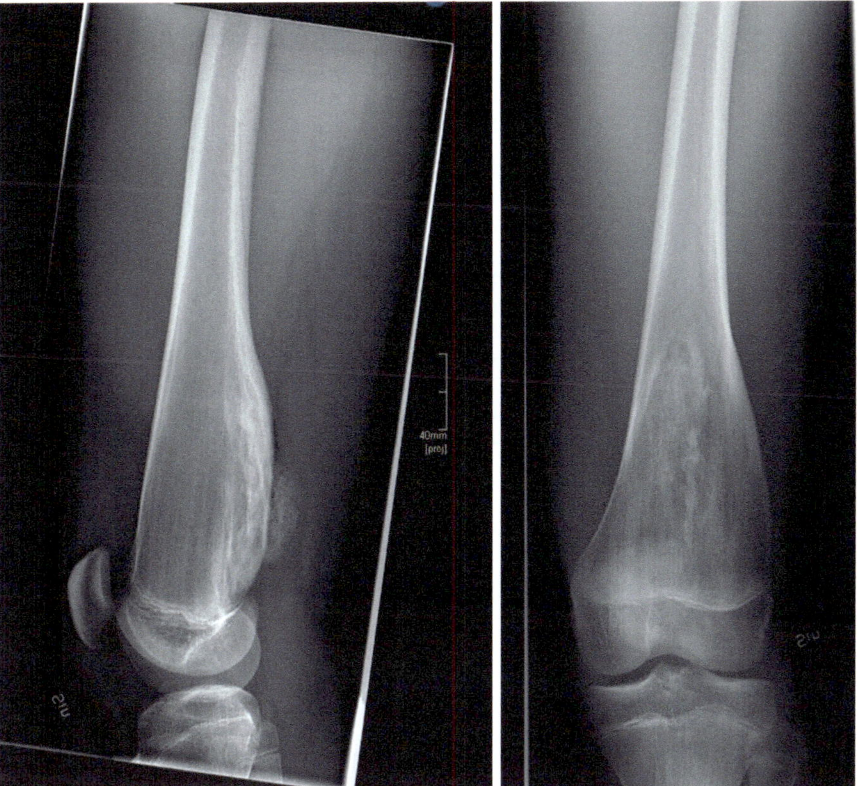

Fig. 8.20 X-ray of the knee

A. a, b, c, d
B. a, b, c
C. a, b, d
D. b, d
E. a, d

144. A 69-year-old patient presents with pain and tenderness in the left hip. X-ray was done (Fig. 8.21). What is the most likely?
   a. metastasis
   b. Paget disease
   c. fibrous dysplasia
   d. chronic osteomyelitis

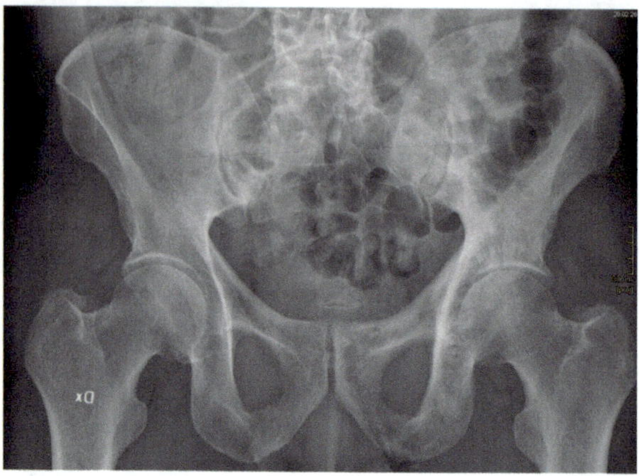

Fig. 8.21 X-ray of the pelvis

A. a, b, c, d
B. a, b, c
C. a, b
D. c
E. b

145. What lesion is most likely in this X-ray of a patient with left ankle pain (Fig. 8.22)?

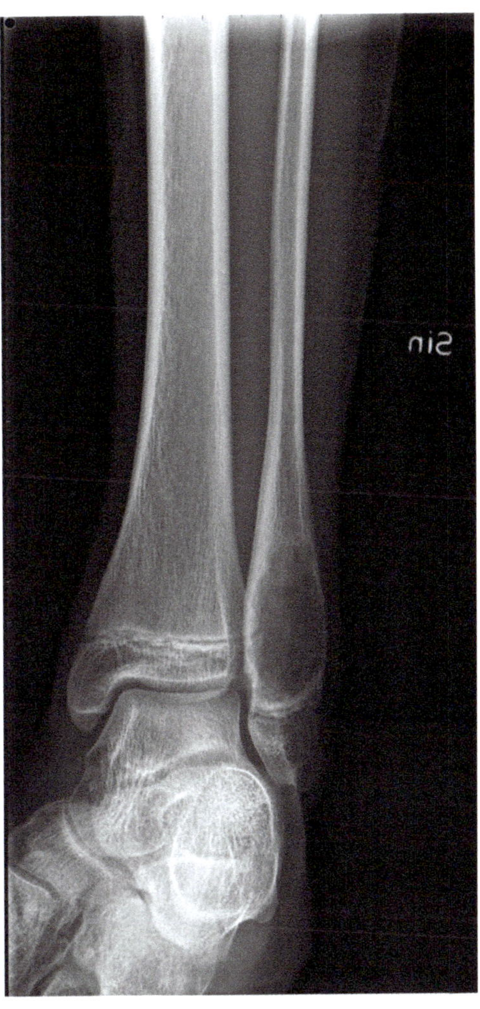

Fig. 8.22 X-ray of the ankle

A. metastasis
B. Ewing sarcoma
C. chondroblastoma
D. giant cell tumour
E. aneurysmal bone cyst

146. What lesion(s) is/are most likely in this X-ray of a patient with knee pain and tenderness (Fig. 8.23)?
    a. Brodie abscess
    b. giant cell tumour
    c. chondroblastoma

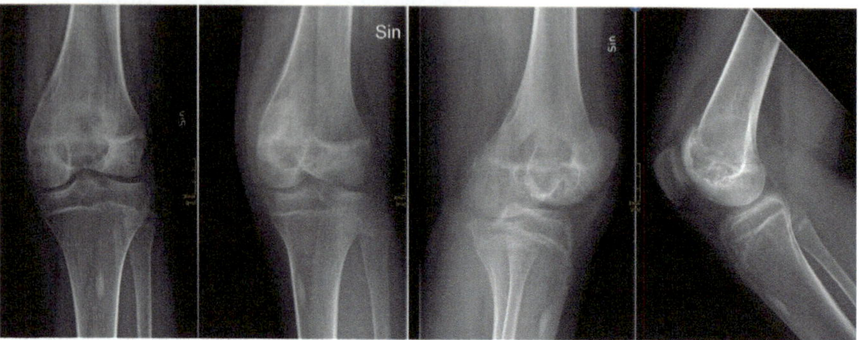

Fig. 8.23 X-ray of the knee

A. a, b, c
B. a, b
C. b, c
D. b
E. c

147. A 49-year-old patient presents with chest pain and a palpable lesion on the left side. X-ray and MRI were performed (Fig. 8.24). Choose the correct option regarding this lesion:
    a. Rib destruction is seen.
    b. Intralesional calcifications are seen.
    c. Heterogenous contrast enhancement is present.

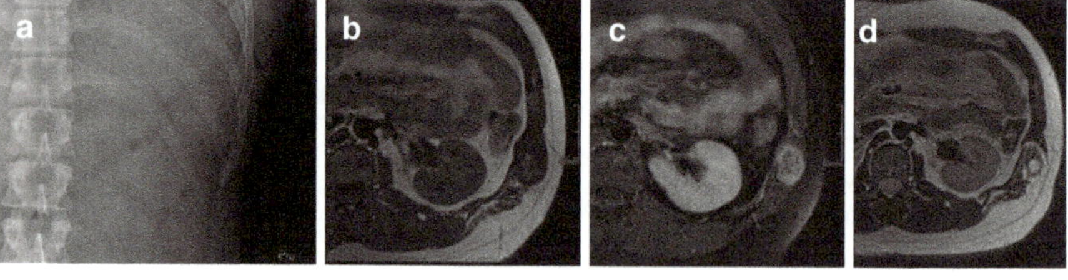

Fig. 8.24 (**a**) X-ray of the ribs; (**b**) T1-weighted image, axial section; (**c**) T1-weighted image, with fat suppression and contrast, axial section; (**d**) T1-weighted image with contrast, axial section

A. a, b, c
B. a, b
C. b, c
D. b
E. c

148. What is the most likely diagnosis regarding the patient from the previous question?
    A. myeloma
    B. metastasis
    C. osteosarcoma
    D. chondrosarcoma
    E. elastofibroma dorsi
149. A 23-year-old patient presents after trauma. X-ray and MRI were performed (Fig. 8.25). What is the correct diagnosis regarding the radiological findings?

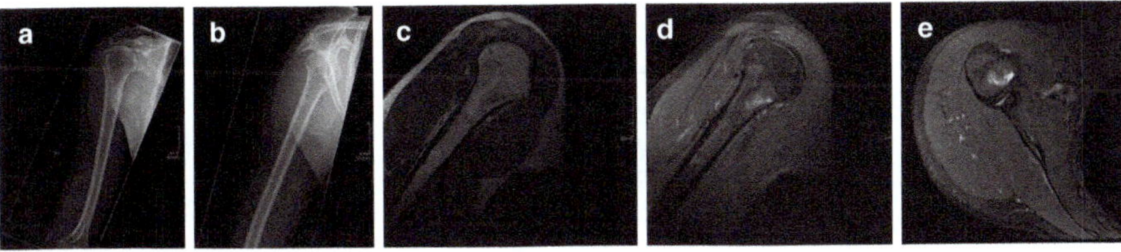

Fig. 8.25 (**a** and **b**) X-ray of the shoulder; (**c**) T1-weighted image, sagittal section; (**d**) proton density-weighted image with fat suppression, sagittal section; (**e**) proton density-weighted image with fat suppression, axial section

    A. aneurysmal bone cyst
    B. non-ossifying fibroma
    C. fibrous dysplasia
    D. giant cell tumour
    E. Paget disease

150. A 40-year-old patient presents with knee pain and a soft tissue mass on the lateral side of the knee. What lesions should be included in the differential diagnosis based on X-ray (Fig. 8.26)?
   a. giant cell tumour
   b. metastasis
   c. chondroblastoma

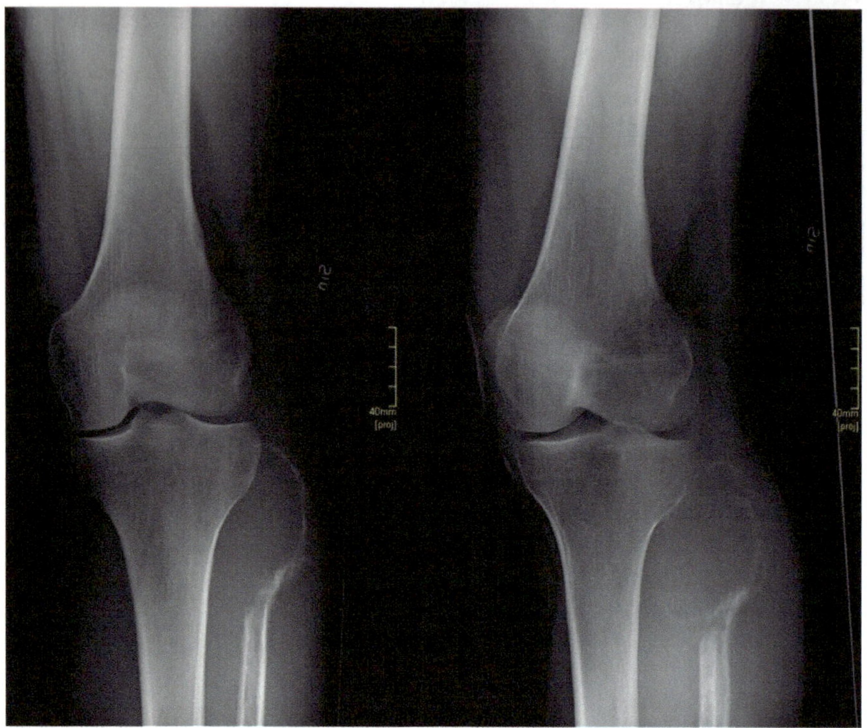

Fig. 8.26 X-ray of the knee

A. a, b, c
B. a, b
C. b, c
D. a, c
E. a

151. A 65-year-old patient presents with bilateral hip pain. X-ray was done (Fig. 8.27). Choose the correct option regarding this patient:

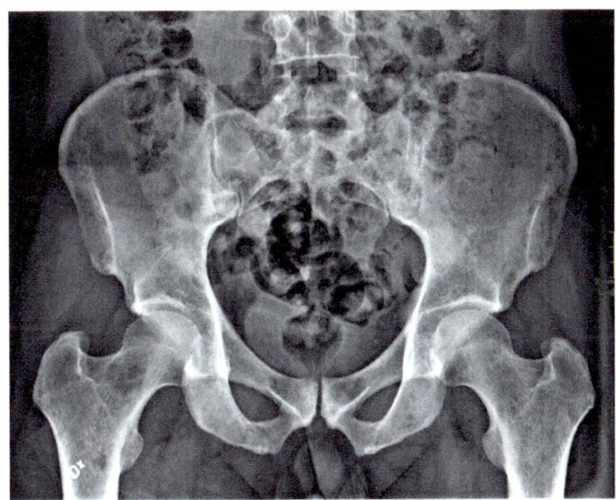

Fig. 8.27 X-ray of the pelvis

A. No abnormality is seen, MRI with contrast is indicated.
B. Osteoarthrosis is most likely cause.
C. Caput necrosis is visible.
D. There are malignant lesions.
E. There are benign lesions.

152. With regard to the patient in the previous question, what is the most likely differential diagnosis?
a. metastases
b. osteonecrosis
c. multiple myeloma
d. aneurysmal bone cyst
A. a, b
B. b, d
C. b, c
D. a, c
E. d

153. A 16-year-old patient presents with knee pain. X-ray was done (Fig. 8.28). What is the most likely diagnosis?

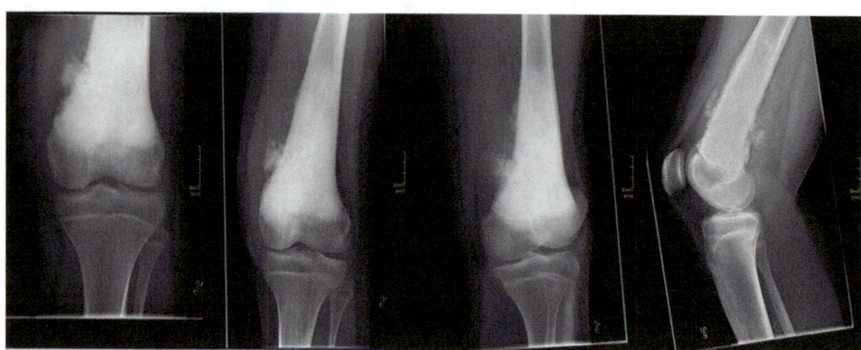

Fig. 8.28 X-ray of the knee

A. osteopetrosis
B. osteomyelitis
C. osteosarcoma
D. Ewing sarcoma
E. Brodie abscess

154. What is the differential diagnosis regarding this X-ray (Fig. 8.29)?
   a. osteomyelitis
   b. stress fracture
   c. cortical desmoid
   d. osteoid osteoma

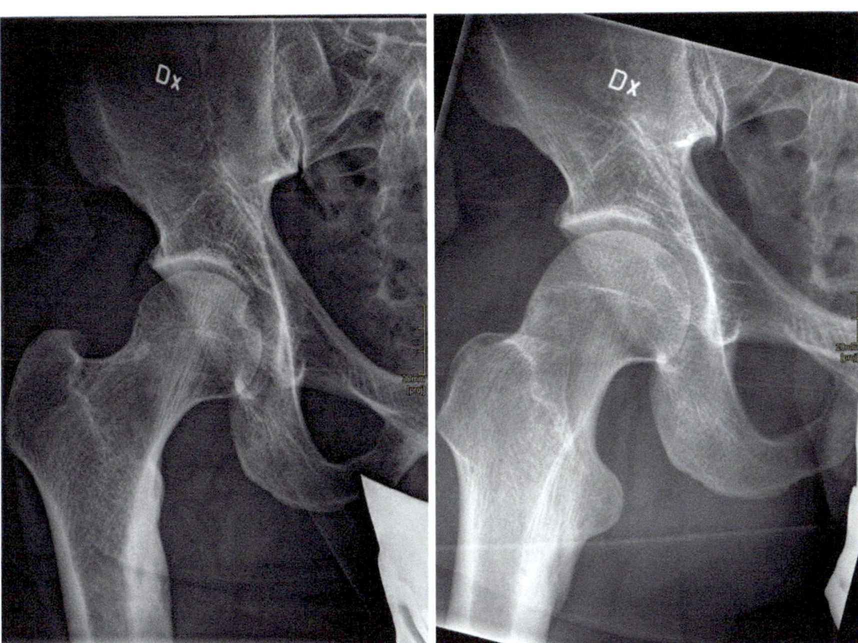

Fig. 8.29 X-ray of the hip

A. a, b, c, d
B. a, b, c
C. a, b
D. c, d
E. a, d

Key to Chapter 8

1. A, B, C, E.
2. B, D, E.
3. A, C, D, E.
4. C.
5. A.
6. E.
7. B, D. Biopsy should not be done because it is hard to distinguished enchondroma from low-grade chondrosarcoma [1].
8. B, C, D. Malignant transformation is not common, if occurs it is seen in flat bones or long tubular bones.
9. A.
10. A, B, C, D, E.
11. A.
12. A, B, C, D. Eosinophilic granuloma may mimic almost all lesions. Osteoma is typical in older age group. Eosinophilic granuloma is typically in patients younger than 30 years.
13. A, B, D.
14. E.
15. E.
16. A.
17. C, D, E.
18. B, C.
19. C, E. In gracile bone, non-ossifying fibroma is located centrally.
20. B, C, D. More than 90% of osteoblastomas are present in the posterior elements.
21. A, B, C. Osteoblastoma has a similar histological appearance as osteoid osteoma.
22. B, D. Myositis ossificans should be separated from bone at least with thin rim of fat. Sacrum is localization of the giant cell tumour; however, it is seen more commonly in older patients.
23. A, B, C, E.
24. A, C, D.
25. B, C, D.
26. C, D. Rare but spectacular disease where the whole bone disappears, scintigraphy usually does not show uptake when bone is totally reabsorbed.
27. B, C, E. Fluid levels may be seen on MRI because secondary aneurysmal bone cyst may be present.
28. A, B.
29. E.
30. C, D.
31. C.
32. A, B, C.
33. A, C, D, E.

34. A, B, E. Differentiating between the enchondroma and low-grade osteosarcoma is very difficult both radiologically and in histopathology. Expansion of bone is usually not present.
35. A, E.
36. A, C, D.
37. C, E.
38. B, D. No matrix is present, no sclerotic reaction or lymphadenopathy is the feature of plasmocytoma.
39. A, B, E.
40. B, C, D.
41. B, C.
42. A, B, C, D, E.
43. A. The most common localization is femur, then proximal tibia and calcaneus.
44. A.
45. A, B. Giant cell tumour matrix contains no calcifications.
46. B, C, D, E.
47. A, B, C.
48. A, B, D.
49. B, C.
50. A, B, C, D, E.
51. A, B, C, E.
52. B. Scintigraphy and PET scanning with the tracer 18F-fluorodeoxyglucose gives variable results due to the potential variable of osteoblastic activity.
53. A, B, D, E.
54. A, B, D. Bony expansion with cortical thinning is due to bone marrow hyperplasia. Rib-within-a-rib appearance is due to subperiosteal extension.
55. A, B, C, D, E. Preserved red bone marrow predispose to infarction and osteomyelitis. Infarction in a bone may cause sclerosis which in consequence results in destruction.
56. A, B, C, D.
57. B.
58. C, E.
59. C, D, E.
60. A, B, C, D, E.
61. A.
62. B.
63. D, E. Geode usually is present in epiphysis and does not cause defect in the cortex. Age does not match with chondroblastoma or solitary bone cyst.
64. C, D.
65. C. Solitary bone cyst is also known as unicameral bone cyst.
66. B.
67. A, B, C, D, E.
68. A, B, E.
69. B, C, D.
70. B. This is pathognomonic appearance of brown tumour.

71. C. Chondroblastoma is very often in humerus however in patients younger than 20 years.
72. B. There three most common benign lesions in patella: most common giant cell tumour (in adult skeleton, most common), chondroblastoma (less common) and aneurysmal bony cyst.
73. A, B, C, E.
74. C, E.
75. A, B, C, D. Epiphyseal lesions are aneurysmal bone cyst, chondroblastoma, enchondroma, geode, giant cell tumour, osteomyelitis, osteoblastoma, osteosarcoma.
76. A, B, C. Diaphyseal lesions are bone infarct, enchondroma, eosinophilic granuloma, Ewing sarcoma, fibrous dysplasia, lymphoma, metastases, myeloma, osteomyelitis, osteoid osteoma, and simple bone cyst [2].
77. A, C. Aneurysmal bone cyst presents as pain especially if cortex is abrupt. Osteoblastoma in spina presents commonly as painful scoliosis.
78. A, B, C. Both benign and malign lesions may contain component of aneurysmal bone cyst with fluid levels.
79. A, B, D, E.
80. B, D, E.
81. A, B, C, E.
82. D, E.
83. A, B.
84. E.
85. A, B, C.
86. A, B. This is a very aggressive reaction seen commonly in osteosarcoma and Ewing sarcoma.
87. B, D, E.
88. B, C, E. It is clear malign lesion thus fibrosus dysplasia should be excluded. Age is not typical for chondrosarcoma.
89. A, C, D, E. The useful mnemonic for common rib lesions is FAME: Fibrous dysplasia, Aneurysmal bone cyst, Metastases/Multiple Myeloma, Enchondroma.
90. A, B, C, D, E. There is a mnemonic "Metastases May Eventually Fracture Bones" which responds to Metastasis, Multiply Myeloma, Enchondroma, Fibrosus dysplasia, and Brown tumour.
91. A, C, D, E.
92. A, B, E.
93. A, B, C, D, E.
94. B.
95. A, D, E.
96. A, B, C, D, E.
97. A, B, C.
98. A, C, D, E.
99. A, B, C, D, E.
100. B, C, D.

101. D, E. Lesions with bony sequestrum: Bordie abscess, eosinophilic granuloma, lymphoma, osteoblastoma, fibrosarcoma, and some metastases.
102. A, B, C, E. Chordoma is a primary malign tumour while myeloma is secondary tumour.
103. A. The most common tumour of scapula is osteochondroma [3].
104. A, C, E.
105. A, B, C, D, E [4].
106. A, B, C, D.
107. A, B, D.
108. C. Calcifications in soft tissue mass with sacrum destructions indicates chordoma. The second most common sacral tumour is giant cell tumour where calcifications are not present. Osteoblastoma is painful lesion and seen in younger patients.
109. A, D. Chondroblastoma is more likely than ganglion. Giant cell tumour could be an alternative in older patients. No clinical evidence regarding osteomyelitis or osteoid osteoma is given.
110. D, E.
111. C, D.
112. B.
113. E.
114. D, E.
115. B.
116. C.
117. E.
118. A, B.
119. A.
120. B. It is the bony island (enostosis). Multiple enostoses is called osteopoikilosis and is classified as the sclerosing bony dysplasia. It is asymptomatic, not degenerated into malignancy and is not correlated with increased risk of fracture.
121. A.
122. D.
123. A, C, E.
124. E.
125. E.
126. E.
127. B, C, D, E.
128. B, C, D, E. Metastasis is located mainly in metaphysis.
129. D. Rapid progress is typical for eosinophilic granuloma.
130. A, C.
131. A, C, D, E.
132. A. Biopsy showed giant cell tumor with aneurysmal bone component.
133. A, B, C, E.
134. A, B, C, D.
135. C, D, E.

136. C.
137. E.
138. E.
139. A, C, D, E.
140. A, B.
141. A.
142. E. Presence of fluid levels is not only seen in aneurysmal bone cyst. There are other lesions containing fluid levels, i.e. chondroblastoma, osteoblastoma, telangiectatic osteosarcoma.
143. A. Histopathology: surface osteosarcoma.
144. E. It is Paget disease.
145. E.
146. E.
147. A.
148. D.
149. C.
150. E.
151. D.
152. D. It is patient with multiple myeloma.
153. C. Histopathology: osteoblastic osteosarcoma.
154. E.

References

1. Murphey MD, Flemming DJ, Boyea SR, Bojescul JA, Sweet DE, Temple HT. Enchondroma versus chondrosarcoma in the appendicular skeleton: differentiating features. Radiographics. 1998;18(5):1213–37; quiz 44–45. https://doi.org/10.1148/radiographics.18.5.9747616.
2. Miller TT. Bone tumors and tumorlike conditions: analysis with conventional radiography. Radiology. 2008;246(3):662–74. https://doi.org/10.1148/radiol.2463061038.
3. Blacksin MF, Benevenia J. Neoplasms of the scapula. AJR Am J Roentgenol. 2000;174(6):1729–35. https://doi.org/10.2214/ajr.174.6.1741729.
4. Eisenberg RL. Bubbly lesions of bone. AJR Am J Roentgenol. 2009;193(2):W79–94. https://doi.org/10.2214/AJR.09.2964.

Soft Tissue Tumours

9

155. What is the most common soft tissue tumour?
   A. sarcoma
   B. liposarcoma
   C. lipoma
   D. schwannoma
   E. neurofibroma
156. Choose the features of lipomas:
   A. Signal on MRI is the same as subcutaneous tissue.
   B. It needs to have a capsule.
   C. Attenuation on CT is usually between −60 and −120 HU.
   D. Low signal on fat suppression sequences.
   E. Small nodularity is commonly present.
157. Choose the correct statement(s) regarding contrast enhancement of lipoma on MRI:
   A. Weak peripheral capsular enhancement may be seen.
   B. Diffuse enhancement of less than 50% of the lipoma is normal.
   C. If nodules are present, less than 50% may show enhancement.
   D. If septa are present, only septal vessels show enhancement.
   E. If a mass-like structure is visible, less than 50% may show enhancement.
158. What is the best imaging tool for the imaging of lipomas?
   A. MRI with contrast
   B. MRI without contrast
   C. ultrasound
   D. CT without contrast
   E. CT with contrast

Supplementary Information The online version contains supplementary material available at (https://doi.org/10.1007/978-3-030-85182-8_9).

P. Szaro, *Musculoskeletal Radiology for Residents*,
https://doi.org/10.1007/978-3-030-85182-8_9

159. Choose worrisome fat-containing tumours:
    A. 5 cm in the retroperitoneal space
    B. with some mineralization
    C. with thick septa
    D. with nodules on the septa
    E. intramuscular
160. Presence of calcifications may be a sign of:
    A. Infarction.
    B. Atypical fat tumour.
    C. Low-grade liposarcoma.
    D. Benign degeneration.
    E. Typical lipoma.
161. Choose the most common localization of lipomas:
    A. superficially in the trunk
    B. intramuscularly in the trunk
    C. superficially in the neck
    D. superficially in the shoulder region
    E. intramuscularly in the shoulder region
162. Choose the most common localization of spindle cell lipoma:
    A. anterior neck in female
    B. posterior neck in female
    C. anterior neck in male
    D. posterior neck in male
    E. anterior neck in both sexes
163. What radiological feature may differentiate low-grade liposarcoma from lipoma?
    A. Contrast administration on MRI.
    B. MRI without contrast.
    C. Ultrasound with contrast.
    D. Ultrasound without contrast.
    E. It is challenging, biopsy is indicated.
164. Choose the features of fat necrosis:
    A. Inhomogeneous signal on MRI.
    B. Calcifications.
    C. Enhancement after contrast administration.
    D. Cystic component.
    E. Fat necrosis is present over pressure points.
165. What is the main difference between a lipoma and lipomatosis?
    A. signal on T1-weighted images
    B. localization
    C. presence of a capsule
    D. contrast enhancement
    E. appearance on CT

166. Choose where lipomatosis may typically be seen:
    A. epidural
    B. mediastinum
    C. shoulder
    D. intraorbital
    E. pelvic
167. What nerve is commonly affected in neural lipomatosis?
    A. radial nerve
    B. ulnar nerve
    C. median nerve
    D. sciatic nerve
    E. femoral nerve
168. Choose the most common localization of lipoma arborescens:
    A. knee joint—popliteal fossa
    B. knee joint—suprapatellar recess
    C. shoulder joint—axillary recess
    D. shoulder joint—intertubercular recess
    E. hip joint—posterior recess
169. Choose the correct statement(s) regarding hibernoma:
    A. Signal on T1-weighted image is like in lipoma.
    B. It is hyperintense on fluid sensitive sequences.
    C. Often is an ill-defined mass.
    D. Malignant transformation is common.
    E. Significant vascularity is a typical feature.
170. What is the most common localization of hibernoma?
    A. shoulder
    B. buttock
    C. arm
    D. thigh
    E. hand
171. Choose the most typical localization of atypical lipomatous tumours:
    A. thorax
    B. leg
    C. foot
    D. buttock
    E. thigh
172. Choose features of an atypical lipomatous tumour:
    A. presence of a capsule
    B. fat signal
    C. presence of nodularity
    D. thickened septa
    E. recurrence after resection

173. Choose features of myxoid liposarcoma:
    A. Fat may be absent.
    B. Heterogenous contrast enhancement.
    C. It is the typical in patients younger than 20 years.
    D. If contrast is not administered, it may resemble a cyst.
    E. Good prognosis.
174. Choose the most common localization of dedifferentiated liposarcoma:
    A. thigh
    B. leg
    C. arm and forearm
    D. pleura and mediastinum
    E. retroperitoneal space
175. What is the most common liposarcoma?
    A. well-differentiated liposarcoma
    B. myxoid liposarcoma
    C. pleomorphic liposarcoma
    D. dedifferentiated liposarcoma
    E. mixed liposarcoma
176. Choose the correct statement(s) regarding Nora's lesion:
    A. The foot is the most common localization.
    B. Ossification is best demonstrated on CT.
    C. It is usually a painful mass.
    D. Usually, benign periosteal reaction is visible.
    E. Apex of the lesion is away from physis.
177. Choose the three most common localizations of fibromatosis:
    A. neck
    B. hand
    C. thorax
    D. penis
    E. foot
178. Choose features of the solitary fibrous tumour:
    A. Pleural localization is common.
    B. Intense contrast enhancement.
    C. Homogenous higher signal on T1-weighted images.
    D. Leiomyoma is in the differential diagnosis.
    E. Conservative treatment is a method of choice.

179. Choose the correct statement(s) regarding undifferentiated pleomorphic sarcoma:
    A. The thigh is the most common localization.
    B. It is usually larger than 5 cm.
    C. It may erode bones.
    D. It may contain necrosis.
    E. Radiologic features are not specific.
180. Choose the common features for dermatofibrosarcoma protuberans:
    A. Localization on trunk is uncommon.
    B. It has form that exists as an exophytic mass.
    C. Skin involvement is common.
    D. Satellite nodules may be present.
    E. Extensive bone destruction is a hallmark.
181. Choose the features of intramuscular myxoma:
    A. It is usually located in small muscles of the hand.
    B. Prominent high signal on T2-weighted images.
    C. Leakage of myxomatous component is common.
    D. Intensive contrast enhancement is typical.
    E. Rim of fat located superior and inferior.
182. Choose features of synovial sarcoma:
    A. Arises from synovial membrane.
    B. Lower extremity is the most common localization.
    C. Calcifications may be present.
    D. Multiloculated tumour with septa.
    E. Cystic component may be dominant.
183. Choose where flow void may be seen:
    A. venous malformation
    B. lymphatic malformation
    C. capillary malformation
    D. angiosarcoma
    E. arteriovenous malformation

184. A 68-year-old patient presenting with thigh and leg swelling and saddle anaesthesia (Fig. 9.1a, b). What is the differential diagnosis?

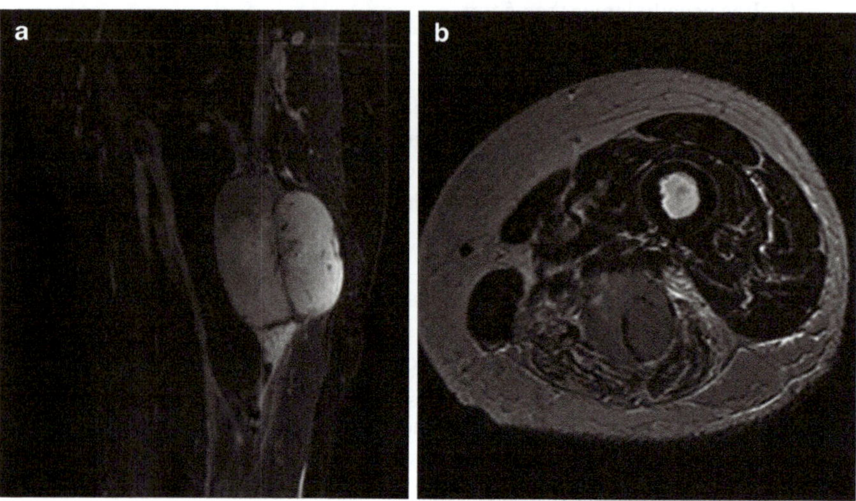

Fig. 9.1 (**a**) Short tau inversion recovery, sagittal section; (**b**) T1-weighted image with contrast

A. sarcoma
B. lipoma
C. atypical lipomatous tumour
D. schwannoma
E. intermuscular ganglion

185. Choose the correct statement(s) regarding the patient from the previous question (Fig. 9.1a, b):
A. Image-guided biopsy is required.
B. No biopsy is needed, patient should be operated on.
C. Homogenic contrast enhancement is a sign of benign character.
D. High signal on STIR is a sign of benign character.
E. If Doppler signal is present on ultrasound, it may exclude malignant character.

186. Choose the correct statement(s) regarding a 67-year-old patient presenting with a swollen and painful arm (MRI Fig. 9.2). The lesion:

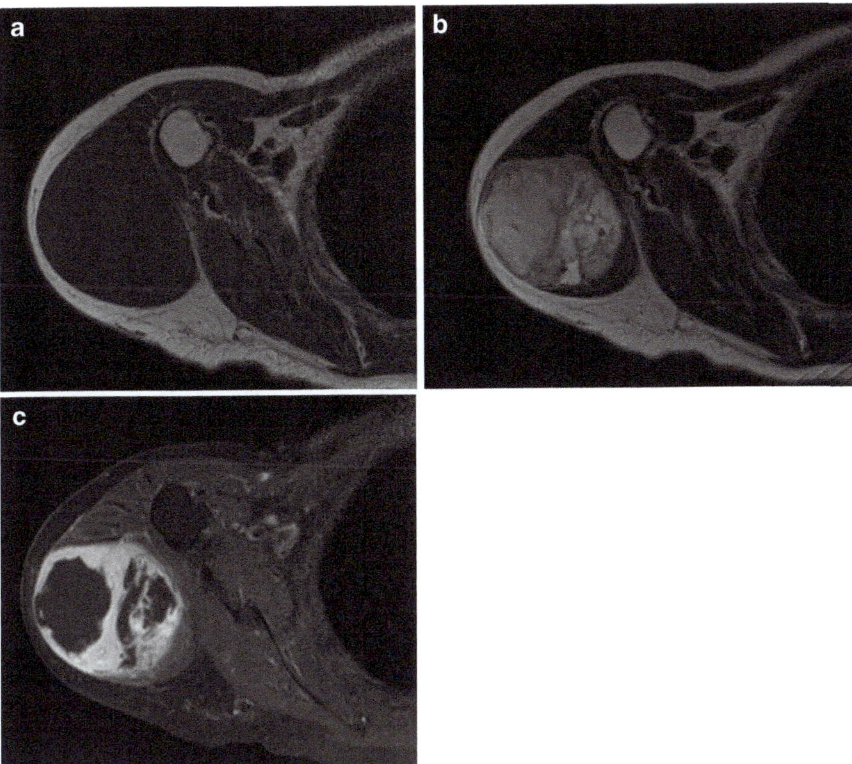

Fig. 9.2 (**a**) T1-weighted image, axial section; (**b**) T2-weighted image, axial section; (**c**) T1-weighted image with contrast enhancement, axial section

A. is located in the posterior compartment
B. contains necrosis
C. is mainly cystic
D. compresses the radial nerve
E. protrudes to the lateral axillary foramen

187. What should be done next with the patient from the previous question (Fig. 9.2a–c)?
A. X-ray
B. CT
C. ultrasound
D. biopsy
E. surgery

188. Based on anamnesis and Fig. 9.2a–c, what is the most likely diagnosis?
    A. nerve tumour
    B. low-grade liposarcoma
    C. pleomorphic sarcoma
    D. intramuscular ganglion with haemorrhage
    E. intramuscular ganglion
189. A 48-year-old patient presents with two palpable tumours on the posterior neck and at the level of the scapula. The first one is painful, while the other is not. MRI was performed (Fig. 9.3a–d). Choose the correct statement(s) regarding the tumour on the posterior neck:

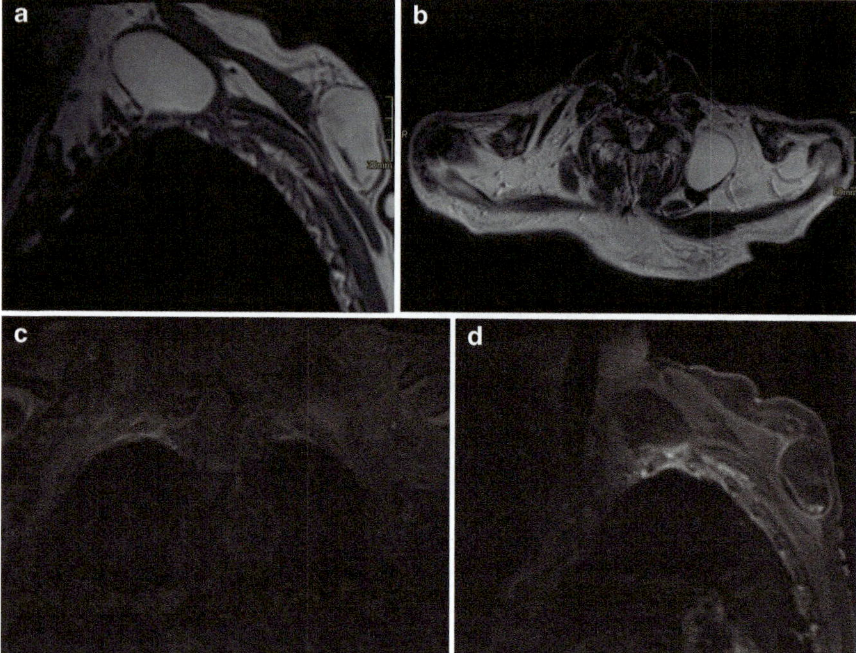

Fig. 9.3 (**a**) T1-weighted image, sagittal section; (**b**) T2-weighted image, axial section; (**c**) T1-weighted image with fat suppression, coronal section; (**d**) T1-weighted image with fat suppression and contrast, coronal section

A. There is a pathological contrast enhancement.
B. The tumour is located in the anterior neck triangle.
C. This structure is located intramuscularly.
D. It has visible bursa formation.
E. It contains mainly fat.

190. An 81-year-old patient presenting with a palpable tumour in the biceps brachii. Ultrasound was performed (Fig. 9.4). What is the differential diagnosis?

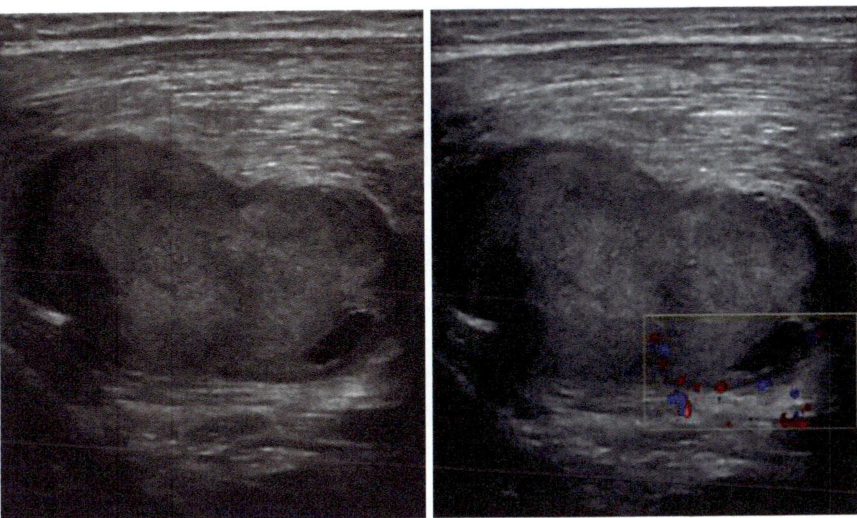

Fig. 9.4 Ultrasound, sagittal section of the biceps brachill

A. low-differentiated liposarcoma
B. pleomorphic sarcoma
C. synovial sarcoma
D. myositis ossificans
E. soft tissue metastasis

191. MRI with contrast was performed (Fig. 9.5a–d); what is the correct statement(s) regarding this patient?

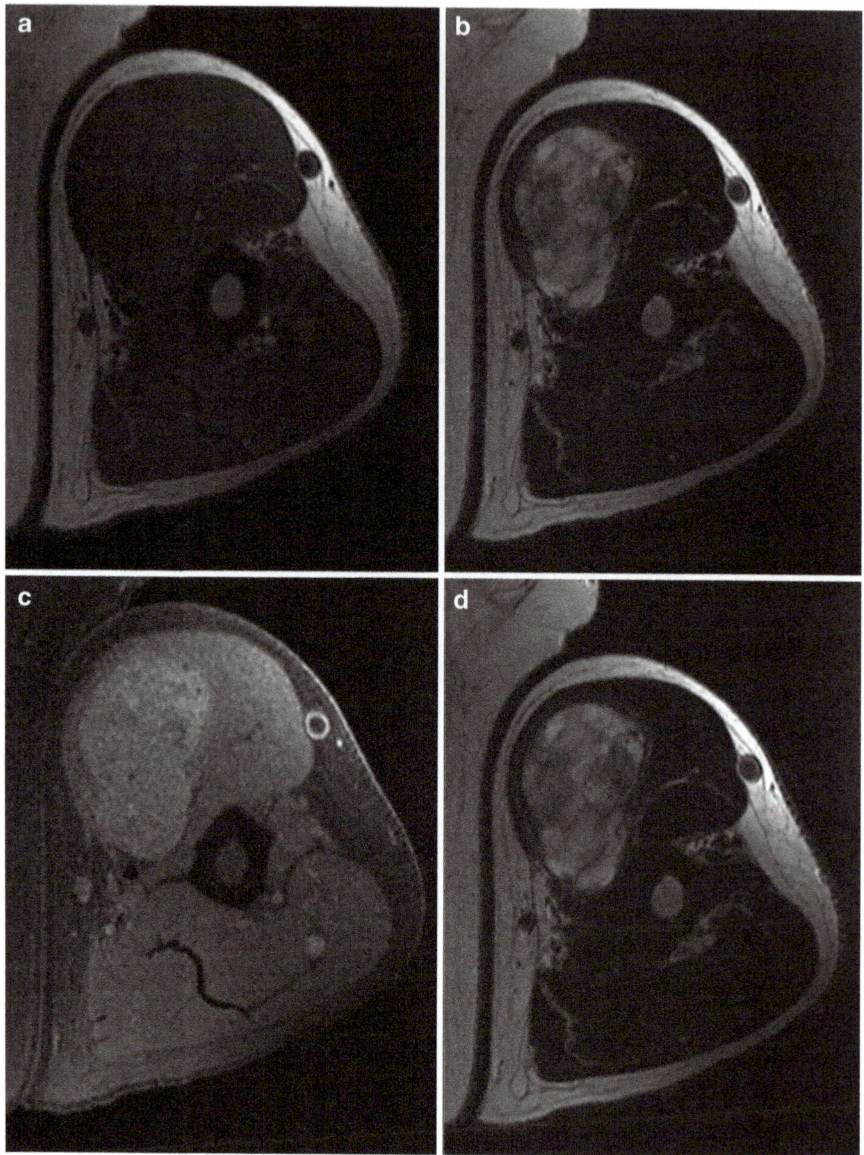

Fig. 9.5 (**a**) T1-weighted image, axial section; (**b**) T2-weighted image, axial section; (**c**) T1-weighted image with fat suppression, axial section; (**d**) T1-weighted image with contrast, axial section

A. Tumour penetrates to the posterior compartment.
B. Tumour is located mainly in the biceps brachii.
C. About one-third of the tumour is necrotic.
D. Tumour character is somewhat unclear.
E. Contrast enhancement is seen.

192. What is needed to make a diagnosis of the tumour?
A. CT with contrast
B. dual energy CT
C. PET/CT
D. biopsy
E. X-ray

193. A 43-year-old patient presenting with leg pain. MRI with contrast was performed (Fig. 9.6a–e). Choose the correct statement(s) regarding the lesion:

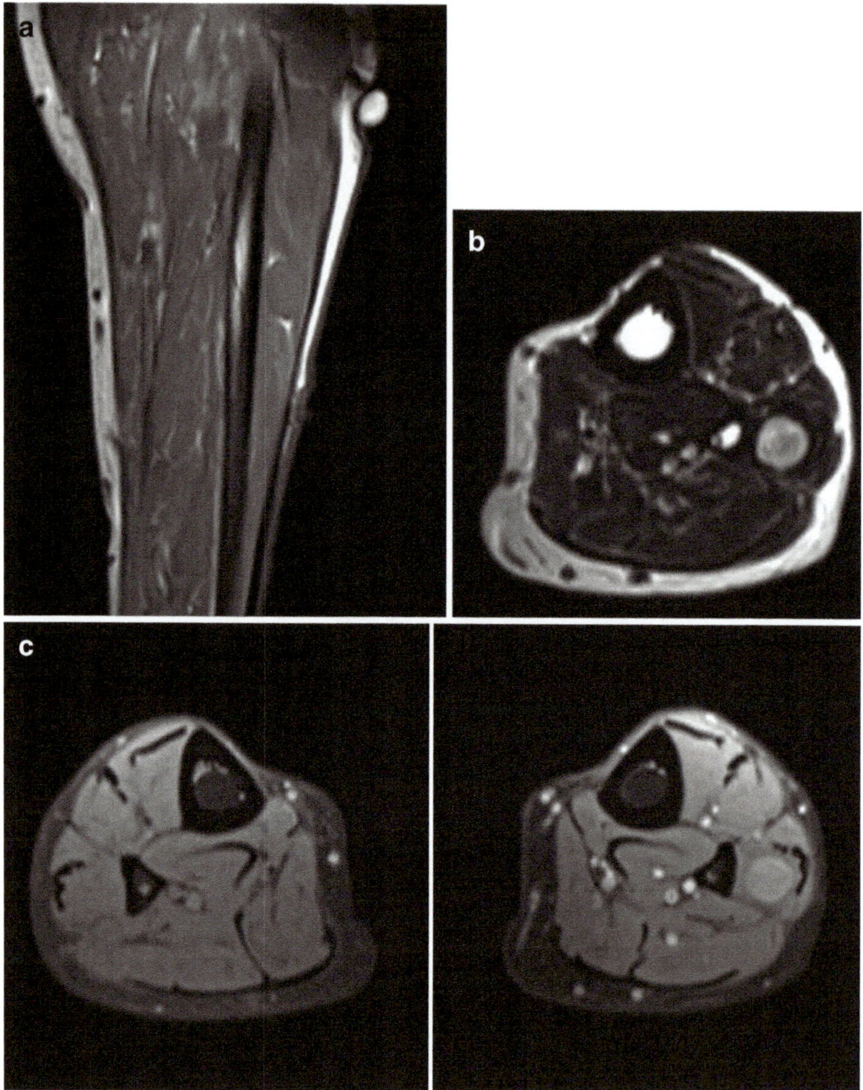

Fig. 9.6 (**a**) T2-weighted image, sagittal section; (**b**) T2-weighted image, axial section; (**c**) T1-weighted image with fat suppression, axial section; (**d**) T1-weighted image with fat suppression and contrast; (**e**) T1-weighted image with contrast, coronal section

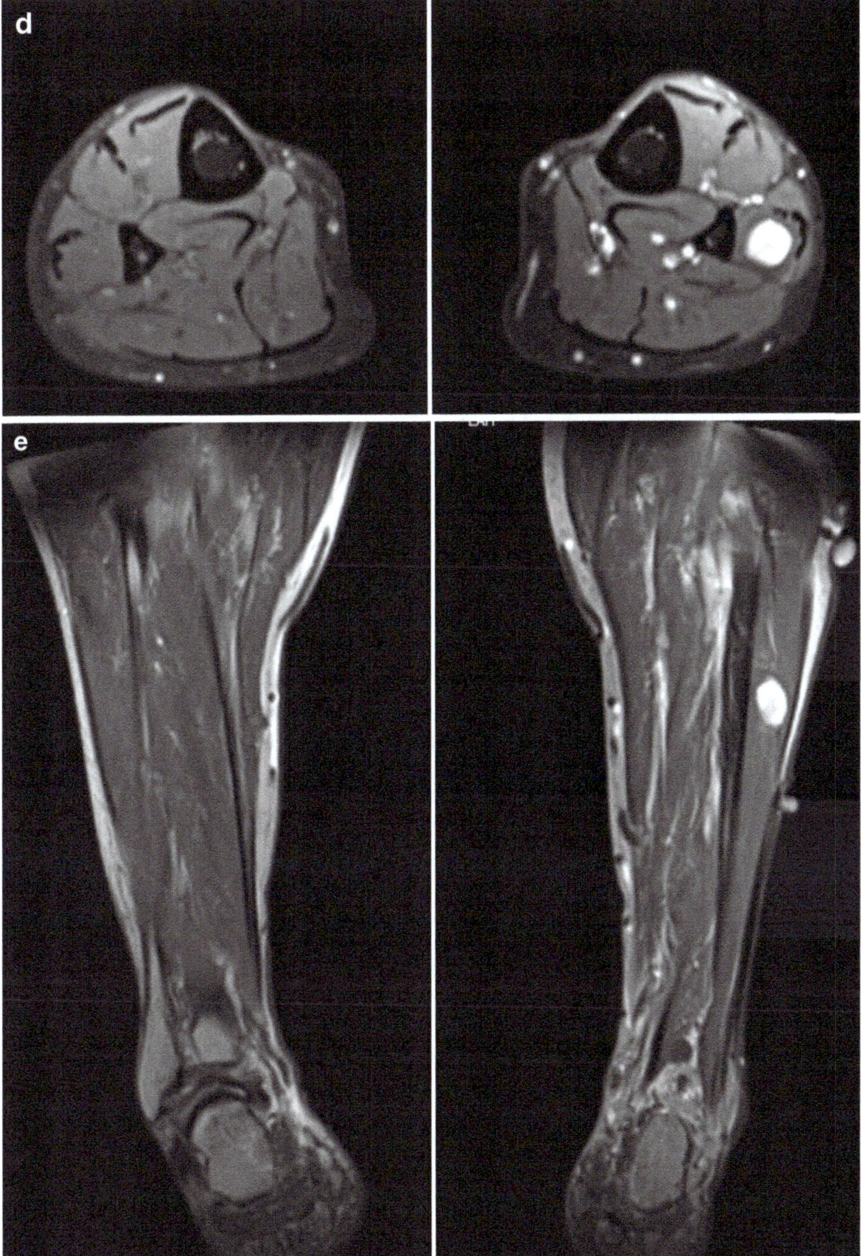

Fig. 9.6 (continued)

A. It is well-defined.
B. It is mainly cystic.
C. Target sign is visible.
D. Fascicular sign is present.
E. Thin peripheral rim of fat is seen.

194. Regarding the patient from the previous question, what is the most likely diagnosis?
   A. schwannoma
   B. neurofibroma
   C. synovial sarcoma
   D. intramuscular ganglion
   E. malignant peripheral nerve sheath tumour
195. A 73-year-old patient presenting with buttock pain. MRI was performed (Videos 9.1 and 9.2). Choose the correct statement(s) regarding this lesion:
   A. It involves the sciatic nerve.
   B. It passes via the greater sciatic foramen.
   C. The levator ani muscle is infiltrated.
   D. The lesion passes the midline.
   E. Sacrum destruction is visible.
196. What is the differential diagnosis regarding the lesion from the previous question (Videos 9.1 and 9.2)?
   A. malignant peripheral nerve sheath tumour
   B. Ewing sarcoma
   C. schwannoma
   D. lymphoma
   E. abscess
197. The patient from the previous question reports fever, night sweats, and weight loss. What is the most likely diagnosis?
   A. malignant peripheral nerve sheath tumour
   B. Ewing sarcoma
   C. schwannoma
   D. lymphoma
   E. abscess

198. A 73-year-old patient presenting with painful mass on the posterior thigh. MRI was performed; T1 with contrast is shown (Fig. 9.7). Choose the correct statement(s) regarding this patient:

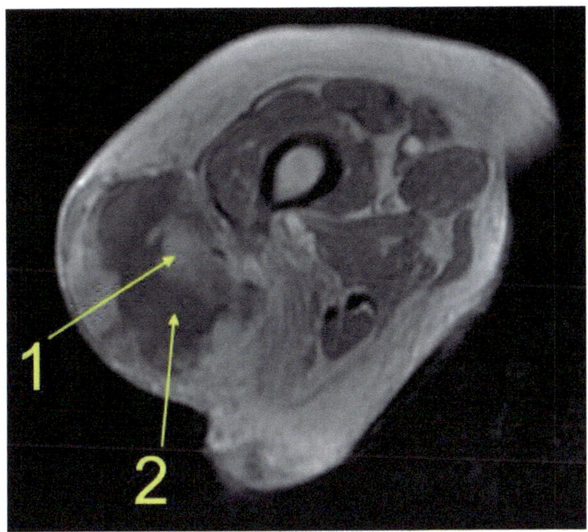

Fig. 9.7 MRI of the arm. T1-weighted image with contrast, axial section

A. 1—represents necrosis, 2—represents solid component
B. 1—represents solid component, 2—represents necrosis
C. 1 and 2 represent solid component.
D. 1 and 2 represent necrosis.
E. It is impossible to say what is necrosis and what is the solid component.

199. A 46-year-old patient with thigh pain. MRI was performed (Videos 9.3, 9.4 and 9.5). Choose the correct statement(s) regarding this patient:
A. Target sign is present on T1-weighted images.
B. Fascicular sign is present on T1-weighted images.
C. Target sign is present on T2-weighted images.
D. Fascicular sign is present on T2-weighted images.
E. Split fat sign is seen on T1-weighted images.

200. What is most likely diagnosis regarding the patient from the previous question (Videos 9.3, 9.4 and 9.5)?
A. malignant peripheral nerve sheath tumour
B. peripheral nerve sheath tumours
C. plexiform neurofibroma
D. lymphoma
E. sarcoma

Key to Chapter 9

155. C. Ca 50% of soft tissue tumours are lipomas [1, 2].
156. A, C, D. Capsule may be absent.
157. A, D. Only discreet capsule and separate enhancement may be seen. Lipoma does not contain any nodularity or mass like structure.
158. B. For lipoma imaging T1 sequence and fat suppression sequence (T2-weighted or STIR) is sufficient. If nodularity, mass like structure or thick septae are present contrast administration is needed because it is not a lipoma [1, 2].
159. A, B, C, D, E.
160. A, B, C, D.
161. A.
162. D.
163. E.
164. A, B, D, E.
165. C.
166. A, B, C, E.
167. C.
168. B.
169. B. Hibernoma contains brow adipose tissue. It is commonly well-defined mass without potential for malign transformation. The presence of vascularity helps to differentiate from lipomatous tumours.
170. D. Ca 30% of hibernomas are present in thigh.
171. E.
172. B, C, D, E.
173. A, B, D. Myxoid liposarcoma occurs commonly in fourth and fifth decade of life; however, it is the most common liposarcoma in patients younger than 20 years. Prognosis is poor, somewhat better in children.
174. E.
175. A. Well-differentiated liposarcoma is also called atypical lipomatous tumour [3].
176. B, C.
177. B, D, E. Hand fibromatosis is called Dupuytren disease, foot fibromatosis Ledderhose disease, penile fibromatosis Peyronie's disease. Localization foot is related to overuse/weight bearing.
178. A, B, D. Leiomyoma is differential diagnosis in intraperitoneal localization.
179. A, B, C, D, E. Radiological features are not specific. Usually, it is a large deep located tumour with non-homogenic signal on T2-weighted, with necrosis and contrast enhancement in the solid parts.
180. B, C, D.
181. B, C, E.

182. B, C, D, E. Synovial sarcoma does not origin from synovial membrane. Only histologically resembles synovial cells. It is usually located deep near large joints. Heterogenous signal correspond to calcifications, hemorrhage, necrosis, and solid component. Cystic appearance is common and sometimes dominant.
183. E.
184. A, D.
185. A.
186. A, B.
187. D.
188. C.
189. E.
190. A, B, C, E.
191. B, C, E.
192. D. Biopsy showed myxofibrosarcoma which is unspecific on MRI. Sometimes, it shows very high signal on T2-weighted or STIR.
193. A, C, E.
194. A.
195. A, B, D, E.
196. A, B, D.
197. D.
198. B.
199. B, D, E.
200. B.

References

1. Wu JS, Hochman MG. Soft-tissue tumors and tumorlike lesions: a systematic imaging approach. Radiology. 2009;253(2):297–316. https://doi.org/10.1148/radiol.2532081199.
2. Kransdorf MJ, Murphey MD. Imaging of soft-tissue musculoskeletal masses: fundamental concepts. Radiographics. 2016;36(6):1931–48. https://doi.org/10.1148/rg.2016160084.
3. Gupta P, Potti TA, Wuertzer SD, Lenchik L, Pacholke DA. Spectrum of fat-containing soft-tissue masses at MR imaging: the common, the uncommon, the characteristic, and the sometimes confusing. Radiographics. 2016;36(3):753–66. https://doi.org/10.1148/rg.2016150133.

Varia

10

201. A 45-year-old patient presenting with knee pain. X-ray showed only effusion. MRI showed lobulated fatty fronds in the suprapatellar recess. Contrast enhancement is superficial and linear. A joint effusion is seen. What is differential diagnosis?
    A. synovitis
    B. lipoma arborescens
    C. pigmented villonodular synovitis
    D. synovial chondromatosis
    E. loose bodies
202. A 32-year-old patient presenting with an enlarged arm. MR showed a tumour in the triceps brachii muscle with signal comparable to subcutaneous tissue on T1-weighted images. On T2-weighted images with fat suppression, the signal of the tumour is non-homogenic with some hyperintense and isointense to subcutaneous fat. What is the differential diagnosis?
    A. lipoma
    B. atypical lipomatous tumour
    C. liposarcoma
    D. lipomatosis
    E. hibernoma

Supplementary Information he online version contains supplementary material available at (https://doi.org/10.1007/978-3-030-85182-8_10).

P. Szaro, *Musculoskeletal Radiology for Residents*,
https://doi.org/10.1007/978-3-030-85182-8_10

203. A 43-year-old patient presenting with painful mass on the index finger. X-ray showed an extra skeletal ossified mass without direct contact with bone. What is the differential diagnosis?
   A. myositis ossificans
   B. osteochondroma
   C. osteolipoma
   D. classical osteosarcoma
   E. chronic haematoma
204. A 39-year-old patient presenting with pain in the scapula. On clinical examination, there is a difference in the position of the lower angle of the scapula. MRI revealed a mass between the thoracic wall and scapula. This localization is common for:
   A. lipoma
   B. exostosis
   C. liposarcoma
   D. elastofibroma
   E. fibrolisarcoma
205. Choose what tumour shows tendency to abut the tendon sheath?
   A. giant cell tumour of tendon sheath
   B. Nora's lesion
   C. fibroma of tendon sheath
   D. lipoma
   E. liposarcoma
206. A 49-year-old patient noticed painful nodules on the soles of the feet. MRI revealed a fusiform mass in the plantar aponeurosis demonstrating low signal on T1-weighted images and discrete higher signal compared to muscles on T2-weighted images. The tumours showed heterogeneous contrast enhancement. What is the most likely diagnosis?
   A. lipoma
   B. liposarcoma
   C. fibromatosis
   D. giant cell tumour of tendon sheath
   E. Nora's lesion
207. Which tumours are located intermuscularly?
   A. schwannoma
   B. pigmented villonodular synovitis
   C. ganglion
   D. nodular fasciitis
   E. neurofibroma

208. Choose which feature is more typical for malignancy in soft tissues?
    A. superficial localization
    B. high signal on T2-weighted images
    C. intramuscular localization
    D. presence of necrosis
    E. diameter more than 6 cm
209. Choose the three most common subcutaneous lesions:
    A. lipoma arborescens
    B. schwannoma
    C. pilomatrixoma
    D. lymphoma
    E. lipoma
210. Choose intra-articular conditions:
    A. pigmented villonodular synovitis
    B. synovial chondromatosis
    C. synovial sarcoma
    D. fibromatosis
    E. metastasis
211. Choose the two most common malignant soft tissue tumours:
    A. undifferentiated pleomorphic sarcoma (malignant fibrous histiocytoma)
    B. liposarcoma
    C. leiomyosarcoma
    D. malignant schwannoma
    E. dermatofibrosarcoma protuberans
212. Choose two the most common benign tumours:
    A. lipoma
    B. fibrosus histiocytoma
    C. nodular fasciitis
    D. haemangioma
    E. fibromatosis
213. A 32-year-old patient presenting with painful distal phalanx of the thumb. MRI revealed on T2-weighted images a well-defined oval subungual tumour with a homogeneously hyperintense signal. What is the most likely diagnosis?
    A. Nora's lesion
    B. glomus tumour
    C. sarcoma
    D. synovial sarcoma
    E. exostosis

214. A 26-year-old patient presenting with a painful mass in the popliteal fossa about 3 cm posterior to the femur. X-ray revealed diffuse calcification, but no osteolysis was noticed. MRI showed an approximately 5 cm non-homogeneous intermuscular, partially cystic lesion somewhat hyperintense tumour on T2-weighted images with fat suppression. After contrast administration, the lesion showed enhancement in the solid component. What the most likely diagnosis?
   A. classic osteosarcoma
   B. myositis ossificans
   C. subacute haematoma
   D. synovial chondromatosis
   E. synovial sarcoma
215. Tumours that showed a high signal on T1-weighted images contain:
   A. methaemoglobin
   B. fat
   C. melanin
   D. diffuse calcifications
   E. proteinaceous material
216. Lesions with low signal on T2-weighted images contain:
   A. calcifications
   B. fibrosis
   C. fluid
   D. haemosiderin
   E. mucinous material
217. A lesion showing a high signal on T1-weighted images and showing no fat suppression may be:
   A. protein-rich ganglion
   B. haematoma
   C. abscess
   D. lipoma
   E. haemangioma
218. Lesion which showed high signal on T1-weighted images with calcifications and partial fat suppression may represent:
   A. lipoma
   B. well-differentiated liposarcoma
   C. haemangioma
   D. low-protein ganglion
   E. synovial sarcoma

219. Choose lesions with low signal on T2-weighted images without calcifications:
    A. plantar fibroma
    B. desmoid
    C. elastofibroma
    D. haemorrhagic tumour
    E. gouty tophi
220. Choose cyst-like tumours with peripheral enhancement:
    A. ganglion
    B. seroma
    C. abscess
    D. bursa
    E. myxoma
221. Choose cyst-like tumours with internal enhancement:
    A. synovial sarcoma
    B. peripheral nerve sheath tumours
    C. bursitis
    D. elastofibroma
    E. tumour with necrosis
222. Choose typical tumour located in the third metatarsal interspace:
    A. schwannoma
    B. neurofibroma
    C. intermetatarsal neuroma
    D. peripheral nerve sheath tumours
    E. malignant peripheral nerve sheath tumours
223. Choose high-flow vascular malformation:
    A. venous malformation
    B. lymphatic malformation
    C. capillary malformation
    D. angiosarcoma
    E. arteriovenous malformation

224. A 25-year-old patient presenting with left hip pain. X-ray was performed (Fig. 10.1). Choose the correct alternative:

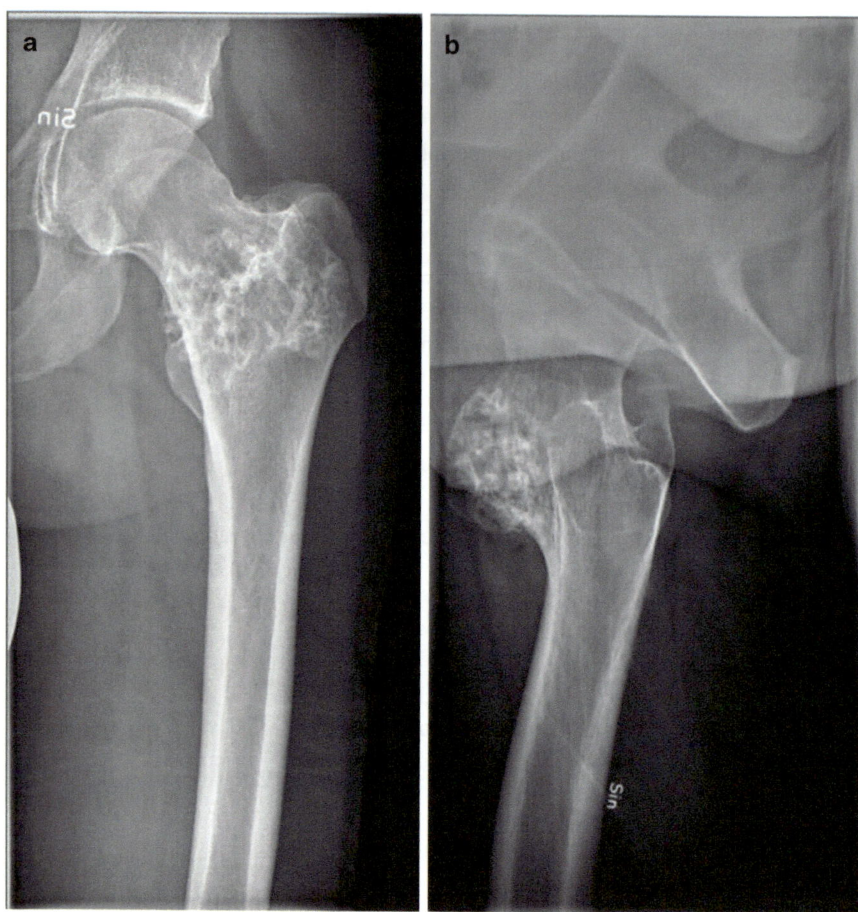

Fig. 10.1 X-ray of the hip (**a** and **b**)

   A. This is a meta-epiphyseal lesion.
   B. The lesion may cause the femoral nerve entrapment.
   C. Popcorn calcifications are visible.
   D. Arc calcifications are present.
   E. MRI is recommended.

225. The patient from the previous question, MRI was performed (Videos 10.1 and 10.2). Choose the correct statement(s) regarding this lesion:
   A. Bursa formation is visible.
   B. MRI was used to assess cartilage thickness.
   C. Oedema in adjacent soft tissues is visible.
   D. Compression of rectus femoris is visible.
   E. Compression of femoral nerve is visible.

226. Fever 38.5 °C, swelling, pain, and tenderness in the proximal tibia is noticed in a 23-year-old patient. X-ray was performed (Fig. 10.2a–d). Choose the correct statement(s) regarding this patient:

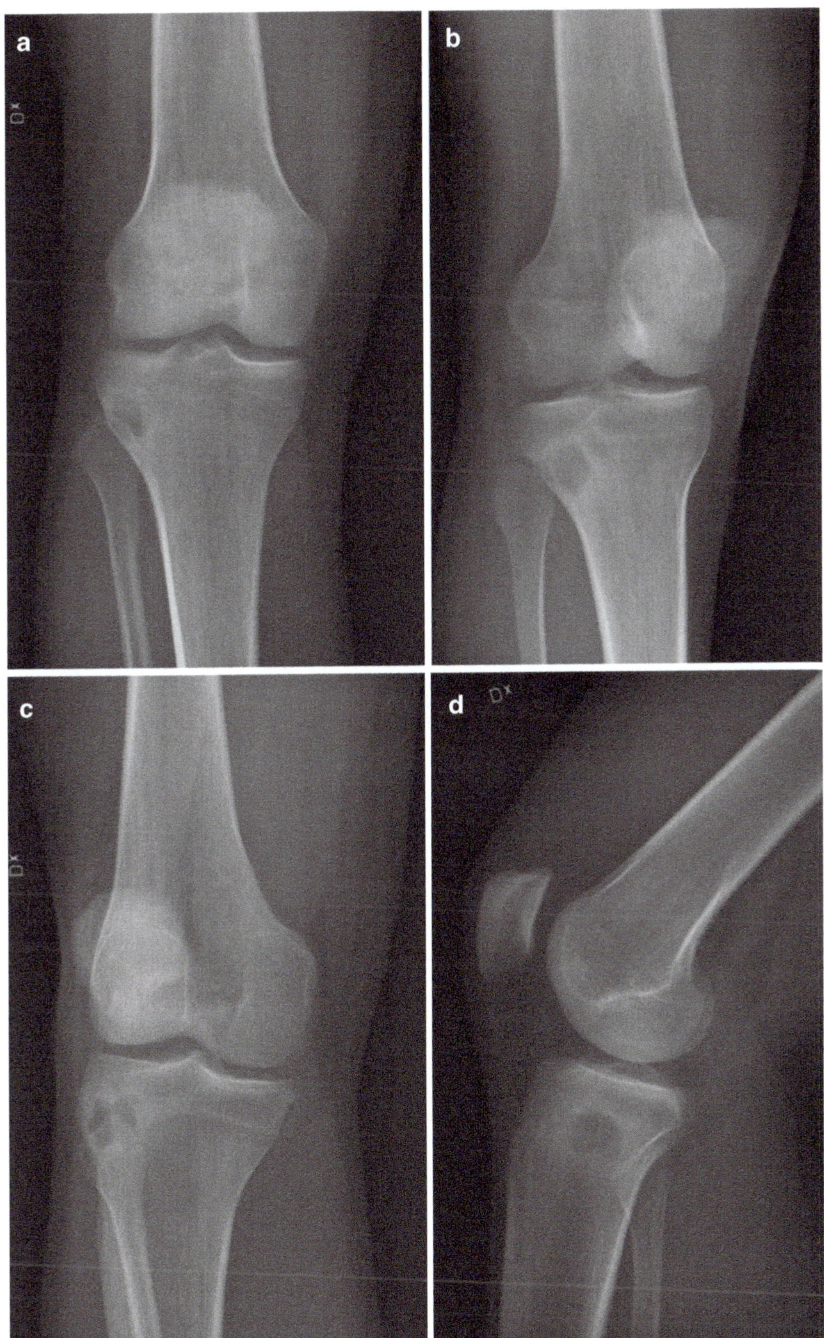

Fig. 10.2 (**a**–**d**) X-ray of the knee

A. Focal destruction in the proximal tibia.
B. Aggressive periosteal reaction is visible.
C. Sclerotic reaction around a radiolucent lesion is visible.
D. Endosteal scalloping is present.
E. Codman's triangle is present.

227. What is the most likely diagnosis?
A. lymphoma
B. osteomyelitis
C. osteosarcoma
D. Ewing sarcoma
E. eosinophilic granuloma

228. The patient from the previous question underwent MRI with contrast (Fig. 10.3a–e). Choose the correct statement(s) regarding MRI:

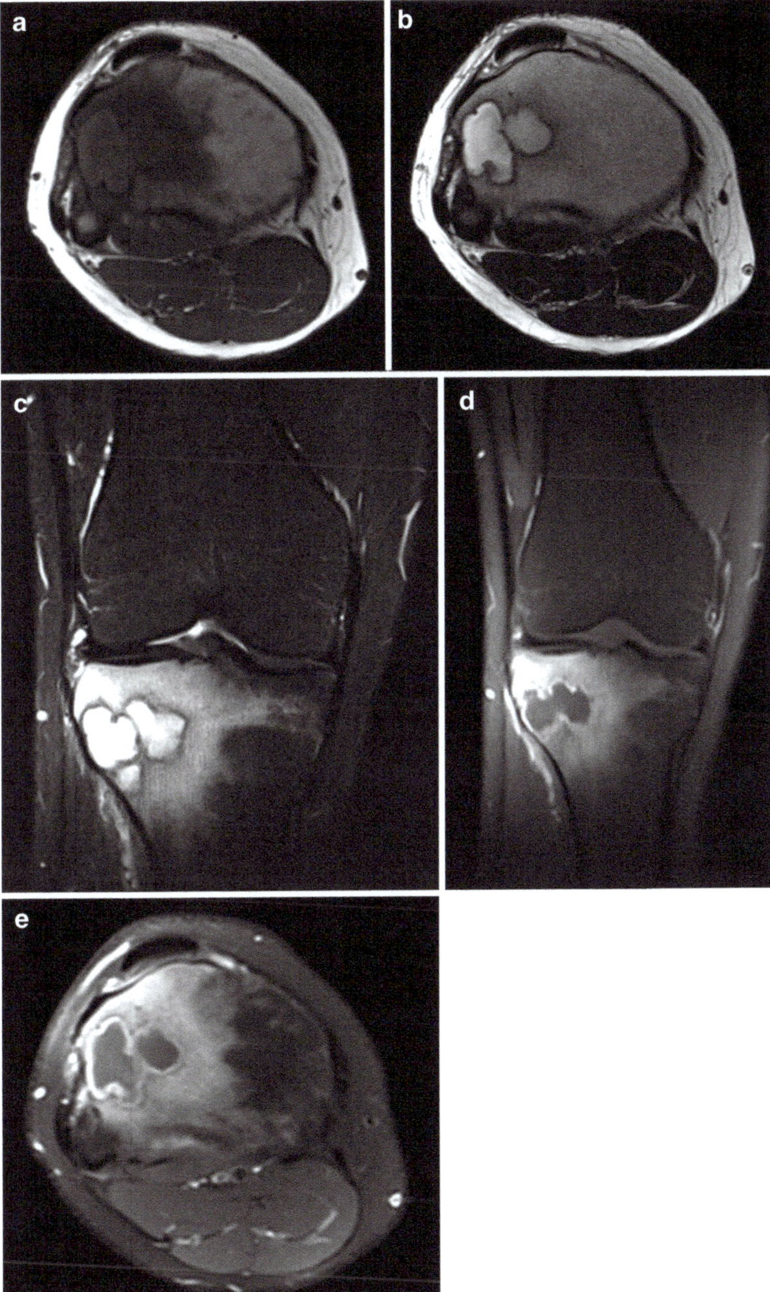

Fig. 10.3 (**a**) T1-weighted image, axial section; (**b**) T2-weighted image, axial section; (**c**) T2-weighted image with fat suppression, coronal section; (**d**) T1-weighted image with fat suppression, coronal section; (**e**) T1-weighted image with fat suppression and contrast, axial section

A. No cortical breakthrough is visible.
B. MRI showed aneurysmal bone cyst.
C. There is an interosseous ganglion with protein containment.
D. There is a solid lesion with mild contrast enhancement.
E. There is a lesion with sclerotic outline and perilesional bone marrow oedema.

229. What lesion is most likely regarding the X-ray (Fig. 10.2a–d) and MRI (Fig. 10.3a–e)?
A. lymphoma
B. osteomyelitis
C. interosseous ganglion
D. aneurysmal bone cyst
E. eosinophilic granuloma

230. A 34-year-old patient with a palpable painful mass on the left hip. CT was performed (Videos 10.3 and 10.4). Choose the correct statement(s) regarding CT:
A. Soft tissue component is present in m. iliacus.
B. Permeative growth is visible in the iliac bone.
C. Geographic destruction is present in the sacrum.
D. Soft tissue component is present in the erector spinae.
E. Soft tissue component is visible in m. gluteus medius and maximus.

231. What is the most likely diagnosis regarding the patient from the previous question?
A. metastasis
B. osteomyelitis
C. osteosarcoma
D. Ewing sarcoma
E. eosinophilic granuloma

232. The patient from the previous question was referred for MRI with contrast (Fig. 10.4a–c). Choose the correct statement(s) regarding this patient:

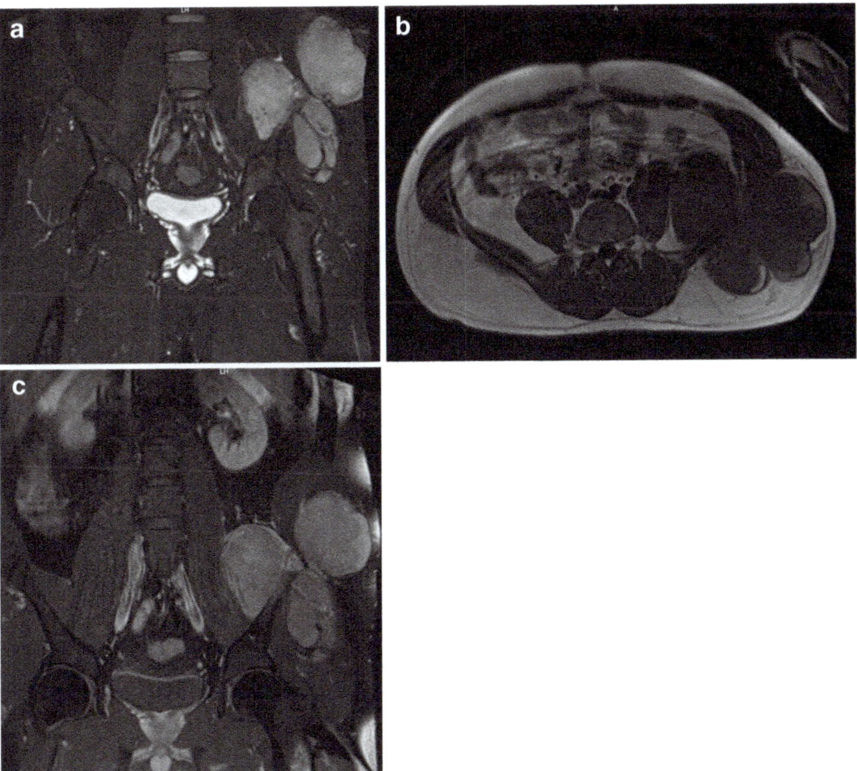

Fig. 10.4 (**a**) Short tau inversion recovery image, coronal section; (**b**) T1-weighted image, axial section; (**c**) T1-weighted image with fat suppression with contrast, coronal section

A. This lesion contains some fat component, which corresponds to high signal on T1-weighted images.
B. Bone marrow infiltration corresponds to an area of lower signal on T1-weighted images.
C. Some calcifications are present, which correspond to lower signal on T1-weighted images.
D. The lesion is benign because it shows only some contrast enhancement.
E. The lesion is probably benign because it is well-defined.

233. Regarding the patient from the previous question, based on CT (Videos 10.3 and 10.4) and MRI (Fig. 10.4a–c), what is the final radiologic diagnosis?
   A. metastasis
   B. osteomyelitis
   C. osteosarcoma
   D. Ewing sarcoma
   E. eosinophilic granuloma
234. A 56-year-old patient presenting with tumour on the posterolateral hip. MRI was performed (Fig. 10.5). What is correct regarding this patient?

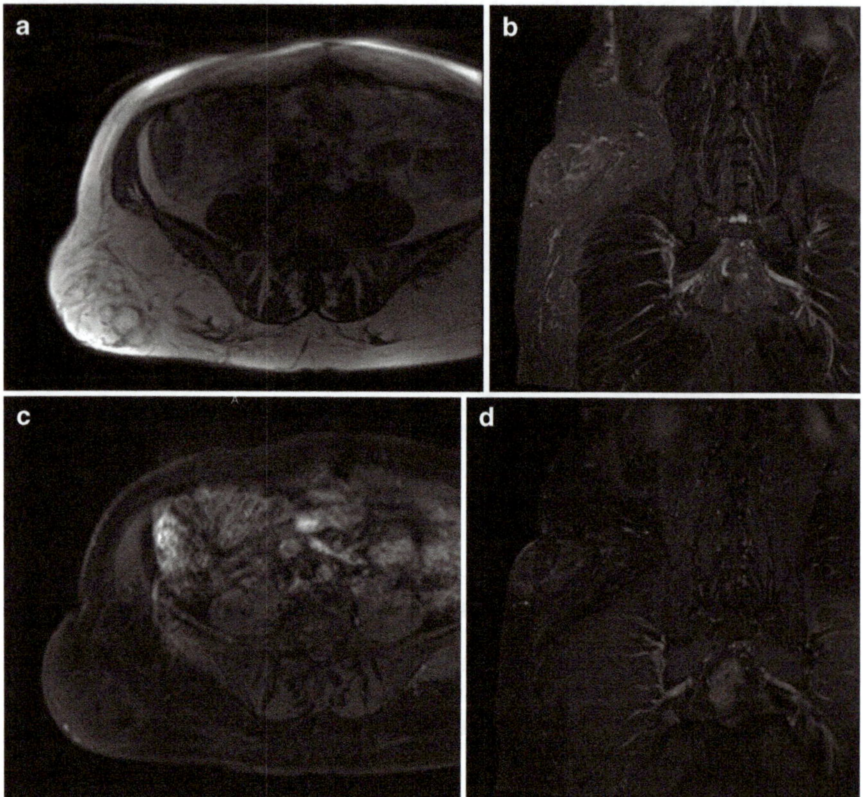

Fig. 10.5 (**a**) T1-weighted image, axial section; (**b**) short tau inversion recovery image, coronal section; (**c**) T1-weighted image with fat suppression, axial section; (**d**) T1-weighted image with fat suppression and contrast, axial section

   A. Irregular margins are seen.
   B. Extensive contrast enhancement is seen.
   C. Mainly fat component is seen.
   D. The entire tumour is fat suppressed.
   E. Tumour infiltrates muscle.

235. What is the most likely diagnosis regarding the patient from the previous question?
    A. myxofibrosarcoma
    B. well-differentiated liposarcoma
    C. low-differentiated liposarcoma
    D. angiolipoma
    E. chondrolipoma

Key to Chapter 10

201. A, B, C. Synovial chondromatosis and loose bodies show usually calcifications.
202. B, C, E.
203. A, B, C, D, E. It is probably bizarre parosteal osteochondromatous proliferation called Nora lesion. Osteolipoma is a lipoma with some degeneration and bone production. Analogously chondrolipoma may contain some cartilage.
204. D.
205. A, C.
206. C. Somewhat higher signal on T2-weighted and contrast enhancement means that this lesion is not mature. Usually, such lesions are painful.
207. A, C, D, E.
208. B, C, D, E.
209. C, D, E. Pilomatrixoma is the skin appendage tumour.
210. A, B. Synovial sarcoma resembles synovium only on histopathology; it is usually located near large joints but not intra-articular.
211. A, B. The other answers present common malignant soft tissue tumours in order of frequency of occurrence.
212. A, B. The other answers present common benign soft tissue tumours in order of frequency of occurrence.
213. B.
214. E. Classic osteosarcoma arises from bone. Myositis ossificans is located intramuscular. Subacute haematoma does not contain calcification or solid part. Synovial chondromatosis is an intra-articular condition.
215. A, B, C, E.
216. A, B, D.
217. A, B, C.
218. B, C.
219. A, B, C, D.
220. A, B, C, D, E.
221. A, B, E.
222. C. Intermetatarsal neuroma is called Morton neuroma.
223. E. Transarterial embolization is indicated in high-flow vascular malformation.

224. A, E.
225. A, B, C.
226. A, C.
227. B.
228. A, E.
229. B.
230. A, B, E.
231. D.
232. B.
233. D.
234. A, C.
235. B.

Part V

Arthritis

Arthritis

11

1. Which of the following are hallmarks of osteoarthritis?
   A. central erosion
   B. marginal erosion
   C. subchondral sclerosis
   D. osteoporosis
   E. joint space narrowing
2. How can osteoporosis change the appearance of osteoarthritis on X-ray?
   A. Sclerosis can be diminished.
   B. Osteophytosis can be diminished.
   C. Osteophytes without sclerosis or joint space narrowing are seen.
   D. Sclerosis is more prominent.
   E. More prominent destruction.
3. Which of the following statements are true?
   A. Osteophytes can be seen both in osteoarthritis and in disseminated idiopathic skeletal hyperostosis (DISH).
   B. Disk space narrowing is typical for osteoarthritis and DISH.
   C. Sclerosis is more typical for osteoarthritis as compared to DISH.
   D. The hallmark of DISH is erosion.
   E. Destruction is seen commonly in both osteoarthritis and DISH.
4. Regarding primary osteoarthritis, which of the following statements are correct?
   A. It is mostly in the hand, knee, hip, and spine.
   B. Typical patient is a middle-aged man.
   C. It is caused by an accumulation of microtrauma over years.
   D. It is a hereditary arthritis.
   E. Typically, osteophytes are not present.

P. Szaro, *Musculoskeletal Radiology for Residents*,
https://doi.org/10.1007/978-3-030-85182-8_11

5. Exceptions to the classic triad of findings in osteoarthritis can be seen in the following localizations:
   A. temporomandibular joint
   B. acromioclavicular joint
   C. metacarpophalangeal joint
   D. pubic symphysis
   E. carpometacarpal joint of thumb
6. Choose the one condition in which geodes are less often seen:
   A. osteoarthritis
   B. rheumatoid arthritis
   C. calcium pyrophosphate dihydrate crystal deposition disease
   D. avascular necrosis
   E. disseminated idiopathic skeletal hyperostosis
7. Choose the radiographic hallmarks of rheumatoid arthritis:
   A. Soft tissue swelling.
   B. Periarticular osteoporosis.
   C. Marginal erosions.
   D. Process is bilaterally symmetrical.
   E. Osteophytes.
8. What are the features of rheumatoid arthritis in large joints?
   A. Marked joint space narrowing.
   B. Marginal erosions might be present.
   C. Marginal erosions might not be present.
   D. Osteophytes.
   E. Subchondral sclerosis.
9. Superior migration of the humerus is a feature of:
   A. rheumatoid arthritis
   B. calcium pyrophosphate deposition
   C. total rupture of the supraspinatus muscle
   D. subacromial bursitis
   E. acromioclavicular dislocation
10. X-ray revealed bilateral erosive arthritis in the carpal bones and the metacarpophalangeal joints with associated periarticular osteoporosis and soft tissue swelling. This description may correspond to (choose one best answer):
    A. gout
    B. psoriatic arthritis
    C. primary osteoarthritis
    D. rheumatoid arthritis
    E. secondary osteoarthritis
11. X-ray revealed joint space narrowing and migration of the femoral head in an axial direction, as well as sclerosis in the superior portion of the joint and osteoporosis. This may correspond to (choose one best answer):
    A. primary osteoarthritis
    B. secondary osteoarthritis
    C. rheumatoid arthritis
    D. gout
    E. psoriatic arthritis

12. X-ray of the index finger showed joint space narrowing, subchondral sclerosis, and osteophytosis in the distal and proximal interphalangeal joints. The MCP joints were unremarkable. This can be a feature of:
    A. gout
    B. rheumatoid arthritis
    C. psoriatic arthritis
    D. osteoarthritis
    E. septic arthritis
13. The hallmarks of spondyloarthropathies are:
    A. marginal erosion
    B. bony ankylosis
    C. new bone formation
    D. predominantly appendicular involvement
    E. extensive spine destruction
14. Which of the following statements regarding rheumatoid arthritis are correct?
    A. Rheumatoid factor is positive in about 85% patients with rheumatoid arthritis.
    B. Rheumatoid factor correlates with activity of inflammation.
    C. Anti-citrullinated protein antibodies are more specific than rheumatoid factor.
    D. X-ray lesions are seen before rheumatoid factor is detectable.
    E. Rheumatoid factor is seen after in patients only with marginal erosions.
15. Choose the features of seronegative arthritis (SA) and rheumatoid arthritis (RA).
    A. Sacroiliac joints are more commonly involved in SA than in RA.
    B. Distal interphalangeal involvement is seen more commonly in RA.
    C. Soft tissue swelling is seen both in SA and RA.
    D. Periarticular osteoporosis is more commonly seen in SA than in RA.
    E. Subluxation is more typical for SA than RA.
16. Which of the following statements are true regarding syndesmophytes in the spine?
    A. Like osteophytes, they run vertically.
    B. They are characteristic findings in erosive arthritis.
    C. They are visible in HLA-B27+ spondyloarthropathies.
    D. Marginal and symmetrical syndesmophytes are seen in ankylosing spondylitis.
    E. They are located at an attachment of a ligament but are not associated with a facet joint.
17. Bilateral symmetric complete fusion of the SI joints is a sign of:
    A. ankylosing spondylitis
    B. arthritis associated with inflammatory bowel disease
    C. psoriatic disease
    D. reactive arthritis
    E. rheumatoid arthritis

18. Usually, asymmetrical bilateral sacroiliac joint involvement is seen in:
    A. ankylosing spondylitis
    B. arthritis associated with inflammatory bowel disease
    C. Reiter syndrome
    D. psoriatic arthritis
    E. gout
19. The sacroiliac joint may be involved in:
    A. ankylosing spondylitis and psoriasis
    B. inflammatory bowel disease
    C. Reiter syndrome and gout
    D. infection
    E. degenerative joint disease
20. Choose the typical features of gout:
    A. osteoporosis
    B. soft tissue nodules
    C. random distribution
    D. well-defined erosions with sclerotic borders and overhanging edges
    E. localization in the metatarsophalangeal joint of the great toe
21. What are three typical features for psoriatic arthritis?
    A. pencil-in-cup deformity
    B. asymmetric sacroiliitis
    C. sausage digits
    D. marginal erosions
    E. periarticular osteoporosis
22. Heterotopic ossifications inside a spinal ligament or of the annulus fibrosus may be seen in:
    A. ochronosis
    B. fluorosis
    C. reactive arthritis
    D. psoriatic arthritis
    E. rheumatoid arthritis
23. Choose the two most common locations of chondrocalcinosis:
    A. meniscus
    B. intervertebral disc
    C. volar plate
    D. symphysis pubis
    E. triangular fibrocartilage complex

24. Osteoarthritis is nearly indistinguishable from calcium pyrophosphate deposition (CPPD). What are features of osteoarthritis (OA) caused by CPPD that will help distinguish it from osteoarthritis caused by other conditions?
    A. Location: in shoulder, elbow, radiocarpal joint, and patellofemoral joint is more typical for calcium pyrophosphate deposition.
    B. Absence of osteophytes is more typical for OA caused by calcium pyrophosphate deposition.
    C. No osteoporosis is more typical for other conditions.
    D. Absence of joint space narrowing is more typical for OA caused by calcium pyrophosphate deposition.
    E. Presence of subchondral sclerosis is more typical for other conditions.
25. Unilateral sacroiliac involvement is seen in (choose one best answer):
    A. osteoarthritis
    B. gout
    C. infection
    D. Reiter syndrome
    E. ankylosing spondylitis
26. Which of the following statements are true regarding collagen vascular diseases?
    A. Erosions are typical features for scleroderma and dermatomyositis.
    B. Soft tissue calcifications are typically seen in scleroderma and dermatomyositis.
    C. Acroosteolysis is seen mostly in scleroderma.
    D. Dystrophic calcifications in subcutaneous tissue are a feature of dermatomyositis.
    E. Pencil-in-cup deformity can be seen in scleroderma and psoriatic arthritis.
27. Which of the following statements are true?
    A. Soft tissue swelling in gout is more irregular and asymmetrical than in rheumatoid arthritis.
    B. Diffuse swelling of the fingers is seen in dactylitis in seronegative inflammatory arthritis.
    C. Uniform joint space loss is more typical for osteoarthritis.
    D. A preserved joint space is seen until the late stages of gout or psoriatic arthritis.
    E. Bony ankylosis is seen most commonly in rheumatoid factor plus arthritis.
28. Choose the one condition when luxation without erosions or cartilage loss is most common:
    A. gout
    B. lupus
    C. psoriatic arthritis
    D. rheumatoid arthritis
    E. calcium pyrophosphate deposition
29. Typical features of Charcot foot are:
    A. joint destruction
    B. dislocation
    C. heterotopic new bone
    D. progressive joint destruction
    E. osteophytes

30. Epiphyseal enlargement with a gracile diaphysis is a feature of:
    A. gout
    B. haemophilia
    C. osteoarthritis
    D. rheumatoid arthritis
    E. juvenile rheumatoid arthritis
31. What features are typical for pigmented villonodular synovitis?
    A. Loose bodies.
    B. Osteophytes.
    C. Localization in the Hoffa fat pad.
    D. Bony erosions with destruction.
    E. The knee is the most frequently affected joint.
32. The "apple core" appearance of bone can be caused by:
    A. gout
    B. rheumatoid arthritis
    C. seronegative arthropathies
    D. synovial chondromatosis
    E. pigmented villonodular synovitis
33. Which of the following statements are true regarding avascular necrosis (AVN)?
    A. The earliest sign of AVN is a joint effusion.
    B. Subchondral lucency is an early X-ray sign.
    C. A patchy or mottled density can be noticeable.
    D. Increased bone density in the normal joint can be seen early on X-ray.
    E. Collapse of the articular surface and joint fragmentation is a late stage.
34. Which of the following statements are true regarding AVN of the hip?
    A. Joint effusion is usually present.
    B. Pain and fever is usually present.
    C. "Double line sign" is visible on MRI.
    D. It begins in the most anterior part of the caput femoris.
    E. Low signal on T1 represents oedema, which can be bordered by a hyperintense line representing blood products.
35. A gull-wing appearance is seen in:
    A. psoriasis
    B. avascular necrosis
    C. rheumatoid arthritis
    D. erosive osteoarthritis
    E. synovial chondromatosis
36. Erosions with overhanging edges are seen in:
    A. gout
    B. psoriasis
    C. rheumatoid arthritis
    D. erosive osteoarthritis
    E. synovial chondromatosis

37. Milwaukee shoulder is a manifestation of:
    A. Charcot joint
    B. septic arthritis
    C. rheumatoid arthritis
    D. vanishing bone disease
    E. destructive shoulder arthropathy
38. What is the most commonly isolated bacteria in septic arthritis?
    A. *Escherichia coli*
    B. Gonococci
    C. Streptococci
    D. *Staphylococcus aureus*
    E. *Haemophilus influenzae*
39. Choose the features of acute septic arthritis:
    A. joint effusion
    B. marginal erosion
    C. cartilage destruction
    D. calcification in soft tissue
    E. juxta-articular osteoporosis
40. Lower signal intensity of the edge of the endplate on T1-weighted images and higher signal on STIR images is seen in (Choose one best answer):
    A. gout
    B. psoriasis
    C. spondylodiscitis
    D. rheumatoid arthritis
    E. ankylosing spondylitis
41. Choose the correct statement(s) regarding amyloid arthropathy:
    A. It frequently manifests as shoulder, hip, or wrist pain.
    B. It is an erosive and destructive osteoarthropathy.
    C. High prevalence of pathologic fractures is noticed.
    D. Large subchondral erosions are common.
    E. Soft tissue deposition with low signal on all MRI sequences.
42. Choose the true statement(s) regarding ankylosing spondylitis:
    A. There is a female predilection.
    B. An association with the HLA B27 gene was noticed.
    C. Asymmetrical bilateral sacroiliitis is usually the first manifestation.
    D. "Bamboo spine" appearance is a pathognomonic radiographic feature.
    E. Subchondral erosions and sclerosis on the iliac side of the sacroiliac joint is seen.
43. A Romanus lesion:
    A. It is the same as an Andresson lesion.
    B. It is seen in ankylosing spondylitis and enteropathic arthritis.
    C. It is an irregularity and erosion involving the endplates.
    D. It is located in the anterior and posterior edges of the vertebral endplates.
    E. It results in the shiny corner sign on MRI.

44. Choose bone-forming arthritis:
    A. rheumatoid arthritis
    B. osteoarthritis
    C. ankylosing spondylitis
    D. psoriatic arthritis
    E. juvenile idiopathic arthritis
45. Paravertebral ossification is seen in:
    A. ankylosing spondylitis
    B. gout
    C. rheumatoid arthritis
    D. psoriatic arthritis
    E. chronic reactive arthritis
46. A soft tissue mass may be seen in:
    A. ankylosing spondylitis
    B. gout
    C. rheumatoid arthritis
    D. psoriatic arthritis
    E. chronic reactive arthritis
47. Choose the correct statement(s) regarding destruction of cartilage:
    A. The pattern of destruction in osteoarthritis is the same as in rheumatoid arthritis and is located peripherally.
    B. Cartilage destruction in rheumatoid arthritis is located peripherally while in osteoarthritis more centrally.
    C. Cartilage destruction in osteoarthritis is located peripherally while in rheumatoid arthritis more centrally.
    D. The pattern of destruction in osteoarthritis is the same as in rheumatoid arthritis and is located centrally.
    E. The pattern of destruction in osteoarthritis is the same as in rheumatoid arthritis and is seen both centrally and peripherally.
48. Ankylosis of the peripheral joints is most commonly seen in:
    A. diffuse idiopathic skeletal hyperostosis
    B. juvenile idiopathic arthritis
    C. rheumatoid arthritis
    D. psoriatic arthritis
    E. gout
49. Choose which two conditions are usually monoarticular:
    A. gout
    B. septic arthritis
    C. haemochromatosis
    D. rheumatoid arthrosis
    E. pigmented villonodular synovitis

50. Bouchard nodes:
    A. They are subchondral cysts in osteoarthritis.
    B. Palpable osteophytes in proximal interphalangeal joints in osteoarthritis.
    C. Palpable osteophytes in distal interphalangeal joints in osteoarthritis.
    D. Palpable erosions in proximal interphalangeal joints in rheumatoid arthritis.
    E. Palpable erosions in distal interphalangeal joints in rheumatoid arthritis.
51. The carpometacarpal joint of the thumb is a typical localization for:
    A. synovial chondromatosis
    B. rheumatoid arthritis
    C. psoriatic arthritis
    D. osteoarthritis
    E. gout
52. The distal interphalangeal joint of the hand is a typically involved in (Choose one best answer):
    A. rheumatoid arthritis
    B. juvenile idiopathic arthritis
    C. psoriatic arthritis
    D. osteoarthritis
    E. gout
53. Choose the typical features of rheumatoid arthritis:
    A. atlantoaxial subluxation
    B. low signal rice bodies on MRI
    C. pencilling of the clavicle
    D. soft tissue calcifications
    E. punch out erosions
54. Hatchet sign refers to:
    A. erosions on the tuberculum majus in ankylosing spondylitis
    B. erosions on the tuberculum minus in ankylosing spondylitis
    C. subchondral geodes in the humeral head in osteoarthropathy
    D. enthesopathy of the supraspinatus in ankylosing spondylitis
    E. Hill-Sachs sign
55. X-ray revealed joint space narrowing and erosions in the distal interphalangeal joint of the index finger and between the carpal bones. The other interphalangeal joints showed significant joint space narrowing. The metacarpophalangeal joints were normal. No erosions were noticed. This patient had spiking fevers and a salmon-coloured rash. What is the most likely diagnosis?
    A. osteoarthritis
    B. psoriatic arthritis
    C. chronic reactive arthritis
    D. adult-onset Still's disease
    E. inflammatory bowel disease arthritis

56. A 56-year-old patient presented with neck pain. CT of the cervical spine revealed significant sclerosis at the endplates of C4–C7. Ossification of the posterior longitudinal ligament was ossified at the C4–C6 levels, which reduces the anterior-posterior diameter of the spinal canal to 8 mm. Foraminal stenosis was noticed at several levels, most significantly at the C5–C6 level bilaterally. Hypertrophy of the uncovertebral joints and facet joints at the C4–C6 levels was noted. Bony hypertrophy posterior to the odontoid process without stenosis at this level was also noted. What is the most likely diagnosis?
    A. spondylodiscitis
    B. ankylosing spondylitis
    C. adult-onset Still's disease
    D. diffuse idiopathic skeletal hyperostosis
    E. osteoarthritis
57. Choose the correct statement(s) regarding diffuse idiopathic skeletal hyperostosis (DISH) and ankylosing spondylitis (AS):
    A. DISH and AS are two names for the same disease.
    B. DISH is seen at a young age, while AS is seen in elderly people.
    C. DISH and AS share involvement of the axial skeleton.
    D. DISH and AS are asymptomatic for a long time.
    E. Vertebral body squaring is seen in AS but not in DISH.
58. Erosions with overhanging edges are considered pathognomonic for:
    A. psoriatic arthritis
    B. ankylosing spondylitis
    C. rheumatoid arthritis
    D. osteomyelitis
    E. gout

59. Which of the following diagnoses is the most likely based on this X-ray (Fig. 11.1)?

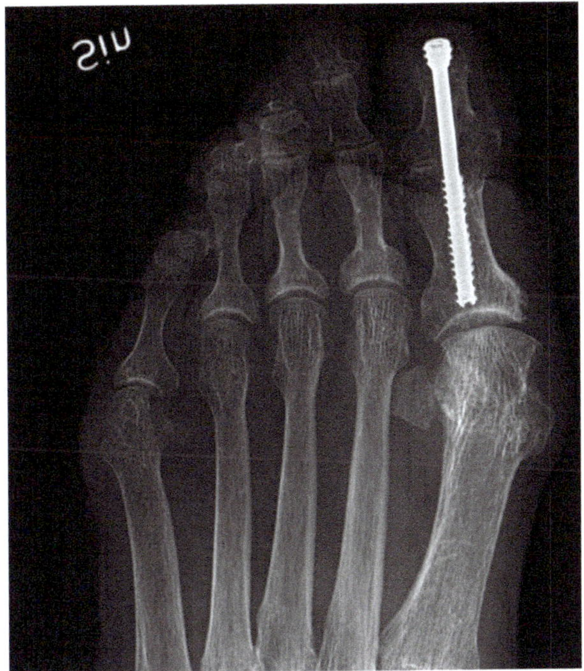

Fig. 11.1 X-ray of the forefoot

A. skeletal manifestation of scleroderma
B. rheumatoid arthritis
C. psoriatic arthritis
D. osteoarthritis
E. gout

60. Which radiological finding(s) can be seen on this X-ray (Fig. 11.2)?
    a. pencil-in-cup deformity
    b. central erosions
    c. acroosteolysis

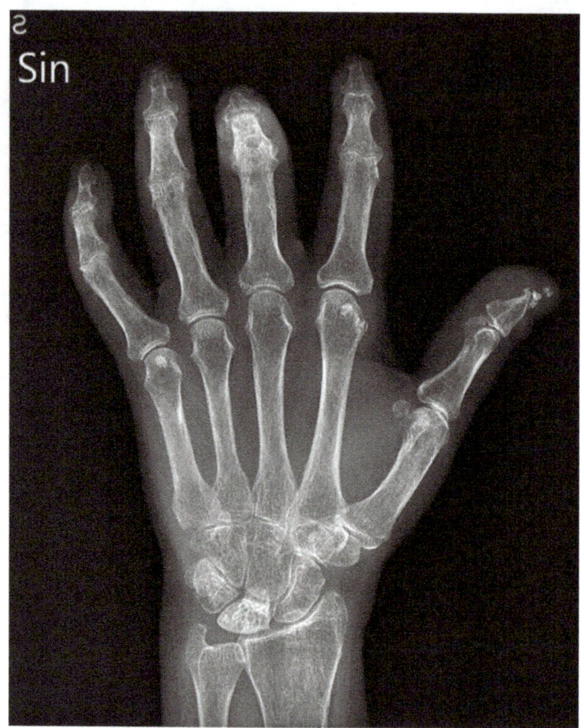

Fig. 11.2 X-ray of the hand

    A. a, b, c
    B. a, b
    C. b, c
    D. a, c
    E. a

61. What is the most likely diagnosis regarding the patient from the previous question?
    A. rheumatoid arthritis
    B. erosive osteoarthritis
    C. psoriatic arthritis
    D. septic arthritis
    E. osteoarthritis

62. Choose the correct comments regarding this X-ray of the hand of a 67-year-old patient with positive rheumatoid factor (Fig. 11.3):
   a. There are degenerative changes in the "a" area.
   b. In area "b," there are rheumatoid arthritis changes.
   c. There are degenerative and rheumatoid arthritis changes in the "a" area.
   d. In the "d" area, post-traumatic and degenerative changes occur.

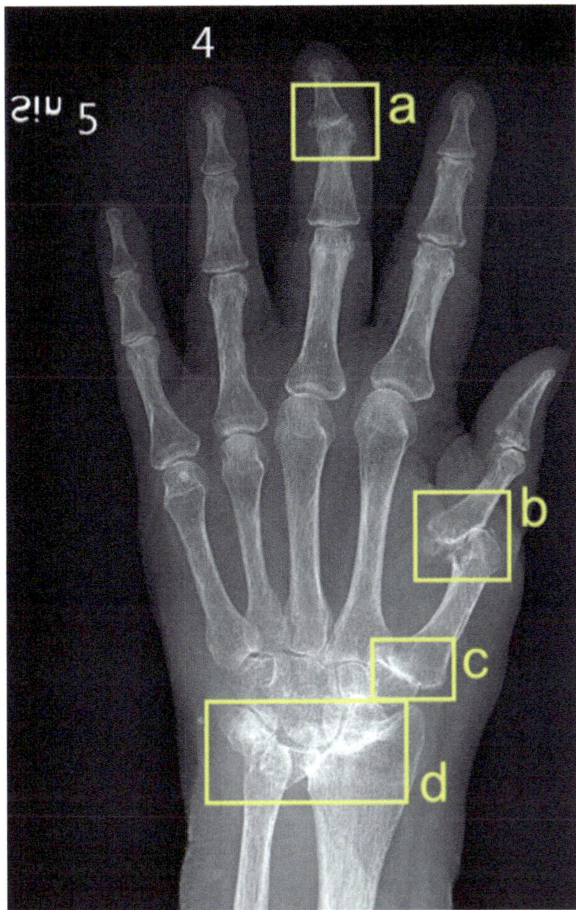

Fig. 11.3 X-ray of the hand

A. a, b, c, d
B. a, b, c
C. a, b
D. c, d
E. d

63. A 47-year-old patient with recurrent tenosynovitis. Dual-energy CT was performed (Fig. 11.4). Choose the correct option regarding this patient:
    a. High attenuation crystal deposition corresponding to monosodium urate.
    b. Localization of abnormality corresponds to rheumatoid arthritis.
    c. MRI is indicated to rule out a diagnosis of gout.
    d. Typical dual-energy CT artefact is seen, no abnormality is noticed.

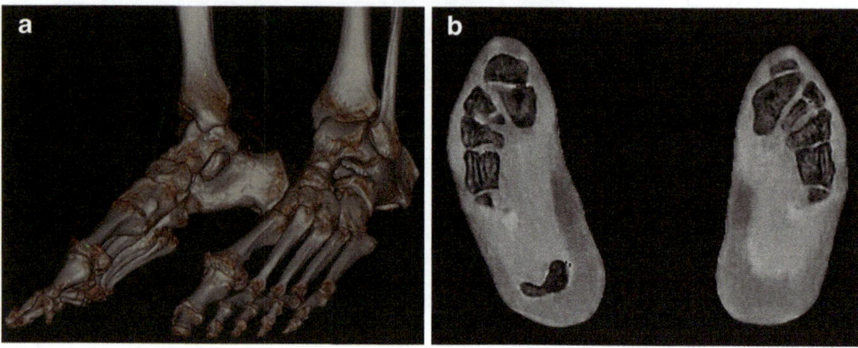

Fig. 11.4 Computed tomography dual energy. (**a**) Volume rendering, (**b**) axial section

A. a, b, c
B. a, b
C. a
D. b, c
E. d

64. A 47-year-old patient presents with painful and swollen feet. Dual-energy CT was performed (Fig. 11.5). What is the most likely diagnosis?

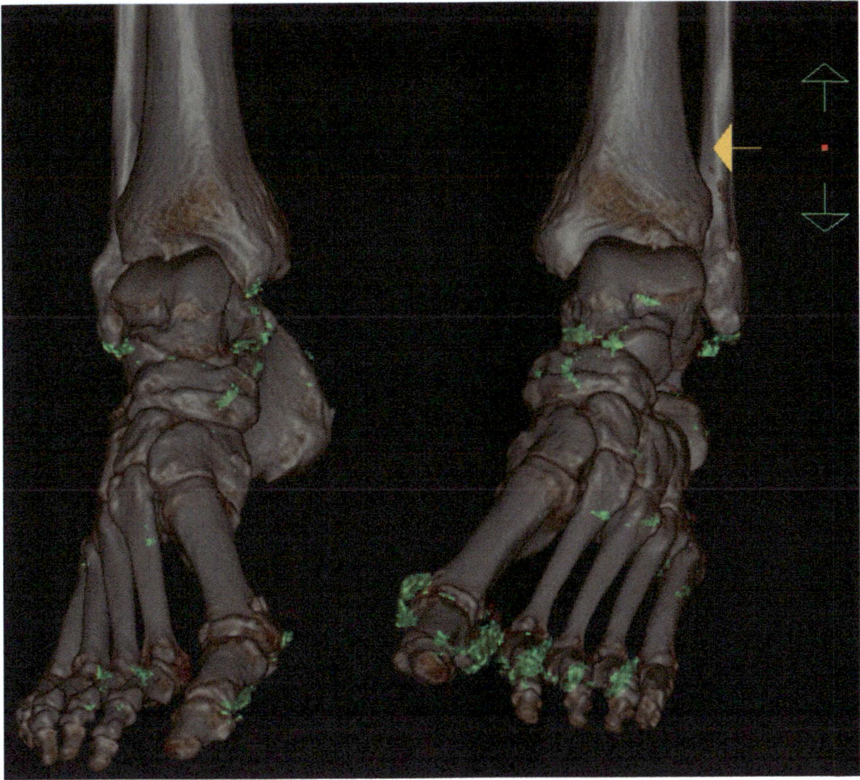

Fig. 11.5 Computed tomography dual energy, volume rendering

A. erosive osteoarthritis
B. rheumatoid arthritis
C. polyarticular gout
D. psoriatic arthritis
E. osteoarthritis

65. A 53-year-old patient presents with a positive rheumatoid factor. In which area can rheumatoid arthritis changes be noticed in Fig. 11.6?

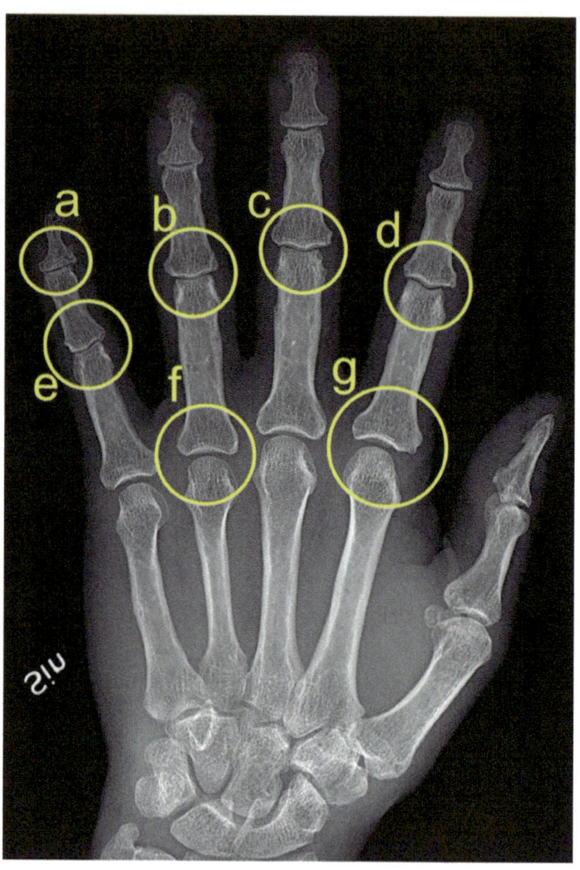

Fig. 11.6 X-ray of the hand

A. a, b, c, d, e, f, g
B. f, g
C. b, c, d, e
D. a, e, b, c, d
E. d, e

66. What would be the differential diagnosis for the patient with low back pain for several months? CT was performed (Fig. 11.7).
    a. ankylosing spondylitis because it is usually bilateral and symmetric
    b. psoriatic arthritis because it is usually bilateral and asymmetric
    c. osteoarthritis because it is usually bilateral and asymmetric
    d. pyogenic septic arthritis because it is usually unilateral

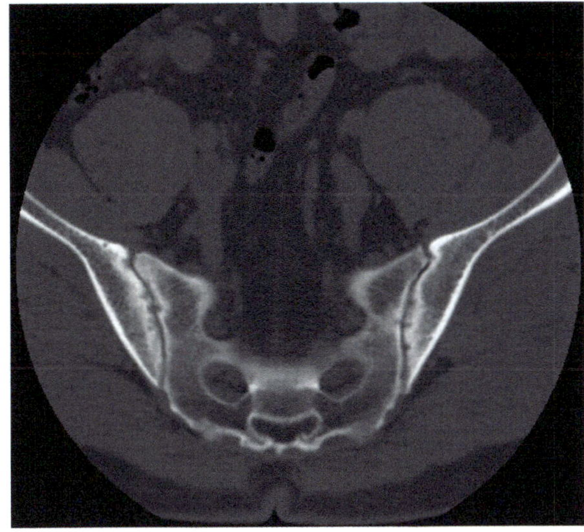

Fig. 11.7 Computed tomography of the sacroiliac joints, axial section

A. a, b, c, d
B. b, c
C. a
D. d
E. b, c, d

67. What radiological findings may be noticed on this MRI of the sacroiliac joints (Fig. 11.8)?
   a. subchondral sclerosis
   b. marrow oedema
   c. joint effusion

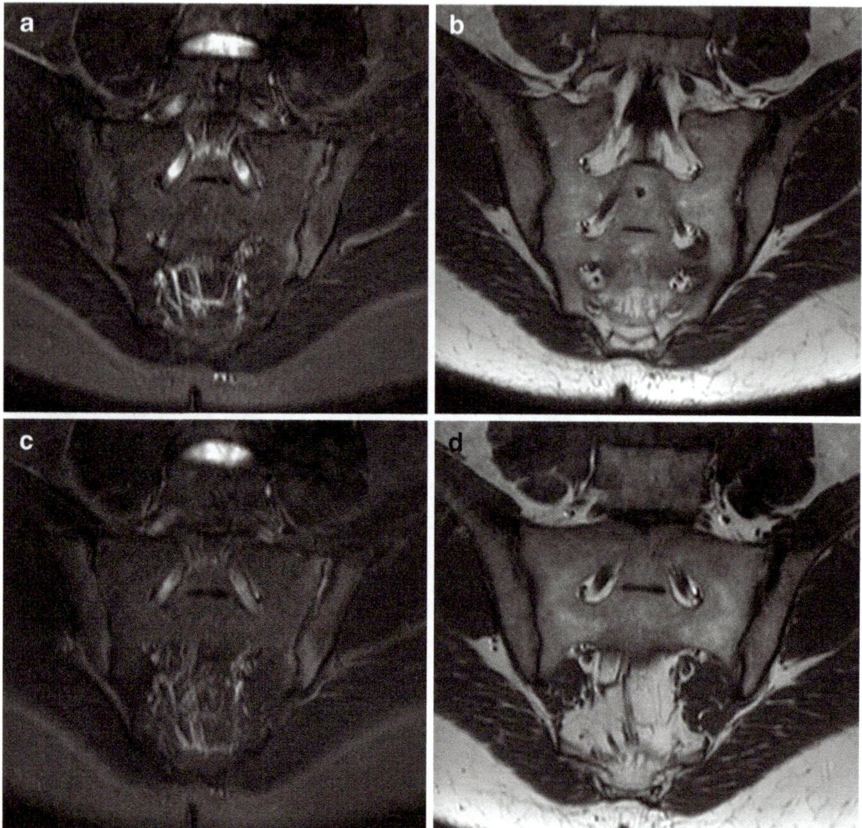

Fig. 11.8 (**a** and **c**) T2-weighted images spectral attenuated inversion recovery, oblique sections; (**b** and **d**) T1-weighted images, oblique sections

A. a, b, c
B. a, b
C. b, c
D. a, c
E. b

68. What would be the differential diagnosis for the patient from the previous question, regarding localization of the lesions?
    A. ankylosing spondylitis
    B. enteropathic arthritis
    C. rheumatoid arthritis
    D. psoriatic arthritis
    E. septic arthritis
69. Pencil-in-cup deformity is seen in:
    A. osteoarthritis
    B. septic arthritis
    C. psoriatic arthritis
    D. rheumatoid arthritis
    E. ankylosing spondylitis
70. Swan neck deformity includes:
    A. flexion of a distal interphalangeal joint
    B. extension of a distal interphalangeal joint
    C. hyperextension of a metacarpophalangeal joint
    D. hyperflexion of a proximal interphalangeal joint
    E. hyperextension of a proximal interphalangeal joint

Key to Chapter 11

1. C, E.
2. A, B.
3. A, C.
4. D.
5. A, B, D.
6. E.
7. A, B, C, D.
8. A, B, C.
9. A, B, C.
10. D.
11. C.
12. D.
13. A, B, C.
14. A, C.
15. A, C.
16. C, D.
17. A, B.
18. C, D, E.
19. A, B, C, D, E.
20. B, C, D, E.
21. A, B, C.
22. A, B, C, D.

23. A, E.
24. A.
25. C.
26. B, C, D, E.
27. A, B, D.
28. B.
29. A, B, C, D.
30. B, E.
31. D, E.
32. D, E.
33. A, B, C, D, E.
34. A, C, D, E.
35. A, C, D.
36. A.
37. E.
38. D.
39. A, C, E.
40. E.
41. A, B, C, D, E.
42. B, D, E.
43. B, C, D, E.
44. B, C, D, E.
45. A, D, E.
46. B.
47. B.
48. B, D.
49. B, E.
50. B.
51. D.
52. D.
53. A, B, C.
54. A.
55. D.
56. E.
57. C, E.
58. E.
59. B.
60. D.
61. C.
62. C.
63. C.
64. C.
65. C.

66. C.
67. B.
68. D.
69. C, D.
70. A, E.

Part VI

Metabolic and Miscellaneous Bone Diseases

Metabolic and Miscellaneous Bone Diseases

12

12.1 Metabolic Bone Diseases

1. Which statement(s) is/are correct regarding bone turn over?
   A. The formation phase of the turnover cycle lasts about 90 days.
   B. Increased bone turnover is related to increased bone resorption and formation.
   C. Vitamin D is a basic for normal bone mineralization.
   D. Imperfect osteoblastic function results in osteoporosis.
   E. Bisphosphonates work by inhibiting osteoclasts.
2. Harris growth arrest lines:
   A. They are the same as looser zones.
   B. They represent pseudofractures.
   C. They represent osteoporotic changes.
   D. They are located in the long bones due to growth arrest.
   E. They are present mainly in the cervical spine.
3. Choose the correct statement(s) regarding osteoporosis:
   A. This is the second most common metabolic disease.
   B. In elderly patients, a T-score less than –2.5 standard deviation of the young adult reference mean is a sign of osteoporosis.
   C. Cortical thickness is reduced.
   D. Horizontal trabeculae in vertebral bodies become more prominent.
   E. Vertebral fractures are the second most common cause of osteoporotic fractures.
4. Choose the causes of primary osteoporosis:
   A. hyperparathyroidism
   B. postmenopausal
   C. homocystinuria
   D. Ehlers-Danlos syndrome
   E. senility

P. Szaro, *Musculoskeletal Radiology for Residents*,
https://doi.org/10.1007/978-3-030-85182-8_12

5. Choose the correct statement(s) regarding osteoporotic vertebral fractures:
   A. Distraction fractures are very common.
   B. Compression of the posterior part of vertebral body is more common than compression of the anterior part.
   C. Most of vertebral fractures are unstable.
   D. They are most commonly located in the thoracic and thoracolumbar regions.
   E. Increased lumbar lordosis may result from osteoporotic fractures.
6. Choose the correct statement(s) regarding vertebroplasty:
   A. It can be used in all vertebral fractures.
   B. It should be done within the first 4–6 months after presenting with pain.
   C. Bone marrow oedema helps to identify vertebra that are amenable to treatment.
   D. Usually, transpedicular injection of cement is used.
   E. Treatment is aimed at reducing pain.
7. Choose potential complications of vertebroplasty:
   A. injection of cement to inferior vena cava
   B. pedicle fracture
   C. pneumothorax
   D. pulmonary fat emboli
   E. infection
8. What is true regarding differentiation between osteoporotic fracture and pathological fracture?
   A. Bony destruction is seen mainly in pathological fractures.
   B. Low-signal intensity line on T1WI and T2WI is more typical for pathological fractures.
   C. Multiple compression fractures are more common in osteoporotic fractures.
   D. Fat signal on T1-weighted images is more typical for osteoporotic fractures.
   E. Bulging of the posterior outline of vertebral body is seen in osteoporotic fractures.
9. Choose the typical localizations of insufficiency osteoporotic fractures:
   A. pubic symphysis region
   B. femoral neck
   C. distal tibia
   D. supraacetabular area
   E. sternum
10. Choose the correct statement(s) regarding insufficiency osteoporotic fractures of the sacrum:
    A. Usually they occur parallel to the sacroiliac joint.
    B. Usually they are not visible on X-ray.
    C. Radionuclide uptake resembles the letter H.
    D. Destruction is usually visible.
    E. Bone marrow oedema is usually not present.

11. Choose the typical MRI features of complex regional pain syndrome:
    A. less prominent vertical trabecular lines
    B. presence of subchondral lobules of fat
    C. more prominent blood vessels
    D. focally increased signal intensity on fluid-sensitive sequences
    E. subchondral line irregularity
12. Choose the correct statement(s) regarding complex regional pain syndrome:
    A. Periarticular patchy osteopenia is visible on X-ray.
    B. Narrowing of the joint space is a feature.
    C. Destruction of articular surfaces is seen.
    D. Immobilization is a known aetiology.
    E. Diffuse osteopenia is a hallmark.
13. Which is true regarding transient osteoporosis of the hip?
    A. Commonly it is located bilaterally.
    B. Acute onset of hip pain is seen.
    C. If untreated, it results in avascular necrosis.
    D. Osteopenia in the proximal end of the femur is typical.
    E. The joint space is commonly reduced.
14. Choose the correct statement(s) regarding generalized osteoporosis:
    A. Erosions of the phalanges may indicate secondary osteoporosis.
    B. Osteoporosis of young adults is seen much more commonly in males.
    C. Lack of estrogen results in decreased trabecular bone.
    D. Juvenile osteoporosis may result from osteogenesis imperfecta.
    E. Glucocorticoids stimulate both osteoblasts and osteoclasts in elderly patients.
15. Choose the correct statement(s) regarding osteogenesis imperfecta:
    A. No callus is usually seen.
    B. Epiphyses are very sclerotic and wide.
    C. It results in mutation of genes of collagen type 1.
    D. Gracile bones and insufficient fractures are signs.
    E. In infancy fractures, it may resemble non-accidental injuries.
16. Primary hyperparathyroidism is caused mainly by:
    A. adenomas
    B. genetic factors
    C. adenocarcinomas
    D. chronic kidney disease
    E. multiple endocrine neoplasia syndrome
17. Choose the most sensitive radiological feature of hyperparathyroidism:
    A. subperiosteal erosions in the radial aspect of the middle phalanx of the index and middle fingers
    B. subperiosteal erosions in the ulnar aspect of the middle phalanx of the index and middle fingers
    C. subperiosteal erosions in the radial aspect of the distal phalanx of the index and middle fingers
    D. subperiosteal erosions in the ulnar aspect of the distal phalanx of the index and middle fingers
    E. acroosteolysis

18. Acroosteolysis is seen in:
    A. scleroderma
    B. osteoporosis
    C. psoriatic arthritis
    D. rheumatoid arthritis
    E. hyperparathyroidism
19. Choose the radiological features of hypoparathyroidism:
    A. acroosteolysis
    B. meniscal calcifications
    C. subcutaneous calcifications
    D. calcifications in the basal ganglia
    E. calcifications in the triangular fibrocartilage complex
20. X-ray revealed shortened and dysplastic fourth and fifth metacarpal bones. Choose one best answer:
    A. gout
    B. psoriatic arthritis
    C. rheumatoid arthritis
    D. pseudohypoparathyroidism
    E. hydroxyapatite deposition disease
21. Choose the typical features of hyperparathyroidism:
    A. brown tumours
    B. rugger jersey spine
    C. ankylosis in sacroiliac joints
    D. osteopenia
    E. chondrocalcinosis
22. Milkman lines:
    A. are visible on X-rays in the long bones due to growth arrest.
    B. are oriented parallel to the involved cortex.
    C. represent cortical infractions.
    D. are a sign of osteonecrosis.
    E. are located commonly in pubic rami and the medial femoral neck.
23. Choose the correct statement(s) regarding osteomalacia:
    A. It may result in insufficient fractures.
    B. Phosphate deficiency may be aetiology.
    C. It may be caused by bisphosphonate therapy.
    D. Thickened vertical bone trabeculae may be seen.
    E. Destruction of non-weight bearing articular surfaces may be seen.
24. Choose the typical radiological features of vitamin D deficiency in the growing skeleton:
    A. gracile long bones
    B. widening of growth plates
    C. narrowing of metaphyseal ends
    D. medial bowing of the tibia and fibula
    E. irregular and blurry outline of the metaphysis

25. Bone within a bone is a radiologic sign of:
    A. Paget disease
    B. osteopetrosis
    C. acromegaly
    D. hypervitaminosis D
    E. hyperparathyroidism
26. Rugger jersey spine is a radiological sign which refers to:
    A. gout
    B. hypoparathyroidism
    C. hyperparathyroidism
    D. rheumatoid arthritis
    E. ankylosing spondylitis
27. X-ray revealed enlargement of the distal phalangeal tufts (radiological sign is the so-called spade tufts). What is the most likely diagnosis?
    A. gout
    B. rickets
    C. acromegaly
    D. rheumatoid arthritis
    E. hyperparathyroidism
28. X-ray of a 64-year-old male with back pain revealed diffuse higher bone density in the lumbar spine and pelvis. What is the differential diagnosis?
    A. myelofibrosis
    B. osteopetrosis
    C. mastocytosis
    D. hyperparathyroidism
    E. prostate cancer metastasis
29. Choose the radiological features of Paget disease:
    A. mixed lytic and sclerotic changes of the calvaria
    B. widening of diploe
    C. increased concavity of the anterior vertebral outline
    D. acetabular protrusion
    E. smooth cortical expansion of pelvic bones
30. Thickened unsystematic oriented bone trabeculae interspersed with a radiolucent and somewhat more regular trabecular bone pattern is seen in:
    A. rickets
    B. myelofibrosis
    C. osteomalacia
    D. Paget disease
    E. hyperparathyroidism

12.2 Miscellaneous Bone Diseases

31. Choose the risk factors for osteonecrosis:
    A. alcoholism
    B. trauma
    C. liver cirrhosis
    D. corticosteroid therapy
    E. sickle cell disease
32. Choose the correct statement(s) regarding the radiological features of osteonecrosis of the femoral head:
    A. Osteopenia is usually seen after the crescent sign.
    B. Osteophytes are commonly seen in the early stages.
    C. X-ray may reveal curvilinear lucent subchondral lines.
    D. Subchondral fracture cleft is usually filled with fluid, which may be seen on MRI.
    E. MRI and scintigraphy are the most sensitive methods to detect early osteonecrosis.
33. Choose the correct statement(s) regarding the double line sign:
    A. It is the same as the crescent sign.
    B. It is located in the subchondral region.
    C. It is commonly seen in osteoporosis.
    D. It is pathognomonic for osteonecrosis.
    E. It demarcates osteochondral fragments.
34. Choose the correct statement(s) regarding the double line sign:
    A. The outer line corresponds to sclerotic bone, while the inner one corresponds to granulation tissue.
    B. The inner line corresponds to sclerotic bone, while the outer one corresponds to granulation tissue.
    C. Both inner and outer lines correspond to sclerotic bone.
    D. Both inner and outer lines correspond to granulation tissue.
    E. It is seen commonly on T2-weighted images.
35. Choose the correct statement(s) regarding the differences between the double line sign and rim sign:
    A. Both the double line sign and rim sign are visible in osteonecrosis.
    B. The double line sign is a typical feature of stress fracture, while the rim sign is seen in osteonecrosis.
    C. The double line sign is seen in osteonecrosis, while the rim sign is seen in osteoporosis.
    D. The double line sign indicates osteonecrosis, while the rim sign indicates an unstable osteochondral fragment
    E. The double line sign indicates an unstable osteochondral fragment, while the rim sign indicates osteoporosis.

36. Choose the correct statement(s) regarding subchondral insufficiency fractures of the knee:
    A. Most common patient is a young male.
    B. Typical localization is weight-bearing of the patella.
    C. Usually, it is manifests with the acute onset of pain.
    D. Subtle subchondral bone marrow oedema is a typical feature on MRI.
    E. It is usually associated with medial meniscal extrusion.
37. Choose the correct statement(s) regarding differences between subchondral insufficiency fracture (SIF) and osteochondritis dissecans (OCD) of the knee:
    A. SIF is seen in older people more often than OCD.
    B. SIF is usually seen in the lateral femoral condyle, while OCD is seen in the medial femoral condyle.
    C. SIF and OCD are located on the weight-bearing surface.
    D. Bone marrow oedema is more extensive in SIF than in OCD.
    E. Articular surface flattening is a feature of SIF, which is not typical for OCD.
38. Choose the radiological features of achondroplasia:
    A. wide tuberosity of the distal phalanx
    B. short pedicles in the lumbar spine
    C. widening of intervertebral discs
    D. wide foramen magnum
    E. shorter long bones
39. X-ray of a patient with a scaphoid fracture also showed an eccentric sclerotic lesion, which is connecting with the cortical bone at the base of the proximal phalanx of the thumb. The lesion has well-defined margins. No periosteal reaction or soft tissue component is visible. What is the most likely diagnosis?
    A. gout
    B. brown tumour
    C. stress fracture
    D. melorheostosis
    E. avascular necrosis
40. A lateral plain film of the spine reveals anterior vertebral body beaking. What is the most likely diagnosis?
    A. fracture
    B. achondroplasia
    C. Down syndrome
    D. Morquio syndrome
    E. ankylosing spondylitis
41. A single layer periosteal reaction is seen in:
    A. stress fracture
    B. osteomyelitis
    C. osteoid osteoma
    D. early fracture healing
    E. Langerhans cell histiocytosis

42. Aggressive periosteal reactions can be seen in:
    A. osteosarcoma
    B. melorheostosis
    C. osteomyelitis
    D. paraosteal osteosarcoma
    E. Langerhans cell histiocytosis
43. What anatomical region is most commonly involved in skeletal sarcoidosis?
    A. skull
    B. scapula
    C. hands
    D. feet
    E. pelvis
44. A 49-year-old male presented with sarcoidosis and low back pain. MRI of the lumbar spine revealed multiple small lesions in the vertebral bodies, which on T1-weighted imaging are hypointense, while on short inversion time and inversion-recovery demonstrated a higher signal. What is differential diagnosis (choose the two best answers)?
    A. metastasis
    B. osteopoikilosis
    C. bone sarcoidosis
    D. avascular necrosis
    E. aggressive osteoporosis
45. A 74-year-old patient with lung cancer presented with painful fingers. X-ray showed periostitis along the shafts of the proximal and distal phalanges of the index and middle fingers. No focal lesion was demonstrated. What is the differential diagnosis (choose the three best answers)?
    A. avascular necrosis
    B. thyroid acropachy
    C. pathological fractures
    D. pachydermoperiostosis
    E. hypertrophic pulmonary osteoarthropathy
46. Choose the correct statement(s) regarding periosteal reaction:
    A. Codman triangle is seen in osteomyelitis.
    B. Hair on end sign is seen in thalassemia major.
    C. Sunburst periosteal reaction is seen in Ewing sarcoma.
    D. Aggressive periosteal reaction can be seen with benign and malignant tumours.
    E. Giant cell tumours and aneurysmal bone cysts do not produce any periosteal reactions.
47. A 32-year-old patient presenting with a painful thigh. X-ray of the area showed a mass adjacent to the posterior cortex, without direct contact with the femur. The mass is calcified peripherally, and no calcifications are visible in the centrum. No periosteal reaction is seen. What is the most likely diagnosis?
    A. myositis ossificans
    B. paraosteal osteosarcoma
    C. dystrophic soft tissue calcification
    D. calcium pyrophosphate dihydrate disease
    E. bizarre parosteal osteochondromatous proliferation

48. Choose the conditions with soft tissue calcifications:
    A. dermatomyositis
    B. milk-alkali syndrome
    C. vitamin D deficiency
    D. chronic venous insufficiency
    E. secondary hyperparathyroidism
49. A 56-year-old patient presented with medial knee pain. X-ray showed medial meniscus calcification. What is the differential diagnosis?
    A. melorheostosis
    B. degenerative joint disease
    C. vitamin D intoxication
    D. chronic venous insufficiency
    E. calcium pyrophosphate deposition disease
50. Chondrocalcinosis may be a manifestation of the following conditions:
    A. hyperparathyroidism
    B. haemochromatosis
    C. hypothyroidism
    D. ochronosis
    E. gout

Key to Chapter 12

Metabolic Bone Diseases

1. A, B, C, D, E.
2. D.
3. B, C.
4. B, E.
5. D.
6. C, D.
7. A, B, C, D, E.
8. A, C, D.
9. A, B, C, D, E.
10. A, B, C.
11. B, C, D.
12. A, D.
13. B, D.
14. A, C, D.
15. C, D, E.
16. A.
17. A.
18. A, C, E.
19. C, D.
20. D.

21. A, B, D, E.
22. B, C, E.
23. A, B, C.
24. B, D, E.
25. A, B, C, D.
26. C.
27. C.
28. A, B, C, E.
29. A, B, D, E.
30. D.

Miscellaneous Bone Diseases

31. A, B, C, D, E.
32. C, D, E.
33. D.
34. A, E.
35. A, D.
36. C, E.
37. A, D, E.
38. B, C, E.
39. D.
40. D.
41. A, B, C, D, E.
42. A, C, D, E.
43. C.
44. A, C.
45. B, D, E.
46. B, C, D.
47. A.
48. A, B, D, E.
49. B, E.
50. A, B, C, D, E.

Part VII

Interventional Radiology in the Musculoskeletal System

Interventional Radiology in the Musculoskeletal System

13

1. Choose contraindication for bone core biopsy:
   A. unicameral bone cyst
   B. spondylodiscitis
   C. non-ossifying fibroma
   D. cortical desmoid
   E. bone metastasis
2. Choose one absolute contraindication of bone core biopsy:
   A. metachronous metastatic cancer
   B. synchronous metastatic cancer
   C. metastasis
   D. primary musculoskeletal tumor
   E. bleeding diathesis
3. Choose indication for bone core biopsy:
   A. diagnosis of spinal metastases in the patients with known primary tumour
   B. diagnosis of spinal metastases in the patients with unknown primary tumour
   C. wedge vertebral fracture in the patient without known tumour
   D. vertebral compression fractures in the patient with osteoporosis without known tumour
   E. determination of infectious agent in spondylodiscitis
4. Choose the correct routes for image-guided spinal biopsy:
   A. transpedicular approach
   B. extra-pedicular posterolateral approach
   C. the intercostovertebral approach
   D. the oropharyngeal approach
   E. the approach through the spinal process

P. Szaro, *Musculoskeletal Radiology for Residents*,
https://doi.org/10.1007/978-3-030-85182-8_13

5. The risk of tract seeding in biopsy of a sarcoma is accounted
   A. 3–5 per 100
   B. 3–5 per 10,000
   C. 3–5 per 100,000
   D. 3–5 per 1,000,000
   E. 3–5 per 10,000,000
6. What trephine needles may be used to obtain an adequate core of bone marrow for histopathology:
   A. 8G
   B. 12G
   C. 16G
   D. 20G
   E. 22G
7. What needles may be used to obtain an adequate core for histopathology of soft tissue component from the tumour:
   A. 12G
   B. 14G
   C. 16G
   D. 18G
   E. 22G
8. The average diagnostic accuracy of spinal bone core biopsies for the investigation of tumours is about:
   A. 50–60%
   B. 60–70%
   C. 70–80%
   D. 80–90%
   E. above 90%
9. Choose the right regarding the amount of biopsy material:
   A. Diagnosis of metastasis may be sufficient with fine-needle aspiration.
   B. Diagnosis of infection may be sufficient with fine-needle aspiration.
   C. Larger core samples should be taken for diagnosing primary spinal tumours.
   D. Risk of a nondiagnostic outcome is when the sample is taken from necrotic areas.
   E. Multiple samples are essential for the diagnosis of lymphoma.
10. The diagnostic accuracy of biopsy for the investigation of infectious spondylodiscitis:
    A. It is the same as spinal bone biopsies for the investigation of tumours.
    B. It is slightly higher than spinal bone biopsies for the investigation of tumours.
    C. It is slightly lower than spinal bone biopsies for the investigation of tumours.
    D. It is much higher than spinal bone biopsies for the investigation of tumours.
    E. It is much lower than spinal bone biopsies for the investigation of tumours.

11. Choose the correct regarding biopsy for the investigation of infectious spondylodiscitis:
    A. Empirical antibiotic treatment may be initiated before biopsy.
    B. 24–48 h before tissue sampling, antibiotics should be stopped.
    C. *Staphylococcus aureus* is the most common pathogen.
    D. Antibiotics should not be stopped before tissue sampling.
    E. Bone core biopsy is contraindicated when spondylodiscitis is suspected.
12. Choose the correct regarding common indications for epidural peri-radicular injections:
    A. lumbosacral radicular pain in the patient who failed conservative therapy
    B. pain relief in the patient with failed back surgery syndrome
    C. spinal canal stenosis and in the patient who is not the candidate for surgical treatment
    D. pain relief in patients with spondylodiscitis
    E. clinical suspicion of metastatic cancer
13. Pulsed radiofrequency ablation is the most effective in:
    A. subacute radiculitis
    B. bone metastasis
    C. spondylodiscitis
    D. chronic radiculitis
    E. disc herniation
14. Corticosteroid injection is the most effective in:
    A. subacute radiculitis
    B. bone metastasis
    C. spondylodiscitis
    D. chronic radiculitis
    E. disc herniation
15. Choose the correct regarding facet joint syndrome treatment:
    A. intra-articular injection of local anaesthetic
    B. intra-articular injection of local anaesthetic with steroid
    C. the medial branch of the dorsal ramus of the spinal nerve blockade
    D. the lateral branch of the dorsal ramus of the spinal nerve blockade
    E. thermal radiofrequency ablation of the medial branch of the dorsal ramus of the spinal
16. Percutaneous disc decompression:
    A. aims to decrease spinal nerve compression
    B. increases intradiscal pressure
    C. may be used in disc sequestration
    D. may be used in disc protrusion
    E. may be used in disc bulge
17. Choose the Indications for percutaneous intervertebral application of cement:
    A. acute burst fracture
    B. aggressive haemangioma
    C. insufficient sacrum fracture
    D. painful vertebral metastases
    E. osteoporotic vertebral compression fractures

18. Choose the correct regarding ablation of tumours:
    A. Pain treatment is a typical indication for thermal ablation.
    B. treatment of osteoid osteoma.
    C. Large pelvic tumours may be treated with alcoholization.
    D. Bowel and bladder symptoms may be complications.
    E. Insulation of carbon dioxide is need.
19. Radiofrequency ablation is successful in the treatment of:
    A. osteoblastoma
    B. chondroblastoma
    C. osteoid osteoma
    D. eosinophilic granuloma
    E. aneurysmal bone cyst
20. Choose indications for embolization of tumours:
    A. thyroid carcinoma metastasis
    B. chordoma
    C. haemangioma
    D. aneurysmal bone cyst
    E. osteoblastoma

Key to Chapter 13

1. A, C, D.
2. E.
3. A, B.
4. A, B, C, D.
5. C.
6. A, B.
7. C, D.
8. E.
9. A, B, C, D, E.
10. E.
11. A, B, C.
12. A, B, C.
13. D.
14. A.
15. A, B, C, E.
16. A, B, D, E.
17. C, D, E.
18. A, B, C, D, E.
19. A, B, C, D.
20. A, B, C, D, E.

Part VIII

Examinations

14 Examination Set 1

(One answer is correct, choose one answer from among A, B, C, D, and E)

1. Congenital spinal stenosis may be seen in:
   A. haemophilia
   B. achondroplasia
   C. ochronosis
   D. osteopetrosis
   E. Morquio syndrome
2. Post-operative changes in the intervertebral disc may enhance:
   A. up to 1 month after surgery
   B. up to 3 months after surgery
   C. up to 6 months after surgery
   D. up to 12 months after surgery
   E. many years

Supplementary Information The online version contains supplementary material available at (https://doi.org/10.1007/978-3-030-85182-8_14).

P. Szaro, *Musculoskeletal Radiology for Residents*,
https://doi.org/10.1007/978-3-030-85182-8_14

3. A 24-year-old patient has pain in the forefoot, which is relieved by aspirin. X-ray was performed (Fig. 14.1). What is the most likely diagnosis?

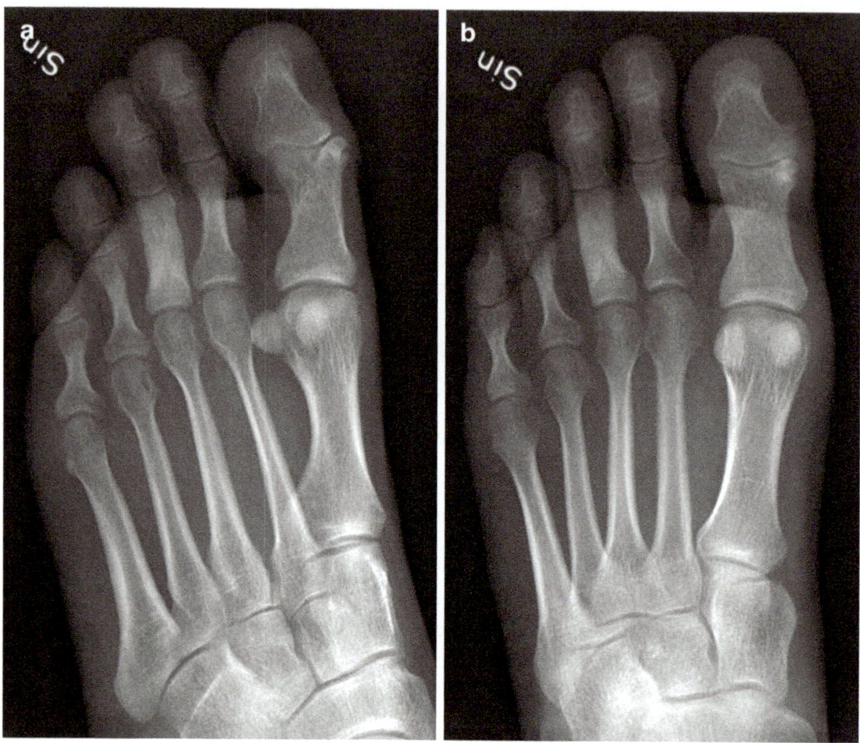

Fig. 14.1 (**a** and **b**) X-ray of the forefoot

A. osteosarcoma
B. stress fracture
C. Brodie abscess
D. cortical desmoid
E. osteoid osteoma

4. A 54-year-old patient presents with a painful tumour on the posterior neck. MRI with contrast was performed (Fig. 14.2). What is the least possible diagnosis based on MRI?

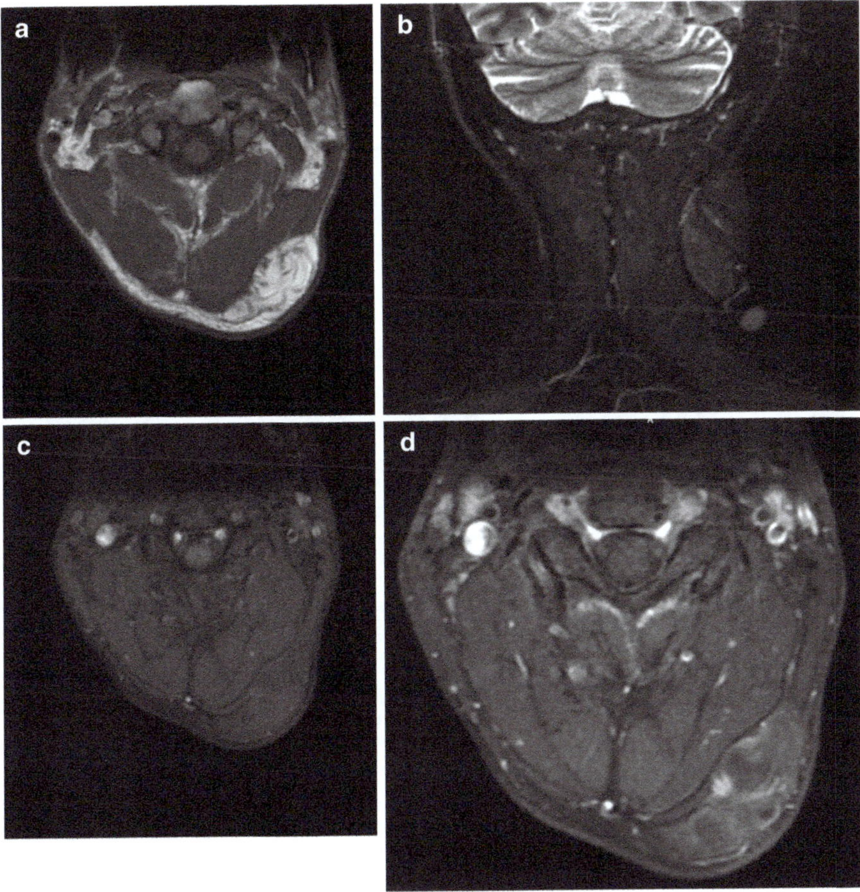

Fig. 14.2 (**a**) T1-weighted image, the axial image; (**b**) short tau inversion recovery, the coronal section; (**c**) T1-weighted image with fat suppression, the axial section; (**d**) T1-weighted image with fat suppression and contrast, the axial section

   A. lipoma with degeneration
   B. hibernoma
   C. poorly differentiated liposarcoma
   D. low-grade liposarcoma
   E. atypical lipomatous tumour

5. A 56-year-old patient presents with a swollen and painful ankle without trauma. X-ray showed no calcifications. MRI was performed (Videos 14.1, 14.2 and 14.3). What is the most likely diagnosis?
   A. pigmented villonodular synovitis
   B. synovial chondromatosis
   C. rheumatoid arthritis
   D. synovial sarcoma
   E. gout

6. A 5-year-old patient presents with a painful and tender thigh. MRI was performed (Fig. 14.3). Choose the correct option regarding the lesion:
   a. Cystic component is visible.
   b. Periosteal reaction is visible.
   c. Cortical breakthrough is present.
   d. This is a solid lesion located in the diaphysis.
   e. Intense contrast enhancement is present.

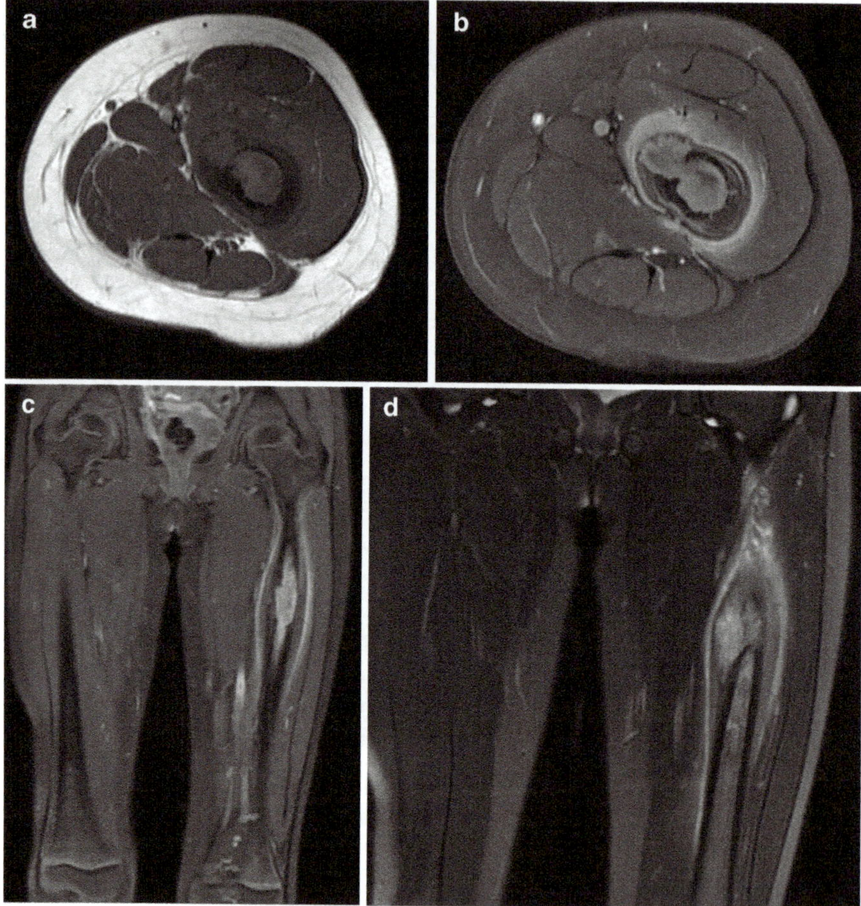

Fig. 14.3 (**a**) T1-weighted image, the axial image; (**b**) T1-weighted image with fat suppression and contrast, the axial section; (**c**) T1-weighted image with fat suppression and contrast, the coronal section; (**d**) T2-weighted image with fat suppression, the coronal section

A. a, b, c, d, e
B. a, c, d, e
C. b, c, d, e
D. a, e
E. c, d

7. A 65-year-old patient noted a slowly growing mass over the previous 8 months. The mass is not painful. Otherwise, the patient has no significant medical history. Choose the correct option regarding this patient:
   a. MRI is indicated.
   b. Infection is most likely.
   c. CT with contrast is indicated.
   d. There is suspicion for malignancy.
   e. X-ray may be omitted because fracture is unlikely.
   A. a, b
   B. b, e
   C. a, d, e
   D. a, d
   E. b, c
8. Regarding the patient from the previous question, what intramuscular lesion is possible?
   a. lipoma
   b. malignant fibrous histiocytoma
   c. liposarcoma
   d. myxoma
   e. fibrous histiocytoma
   A. a, b, c, d, e
   B. a, b, e
   C. b, c, d, e
   D. b, e
   E. b, d, e
9. Choose the correct option regarding the lesions from the previous question:
   a. Lipoma shows isointense signal to subcutaneous fat.
   b. Malignant fibrous histiocytoma is the most common malignant intramuscular tumour.
   c. Fat signal is visible in low differentiated liposarcoma.
   d. Fibrous histiocytoma is usually located subcutaneously.
   A. a, b
   B. a, c
   C. c, d
   D. a, b, d
   E. a, b, c, d
10. Choose the correct option regarding soft tissue tumours:
   a. Malignancies are deep and large.
   b. More than 50% of benign tumours exceed 6 cm in diameter.
   c. Less aggressive biologic character is visible in superficial sarcomas.
   d. A connective tissue capsule is a typical feature of benign lesions.
   A. a, c
   B. b, d
   C. a, b, c
   D. a, c, d
   E. a, b, c, d

11. The origin of the sartorius muscle is the:
    A. anterior superior iliac spine
    B. anterior inferior iliac spine
    C. iliac crest
    D. greater trochanter
    E. lesser trochanter
12. What shoulder ligament may be found at the level of the subscapularis tendon?
    a. superior glenohumeral ligament
    b. middle glenohumeral ligament
    c. anterior bundle of the inferior glenohumeral ligament
    d. posterior bundle of the inferior glenohumeral ligament
    A. a, b, c, d
    B. a, b, c
    C. a, b
    D. c, d
    E. d
13. Choose the correct description of the sagittal section of MRI (Fig. 14.4):

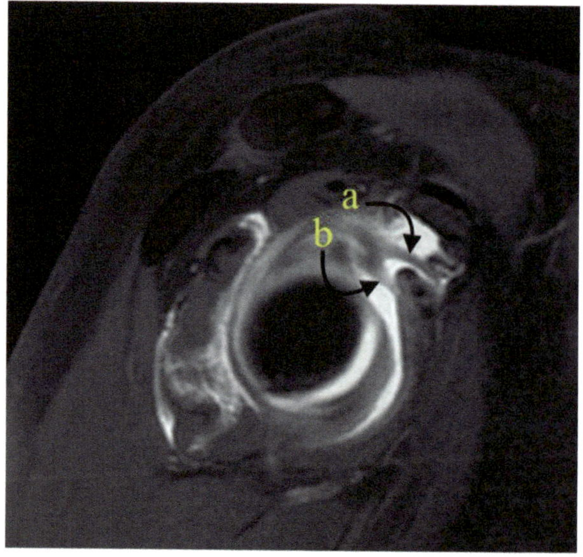

Fig. 14.4 T1-weighted image with intra-articular contrast; the sagittal section

    A. a—superior glenohumeral ligament, b—middle glenohumeral ligament
    B. a—coracoacromial ligament, b—superior glenohumeral ligament
    C. a—superior glenohumeral ligament, b—coracohumeral ligament
    D. a—coracohumeral ligament, b—superior glenohumeral ligament
    E. a—middle glenohumeral ligament, b—inferior glenohumeral ligament

14. Choose the correct name of the structure labelled on the axial section of MRI (Fig. 14.5):
    1. superior glenohumeral ligament
    2. middle glenohumeral ligament
    3. inferior glenohumeral ligament
    4. coracohumeral ligament
    5. subscapularis tendon
    6. labrum

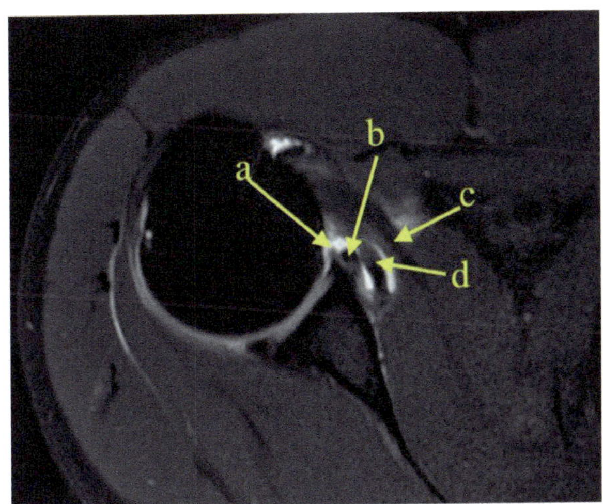

Fig. 14.5 T1-weighted image with intra-articular contrast; the axial section

    A. a—3, b—2, c—5, d—2
    B. a—6, b—3, c—2, d—5
    C. a—6, b—2, c—2, d—3
    D. a—6, b—3, c—5, d—3
    E. a—3, b—6, c—5, d—3
15. The Rolando fracture is a fracture of the:
    A. proximal humerus
    B. intercondylar eminence
    C. base of the first metacarpal
    D. base of the fifth metatarsal
    E. scaphoid tuberculum
16. In mallet finger, the:
    A. Fracture is noted at the base of the proximal phalanx.
    B. Fracture is noted at the lateral outline of the base of the distal phalanx.
    C. Fracture is noted at the medial outline of the base of the distal phalanx.
    D. Fracture is noted at the anterior outline of the base of the distal phalanx.
    E. Fracture is noted at the posterior outline of the base of the distal phalanx.

17. Choose the correct option regarding perilunate dislocations:
    A. Disruption of the line is made by tracing the proximal articular surfaces of the radius and capitate.
    B. It is usually due to a hyperextended and ulnarly deviated hand.
    C. Scaphoid fracture is usually seen in about 20% of cases.
    D. If untreated, a high risk of radial nerve palsy is seen.
    E. It is a synonym for lunate dislocations.
18. The extra-articular fracture of the distal radius with dorsal subluxation is called a:
    A. Barton fracture
    B. Colles fracture
    C. Smith fracture
    D. Rolando fracture
    E. Bennett fracture
19. Falling onto an outstretched hand is a common mechanism for a(n):
    a. Barton fracture
    b. Galeazzi fracture-dislocation
    c. Essex-Lopresti fracture-dislocation
    A. a, b, c
    B. a, b
    C. a, c
    D. b, c
    E. b
20. Choose the correct option regarding scaphoid bone fractures:
    A. Most of fractures involve the proximal pole.
    B. It accounts for 30–40% of all carpal bone fractures.
    C. The Terry Thomas sign is the same as the humpback sign.
    D. Slight sclerosis of the proximal fragment is the first sign of avascular necrosis.
    E. Slight sclerosis of the distal fragment is the first sign of avascular necrosis.
21. An AP view of the wrist showed sclerosis, volume reduction, and abnormal shape of the lunate bone. No other abnormality is seen. Negative ulnar variance is noted. What is the most likely diagnosis?
    A. perilunate dislocation
    B. radial impaction syndrome
    C. ulnar impaction syndrome
    D. lunate bone fracture
    E. lunatomalacia

22. Higher signal on T2-weighted images may be seen in:
    a. the acute phase of Kienböck disease
    b. the chronic phase of Kienböck disease
    c. a fracture
    d. a complex regional pain syndrome
    A. a, b, d
    B. b, c, d
    C. a, c, d
    D. b, c, d
    E. a, b, c, d
23. A 44-year-old patient fell during a match. X-ray showed that the anterior fat pad was elevated and anteriorly displaced. No obvious bone deformity, luxation, or loose body was revealed. Choose the correct option regarding this patient:
    A. CT is required to rule out a caput radii fracture.
    B. MRI is required to rule out a caput radii fracture.
    C. Ultrasound is required to rule out a caput radii fracture.
    D. Control X-ray in 3 weeks is recommended.
    E. No further diagnostic testing is required.
24. A 73-year-old female presents complaining of pelvic pain. CT revealed vertically orientated sclerosis in the whole right part of the sacrum. Choose the correct option regarding this patient:
    A. It is a picture of a fracture.
    B. It is a typical picture of a malignancy.
    C. It is a clear picture of osteomyelitis.
    D. It is an unclear lesion, bone core biopsy is recommended.
    E. It is an unclear lesion, further diagnostic MRI is required.
25. A young runner presents with a complaint of pubic pain. X-ray showed sclerosis with erosion. What is the correct diagnosis for this patient?
    A. Osteoarthritis.
    B. Osteomyelitis.
    C. Rheumatoid arthritis.
    D. Spondyloarthropathy.
    E. It is an unclear finding and MRI is indicated.
26. Choose the abnormal value of an angle between a line across the anterior process extending to the apex of the calcaneus intersecting with a line from the posterior portion of the calcaneus to the apex.
    A. 15°
    B. 25°
    C. 30°
    D. 35°
    E. 40°

27. An increased space between the base of the first and second metatarsal bones:
    A. It is an indirect sign of peroneus longus rupture.
    B. It is a sign of aneurysm of the metatarsal artery.
    C. It is sign of a Lisfranc ligament tear.
    D. It is a hallmark of Morton neuroma.
    E. It may be seen in bursitis.
28. Thirty-two-year-old runner presents with tibial pain. X-ray showed irregular somewhat diffuse sclerosis in the posterior part of the proximal tibia. Adjacent periostitis is seen. Choose the correct comment:
    A. Bone core biopsy is recommended.
    B. CT is indicated to better visualize soft tissue.
    C. Ultrasound is indicated to characterize the periosteum.
    D. CT is indicated to better visualize the periosteum.
    E. MRI is indicated for better characterizing the lesion.
29. Regarding the patient from the previous question, what is the most likely diagnosis?
    A. osteosarcoma
    B. stress fracture
    C. Ewing sarcoma
    D. muscle rupture
    E. osteoid osteoma
30. Choose the abnormal values for the distance between the anterior arch of the atlas to the odontoid process in adults:
    a. 1.5 mm
    b. 2.5 mm
    c. 4.5 mm
    d. 5.5 mm
    A. a, b, c
    B. b, c, d
    C. a, b
    D. c, d
    E. d
31. A fracture of the spinous process of a lower cervical vertebra is called a:
    A. seatbelt injury
    B. Jefferson fracture
    C. Hangman fracture
    D. clay-shoveler fracture
    E. pseudo-Jefferson fracture

32. Choose the features of a flexion teardrop fracture:
    a. Widening of the interspinous processes.
    b. Most frequently, it occurs in the upper cervical spine.
    c. Cervical kyphosis.
    d. It is not considered as severe as an extension teardrop fracture.
    A. a, b, c
    B. a, c
    C. b, d
    D. a, b, d
    E. a, b, c, d
33. Spondylolysis is a break or defect in the:
    A. lamina of the arch
    B. vertebral body
    C. spinous process
    D. transverse process
    E. interarticular part of the lamina
34. A sclerotic and collapsed vertebral body of L4 with a horizontal cleft of gas within the endplate is the appearance of:
    A. acute compression
    B. avascular necrosis
    C. disc degeneration
    D. a burst fracture
    E. osteomyelitis
35. Geodes are present in the following conditions:
    a. calcium pyrophosphate dihydrate crystal deposition disease
    b. rheumatoid arthritis
    c. osteoarthritis
    A. a, b, c
    B. a, b
    C. c, d
    D. only c
    E. a, c
36. Choose the exceptions to the classic triad of findings seen in osteoarthritis:
    a. temporomandibular joint
    b. acromioclavicular
    c. shoulder joint
    A. a, b, c
    B. a, b
    C. b, c
    D. a, c
    E. a

37. Choose the most common localization of primary osteoarthritis:
    A. second through fifth distal interphalangeal joints in the hand
    B. second through fifth proximal interphalangeal joints
    C. second through fifth metacarpophalangeal joints
    D. carpometacarpal joint of the thumb
    E. second through fifth carpometacarpal joints
38. Choose the radiological hallmarks of rheumatoid arthritis:
    A. subchondral sclerosis and osteophytes
    B. marginal erosions and subchondral sclerosis
    C. marginal erosions and periarticular osteoporosis
    D. joint space narrowing and periarticular osteoporosis
    E. central subchondral erosions and marginal sclerosis
39. A 56-year-old female presents with hand swelling. X-ray showed erosions in both the carpal bones and metacarpophalangeal joints and soft tissue swelling. What is the most likely diagnosis?
    A. systemic lupus erythematosus
    B. rheumatoid arthritis
    C. scleroderma
    D. osteoarthritis
    E. psoriasis
40. Geodes are typically found in:
    a. psoriatic arthritis
    b. rheumatoid arthritis
    c. degenerative joint disease
    A. a, b, c
    B. a, b
    C. b, c
    D. a, c
    E. a
41. Joint destruction with subluxation and clumps of ossification neighbouring the joint is the classic appearance of:
    A. gout
    B. Charcot joint
    C. early psoriatic arthritis
    D. late rheumatoid arthritis
    E. calcium pyrophosphate dihydrate crystal deposition
42. What is the second most common site of avascular necrosis?
    A. femoral head
    B. talus
    C. humeral head
    D. scaphoid
    E. head of the second metatarsal bone

43. X-ray revealed significant cortical narrowing at the metacarpal cortex in a 55-year-old female. What is the most likely diagnosis?
    A. metastasis
    B. osteoporosis
    C. Brown tumour
    D. osteosarcoma
    E. Ewing sarcoma
44. Choose the X-ray feature/-s of hyperparathyroidism:
    a. subperiosteal bone resorption at the radial aspect of the middle phalanges of the hand
    b. enlargement of the tuberosity of the distal phalanges (acromegalia)
    c. sclerotic bands at the vertebral body endplates
    A. a, b, c
    B. a, b
    C. b, c
    D. a, c
    E. a
45. A 16-year-old patient presents with knee pain. MRI was done (Fig. 14.6). What is the correct statement regarding the lesion marked with the arrow?

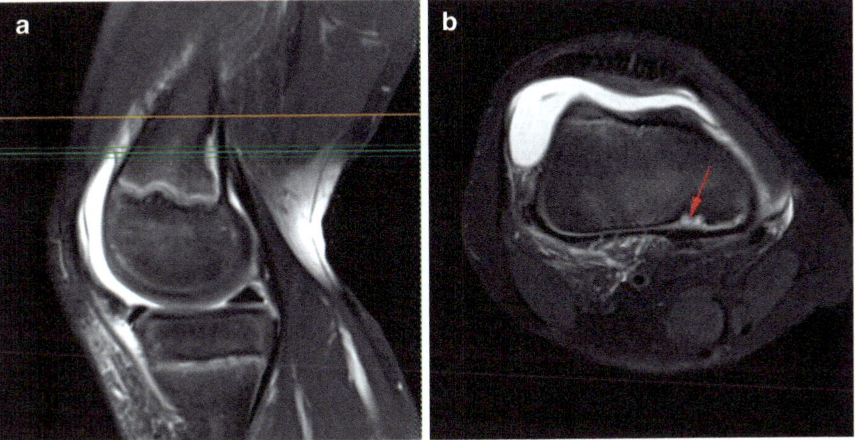

Fig. 14.6 Proton density-weighted images with fat suppression. (**a**) Sagittal section, (**b**) axial section

    A. It is a non-specific malignant lesion, CT is indicated.
    B. it is a cortical avulsive irregularity.
    C. It is a fibrous cortical defect.
    D. It is an osteosarcoma.
    E. It is a Ewing sarcoma.

46. A 24-year-old patient presents with foot pain after trauma. X-ray was done (Fig. 14.7). Choose the correct option regarding this patient:

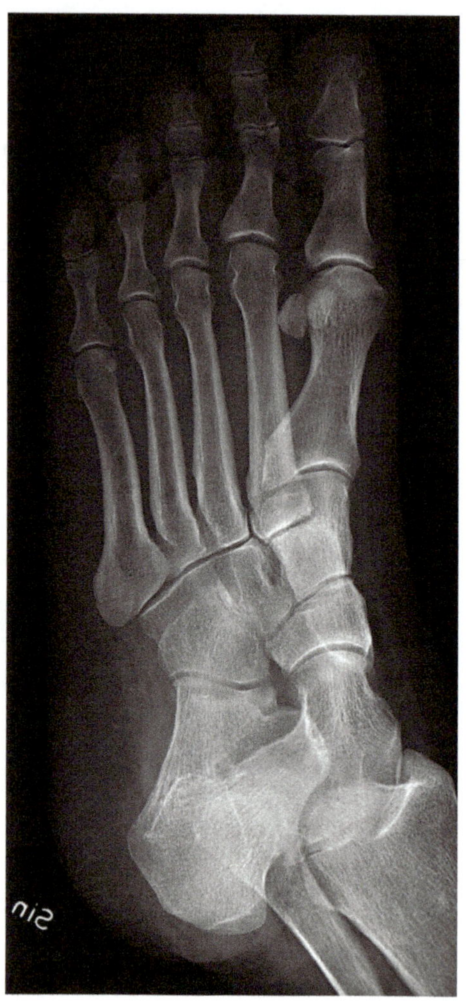

Fig. 14.7 X-ray of the foot

A. No fracture is seen.
B. Osteomyelitis is seen.
C. Stress fracture is seen.
D. Jones fracture is seen.
E. Avulsion fracture is seen.

47. A 23-year-old patient presents with ankle pain. X-ray was done (Fig. 14.8). What is correct with regard to the differential diagnosis?
    a. giant cell tumour
    b. intraosseous ganglion
    c. aneurysmal bone cyst
    d. chondroblastoma

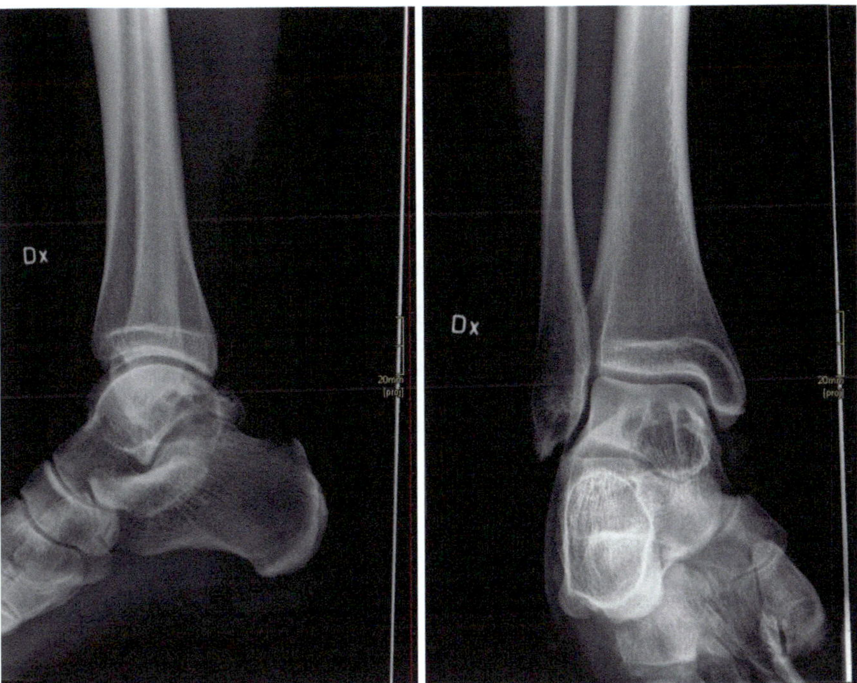

Fig. 14.8 X-ray of the ankle

A. a, b, c, d
B. a, b, c
C. b, c
D. a, d
E. d

48. A 34-year-old patient presents with lumbar pain. CT was performed (Fig. 14.9). What is the most likely diagnosis?

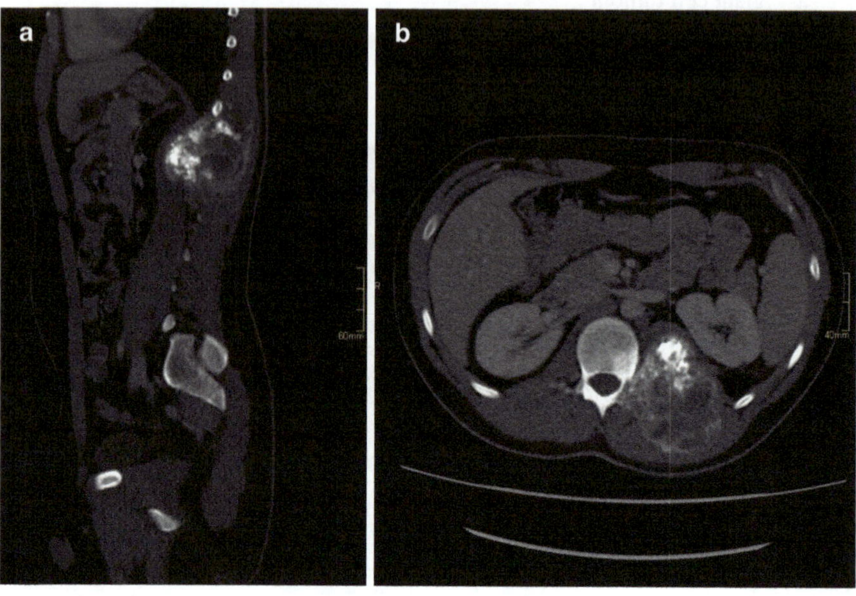

Fig. 14.9 Computed tomography of the abdomen. (**a**) Sagittal section, (**b**) axial section

A. osteomyelitis
B. osteosarcoma
C. Ewing sarcoma
D. osteoblastoma
E. chondroblastoma

49. A 33-year-old patient presents with hip pain after trauma. X-ray was performed (Fig. 14.10). What is correct regarding this patient?
    a. It is a classical fracture, no tumour is seen.
    b. It is a pathologic fracture.
    c. It is a benign lesion.
    d. It is a malignant lesion.
    e. It is non-specific, MRI is indicated.
    f. No fracture is seen.

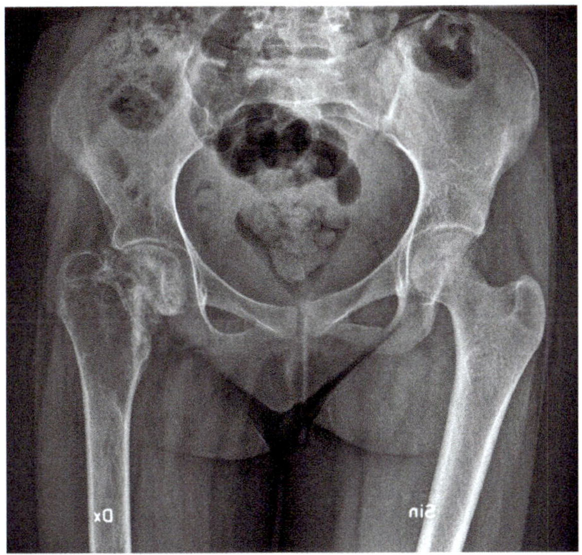

Fig. 14.10 X-ray of the pelvis

A. a
B. b, c
C. b, d
D. b, e
E. d, f

50. What is correct regarding the X-ray (Fig. 14.11)?
    a. metastasis
    b. septic arthritis
    c. avascular necrosis
    d. rheumatoid arthritis

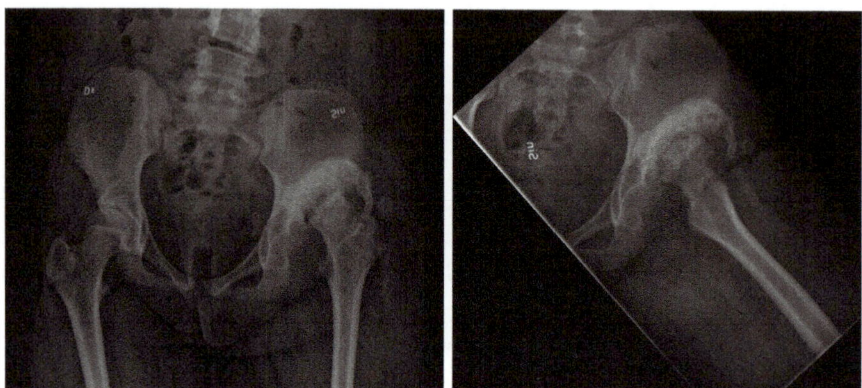

Fig. 14.11 X-ray of the pelvis

A. a, b, c, d
B. a, b, c
C. b, c, d
D. b, d
E. b

51. What is the possible differential diagnosis of the X-ray of an 83-year-old patient (Fig. 14.12)?
    a. fibrous dysplasia
    b. Paget disease
    c. osteomyelitis
    d. metastasis
    e. myeloma

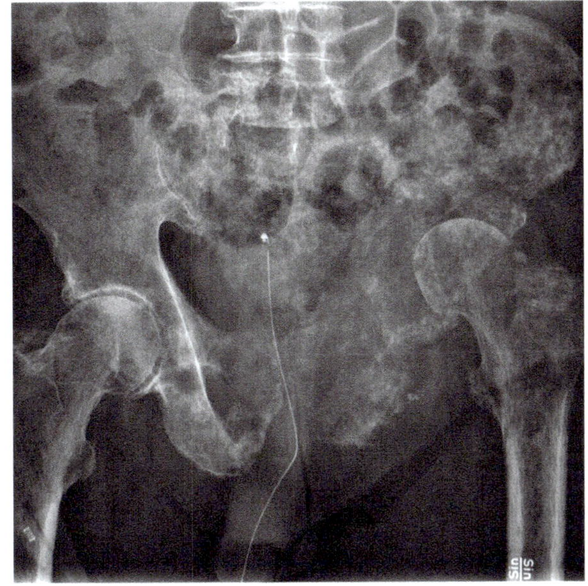

Fig. 14.12 X-ray of the pelvis

A. a, b, c, d, e
B. a, b, c, d
C. b, c, d, e
D. a, d
E. d, e

52. What is the most likely diagnosis regarding the X-ray of a 56-year-old patient after trauma (Fig. 14.13)?

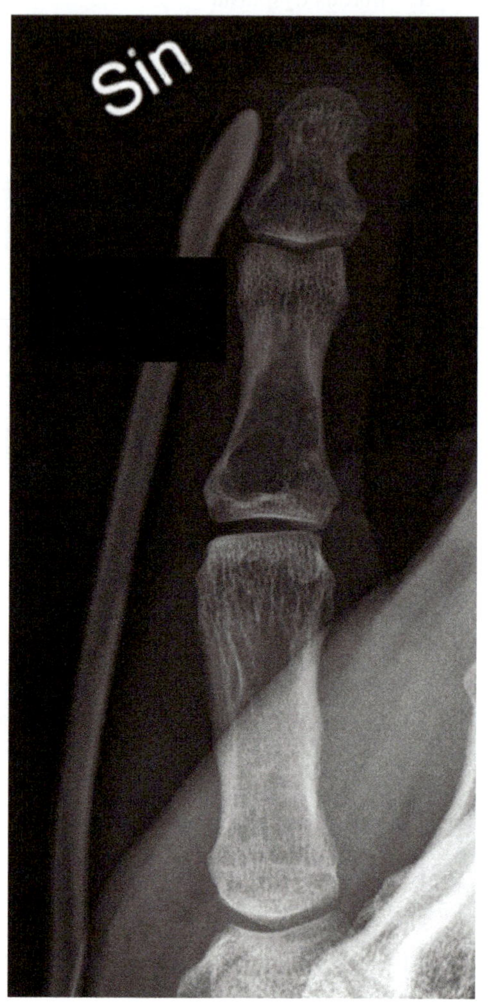

Fig. 14.13 X-ray of the thumb

A. intraosseous ganglion
B. enchondroma
C. metastasis
D. myeloma
E. geode

53. A 32-year-old patient presenting with thigh pain. CT was performed (Fig. 14.14). What is the most likely diagnosis based on CT?

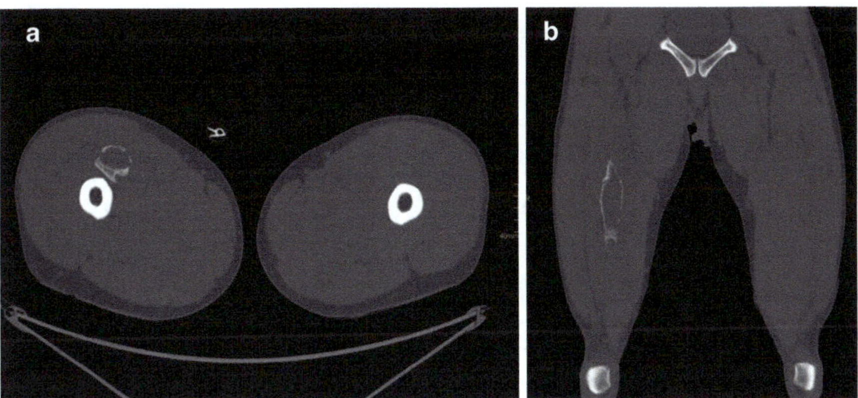

Fig. 14.14 Computed tomography of the thighs (**a** and **b**)

A. It is a non-specific lesion, MRI is indicated.
B. Myositis ossificans.
C. Ewing sarcoma.
D. Osteosarcoma.
E. Schwannoma.

54. The patient from the previous question was referred for MRI. What is the most likely diagnosis regarding CT (Fig. 14.14) and MRI (Fig. 14.15)?

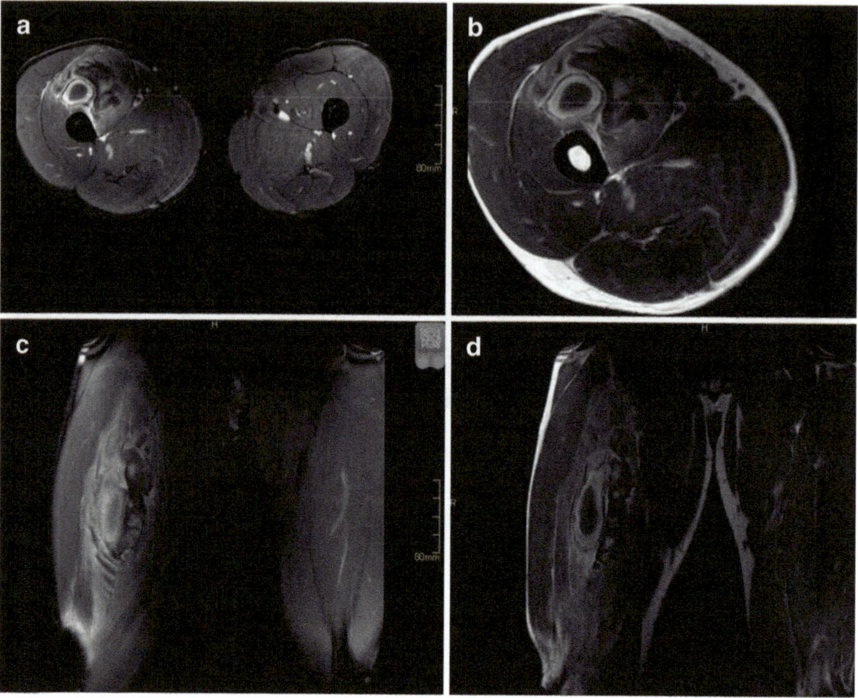

Fig. 14.15 (**a**) T1-weighted image with fat suppression and contrast, axial section; (**b**) T2-weigthed image, axial section; (**c**) T1-weighted image with fat suppression and contrast, coronal section; (**d**) T1-weighted image with contrast, coronal section

A. Intramuscular abscess and pyogenic myositis.
B. Myositis ossificans and haematoma.
C. Biopsy is indicated.
D. Ewing sarcoma.
E. Osteosarcoma.

55. What of the following diagnoses is the most likely based on X-ray (Fig. 14.16)?

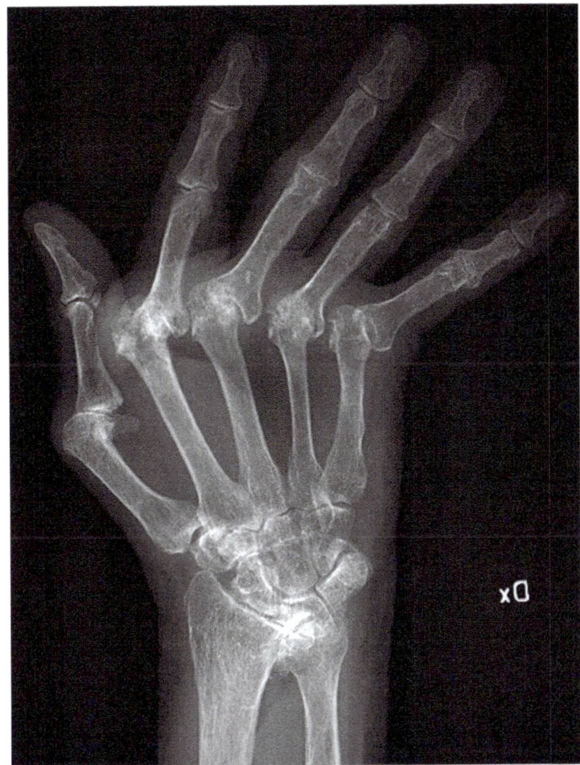

Fig. 14.16 X-ray of the hand

A. skeletal manifestation of scleroderma
B. rheumatoid arthritis
C. psoriatic arthritis
D. osteoarthritis
E. gout

Key to Chapter 14

1. B.
2. E.
3. E.
4. C.
5. A.
6. C.
7. D.
8. A.
9. D.
10. A.
11. A.
12. B.
13. A.
14. D.
15. C.
16. E.
17. B.
18. B.
19. A.
20. E.
21. E.
22. C.
23. E.
24. A.
25. A.
26. A.
27. C.
28. E.
29. B.
30. D.
31. D.
32. B.
33. E.
34. B.
35. A.
36. B.
37. D.
38. C.
39. B.
40. C.
41. B.
42. C.
43. B.

44. D. Enlargement of the tuberosity of the distal phalanges is seen in acromegalia.
45. B.
46. E.
47. A.
48. B.
49. B. Histopathology: fibrosus dysplasia.
50. E.
51. E.
52. B.
53. B.
54. B.
55. B.

15 Examination Set 2

(One answer is correct, choose one answer from among A, B, C, D, and E)

1. Spinoglenoid cysts may compress the:
   A. radial nerve
   B. axillary nerve
   C. subscapular nerve
   D. dorsal scapular nerve
   E. suprascapular nerve
2. An intra-articular disc is usually present in the:
   a. sternoclavicular joint
   b. acromioclavicular joint
   c. temporomandibular joint
   A. a, b, c
   B. b, c
   C. a, c
   D. b
   E. c
3. A typical pitfall in diagnosing an osteochondral lesion in the elbow is the pseudodefect of the:
   A. caput radii
   B. trochlea
   C. capitellum
   D. olecranon
   E. medial epicondyle

P. Szaro, *Musculoskeletal Radiology for Residents*,
https://doi.org/10.1007/978-3-030-85182-8_15

4. Choose the correct option regarding the ulnar collateral ligament of the elbow:
   a. The anterior bundle inserts on the medial outline of the coronoid process.
   b. The posterior bundle is located deep to the ulnar nerve.
   c. The transverse bundle provides most of the stability.
   A. a, b, c
   B. b, c
   C. a, c
   D. a, b
   E. b
5. What is the most typical radiological feature of an annular fissure?
   A. hyperintense on T1-weighted image
   B. hypointense on T1-weighted image
   C. hyperintense on T2-weighted image
   D. hypointense on T2-weighted image
   E. Hyperdense on computed tomography
6. A 35-year-old runner presents with increasing right leg pain. The pain started 3 weeks ago after energetic training. Which modality is the best to assess the possible pathology?
   A. X-ray
   B. computed tomography with contrast
   C. ultrasound
   D. MRI without contrast
   E. MRI with contrast
7. What ligament is orientated vertically?
   A. the anterior talofibular ligament
   B. the posterior talofibular ligament
   C. the calcaneofibular ligament
   D. the bifurcate ligament
   E. the talonavicular ligament
8. The anterior tibial nerve is innervated by the:
   A. common peroneal nerve
   B. superficial fibular nerve
   C. deep fibular nerve
   D. sciatic nerve
   E. tibial nerve

9. Choose the correct description of the ligaments (Fig. 15.1):

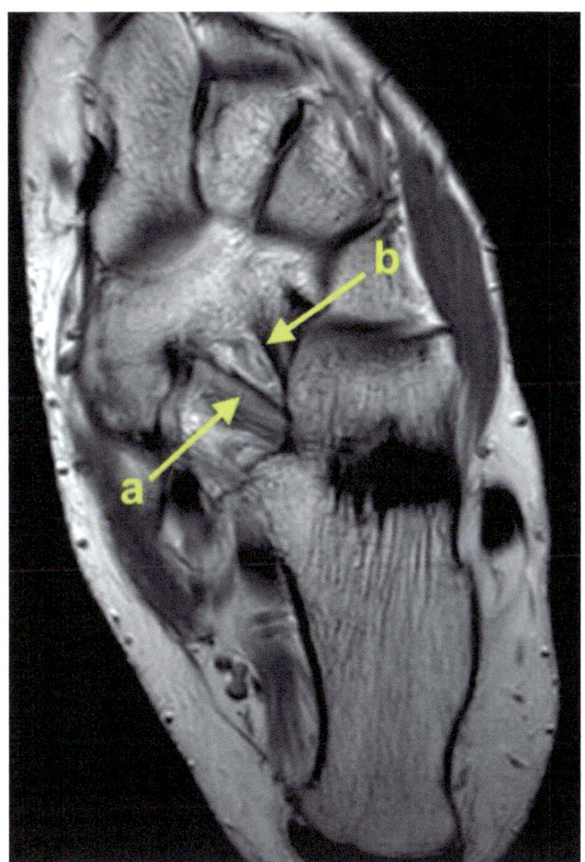

Fig. 15.1 Proton density image, axial section

A. a and b—bifurcate ligament
B. a—bifurcate ligament, b—lateral calcaneonavicular ligament
C. a—superomedial ligament, b—inferoplantar longitudinal ligament
D. a—inferoplantar longitudinal ligament, b—medioplantar oblique ligament
E. a—medioplantar oblique ligament, b—inferoplantar longitudinal ligament

10. The nerve marked by the arrow in Fig. 15.2 supplies the following muscles:
    a. gluteus maximus, gluteus medius, gluteus minimus
    b. gastrocnemius and semitendinosus
    c. iliopsoas

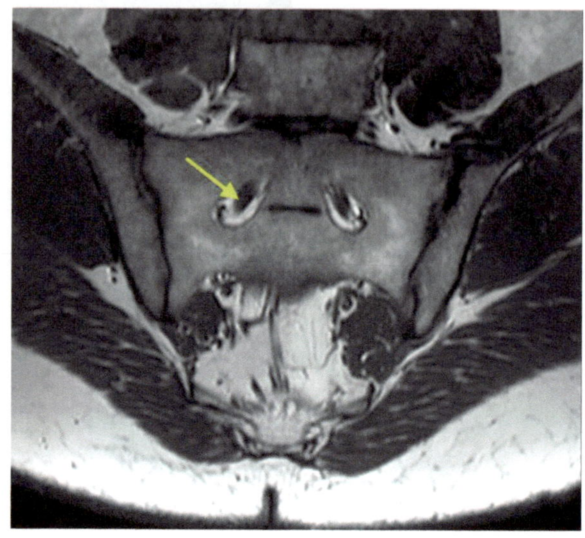

Fig. 15.2 T1-weighted image, oblique section

A. a, b, c
B. b, c
C. a, c
D. a, b
E. b

11. Which nerve passes via the foramen marked in Fig. 15.3?

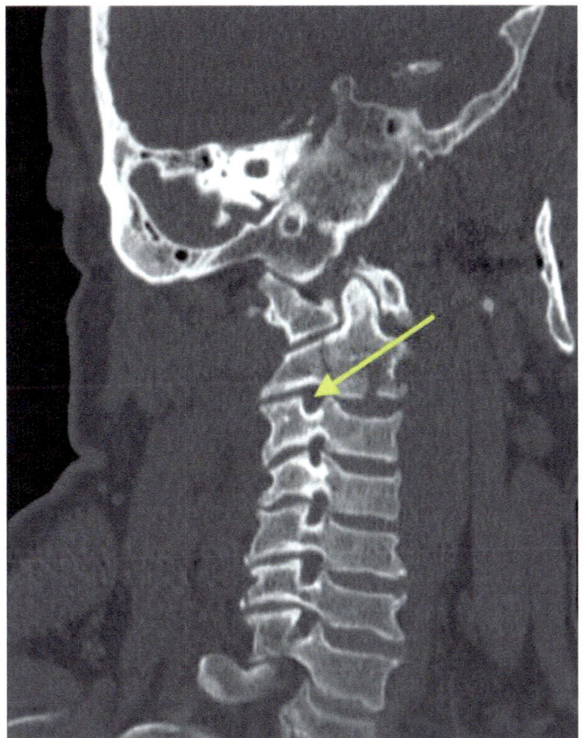

Fig. 15.3 Computed tomography, oblique section

A. C1
B. C2
C. C3
D. C4
E. greater occipital nerve

12. Anterior dislocation of the humeral head may cause:
    a. Perthes lesion
    b. soft tissue Bankart lesion
    c. glenolabral articular disruption

    A. a, b, c
    B. b, c
    C. a, c
    D. a, b
    E. b

13. Choose the common sites of avulsion fractures:
    a. patellar apex
    b. ischial tuberosity
    c. lateral tibial plateau
    d. medial tibial plateau
    A. a, b, c, d
    B. a, b, c
    C. b, c, d
    D. a, d
    E. b, c
14. What condition is a known cause of stress fractures?
    a. osteomalacia
    b. Paget disease
    c. hyperparathyroidism
    d. osteopoikilosis
    A. a, b, c, d
    B. a, b, c
    C. b, c, d
    D. a, d
    E. b, c
15. A 17-year-old patient presents with a painful elbow. MRI showed focal subchondral bone marrow oedema in the anterior part of the capitellum. What is the most likely diagnosis?
    A. stress fracture
    B. insufficient fracture
    C. rheumatoid arthritis
    D. osteochondritis dissecans
    E. anatomical variant of the capitellum
16. What acromial type is a known risk factor for subacromial impingement?
    A. types 1 and 2
    B. type 2
    C. types 2 and 3
    D. type 3
    E. types 3 and 4

17. A 35-year-old patient presents with shoulder pain after minor trauma. What is the most likely diagnosis regarding Fig. 15.4?
    a. intrasubstance tear
    b. tendinopathy
    c. calcification
    d. bursal side tear

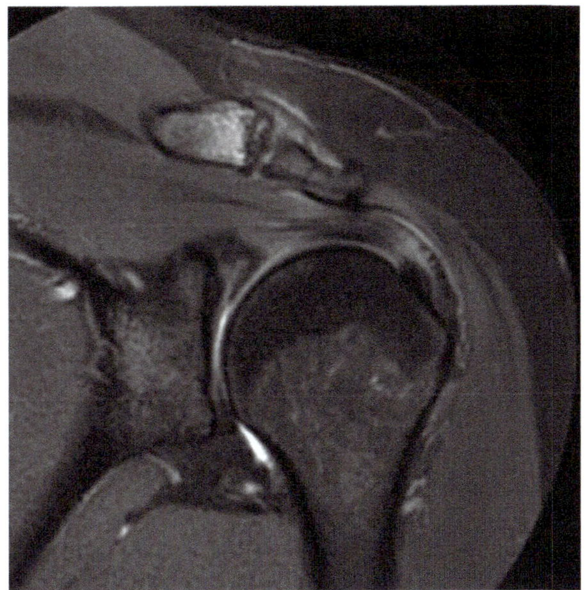

Fig. 15.4 T2-weighted image with fat suppression, coronal section

A. a, b, c
B. b
C. c, d
D. b, d
E. a, d, c

18. What is the most likely diagnosis regarding the patient from Fig. 15.5?

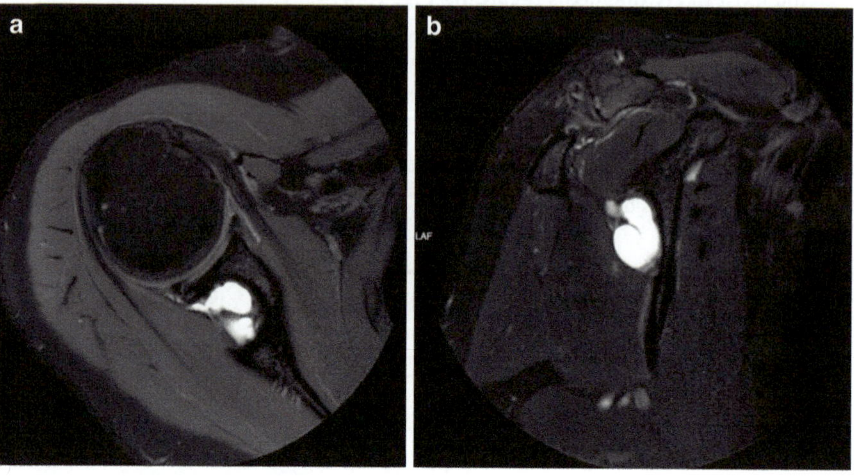

Fig. 15.5 (**a**) T2-weighted image with fat suppression, axial section; (**b**) T2-weighted image with fat suppression, sagittal section

A. Spinoglenoid notch ganglion with compression to the suprascapular nerve.
B. Spinoglenoid notch ganglion without compression to the suprascapular nerve.
C. Myxoid tumour, further diagnostic testing with contrast is indicated.
D. MRI with intra-articular contrast is indicated to check if a connection with the joint space is present.
E. Intramuscular ganglion with compression to the dorsal scapular nerve.

19. What is the anterior boundary of the rotator interval?

a. superior glenohumeral ligament
b. coracohumeral ligament
c. supraspinatus tendon
d. coracoid process

A. a, b
B. b, c
C. c
D. d
E. a, b, c

20. Choose the correct option regarding anatomical variants of the labrum:
    a. The sublabral foramen is when the anterosuperior labrum is not attached to the glenoid.
    b. Buford complex: the middle glenohumeral ligament is thick, while the anteroinferior labrum is congenitally absent.
    c. Reverse Buford complex: the inferior glenohumeral ligament is thick, while the posterior-inferior labrum is congenitally absent.
    A. a, b
    B. a
    C. b, c
    D. b
    E. c
21. What is the most likely diagnosis regarding the lesion showed by the arrow in Fig. 15.6?

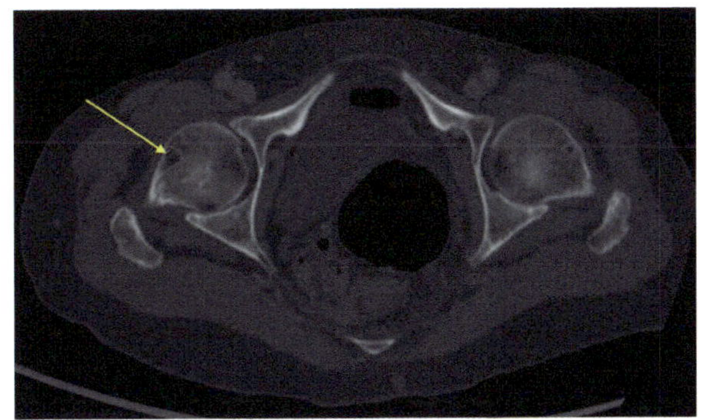

Fig. 15.6 Computed tomography of the pelvis

    A. intraosseus ganglion
    B. osteoid osteoma
    C. osteoblastoma
    D. Brodie abscess
    E. Pitt pit
22. A perforation of the triangular fibrocartilage and bone marrow oedema in the lunate may indicate:
    A. scapholunate advanced collapse
    B. avascular scaphoid necrosis
    C. Madelung deformity
    D. ulnar abutment
    E. osteoarthritis

23. Choose the correct option regarding the wrist:
    a. Thickening of the ulnar joint capsule that is inconsistently present distal of the styloid process is called a meniscal homologue.
    b. The anterior wrist ligaments are stronger than the posterior ligaments; thus, they are major stabilizers of the wrist.
    c. The lunate inclines dorsally in relation to the radius when the wrist is placed in radial deviation.
    A. a, b
    B. b, c
    C. c
    D. a
    E. a, b, c
24. Choose the correct option regarding gamekeeper's thumb or skier's thumb:
    a. The ulnar collateral ligament is located deep into the adductor aponeurosis.
    b. The ulnar collateral ligament being retracted proximally and displaced superficial to the adductor aponeurosis is seen in more than two-thrid of cases.
    c. Chronic laxity may be caused by the interposition of the adductor aponeurosis between the torn ulnar collateral ligament and MCP-1.
    A. a, b
    B. b, c
    C. c
    D. a, c
    E. a, b, c
25. Choose the correct option regarding idiopathic transient osteoporosis of the hip:
    a. It is usually a self-limited entity, which most often affects middle-aged women.
    b. Usually, there is no trauma in anamnesis and spontaneous resolution is observed in 6–8 months.
    c. This condition is common in children 4–10 years old, which may lead to growth arrest.
    A. a, b
    B. b, c
    C. b
    D. a, c
    E. a, b, c
26. Choose the typical age and gender for slipped capital femoral epiphysis:
    a. boy aged 12
    b. girl aged 14
    c. boy aged 6
    d. girl 6
    A. a, b, c
    B. a, b
    C. c, d
    D. b, d
    E. a, c, d

27. The fovea centralis (fovea capitis femoris) is typically located in:
    A. the superior outline of the femoral head
    B. the inferior outline of the femoral head
    C. the anterior outline of the femoral head
    D. the posterior outline of the femoral head
    E. the medial outline of the femoral head
28. Choose the correct option regarding femoroacetabular impingement:
    a. Major cause of early hip osteoarthrosis.
    b. The cam type is more common in middle-aged women.
    c. os acetabuli has an association with pincer type.
    A. a, b, c
    B. a, b
    C. b, c
    D. b
    E. a, c
29. The double posterior cruciate ligament sign is seen in a:
    A. horizontal meniscal tear on sagittal section
    B. vertical meniscal tear on sagittal section
    C. radial meniscal tear on sagittal section
    D. vertical meniscal tear on coronal section
    E. horizontal meniscal tear on coronal section
30. An extruded meniscus results from:
    a. longitudinal rupture
    b. horizontal rupture
    c. radial rupture
    d. degeneration
    A. a, b, c, d
    B. a, d
    C. c, d
    D. b, d
    E. a, c, d
31. In the Wrisberg variant of a discoid lateral meniscus:
    A. The anterior horn is not present.
    B. The posterior horn is not present.
    C. Lacks posterior ligament attachments.
    D. The only attachment to the posterior horn is the Humprey ligament.
    E. It is less prone to undergo degeneration than the classic discoid meniscus.
32. A 17-year-old football player presents with the anterior knee pain. MRI revealed only oedema in Hoffa's fat pad just inferior to the patellar apex. What is your diagnosis?
    A. bursitis
    B. fat necrosis
    C. impingement
    D. jumper's knee
    E. pigmented villonodular synovitis

33. A fluid collection separating the subcutaneous fat from fascia:
    a. It may result from shearing force.
    b. It is called a Morel-Lavallée lesion
    c. It results from fat necrosis.
    A. a, b, c
    B. a, b
    C. b, c
    D. b
    E. a, c
34. A 23-year-old patient presents after knee trauma. X-ray showed no fracture. MRI revealed reticular high-signal intensity on STIR at the level of the central part of the femoral condyle and posterolateral tibial plateau. This is a pattern seen with:
    A. clip injury
    B. pivot shift
    C. hyperflexion
    D. hyperextension
    E. dashboard injury

35. A 45-year-old patient presents with knee pain 6 months after ACL reconstruction. What is the most likely diagnosis based on T2-weighted imaging (Fig. 15.7)?

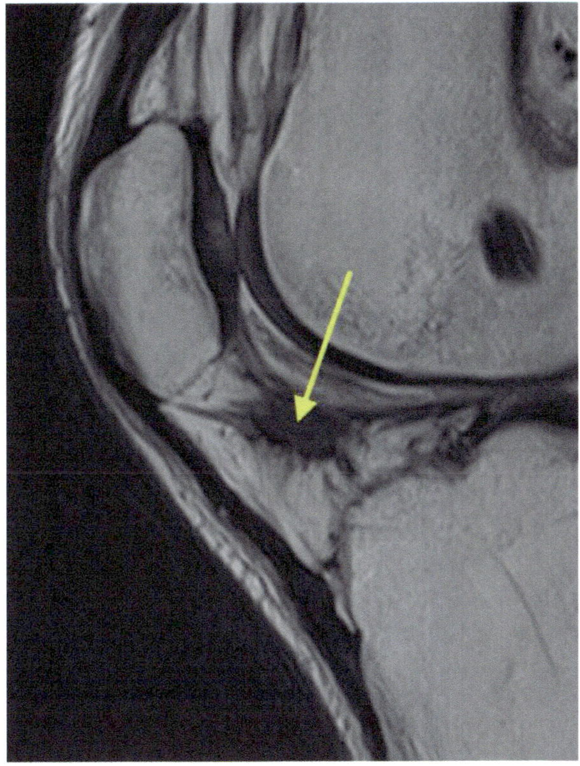

Fig. 15.7 Proton density-weighted, sagittal section

A. fat necrosis
B. arthrofibrosis
C. cyclops lesion
D. lipoma arborescens
E. pigmented villonodular synovitis

36. A 65-year-old patient presents with knee pain after trauma. MRI was done (Fig. 15.8), what option is correct regarding this patient?
    a. osteochondral fracture
    b. chondral delamination
    c. horizontal meniscal tear
    d. radial meniscal tear
    e. subchondral insufficient fracture

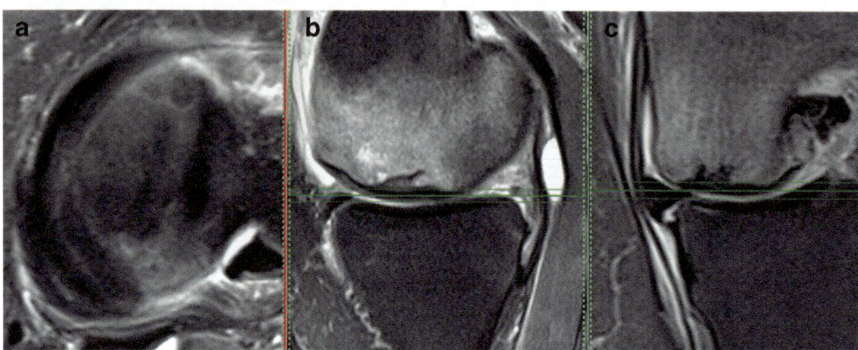

Fig. 15.8 Proton density weighted with fat suppression. (**a**) Axial section, (**b**) sagittal section; (**c**) coronal section

A. a, b, c, e
B. a, b, d, e
C. a, c
D. a, c, d
E. d, e

37. A 41-year-old patient presents after trauma. MRI showed (Fig. 15.9):

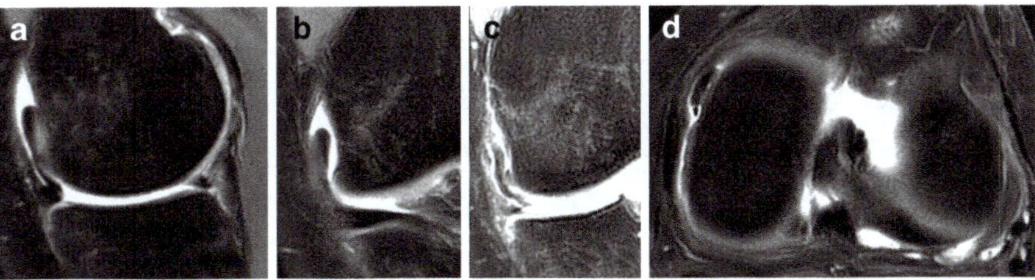

Fig. 15.9 Proton density weighted with fat suppression. (**a**) Sagittal section, (**b** and **c**) coronal sections; (**d**) axial section

   A. longitudinal meniscal tear
   B. horizontal meniscal tear
   C. radial meniscal tear
   D. bucket handle tear
   E. flipped meniscus

38. Which tendons cross in the plantar side of the foot?
   A. peroneus brevis and peroneus longus
   B. tibialis posterior and flexor digitorum longus
   C. tibialis anterior and extensor digitorum longus
   D. flexor digitorum longus and flexor hallucis longus
   E. extensor digitorum longus and extensor hallucis longus

39. Asymptomatic ankle fluid is commonly present in the:
   A. flexor hallucis longus
   B. flexor digitorum longus
   C. extensor hallucis longus
   D. extensor digitorum longus
   E. peroneus brevis and peroneus longus synovial sheath

40. A 56-year-old patient presents with a non-tender lump on the scapular region. MRI was done (Fig. 15.10). What is the most likely diagnosis?

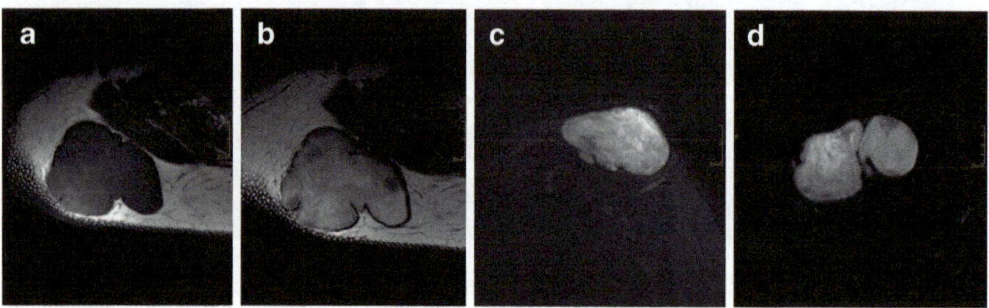

Fig. 15.10 (**a**) T1-weighted image, axial section; (**b**) T2-weighted image, axial section; (**c**) T1-weighted image with fat suppression and contrast, sagittal section; (**d**) T1-weighted image with fat suppression and contrast, coronal section

A. lipoma
B. ganglion cyst
C. myxoid tumour
D. neurofibroma
E. epidermal inclusion cyst

41. Choose the correct option regarding the lesion seen in Fig. 15.11:
    a. lytic lesion in the metaphysis.
    b. Cortical breakthrough is seen.
    c. Permeative bone destruction.
    d. No periosteal reaction is present.

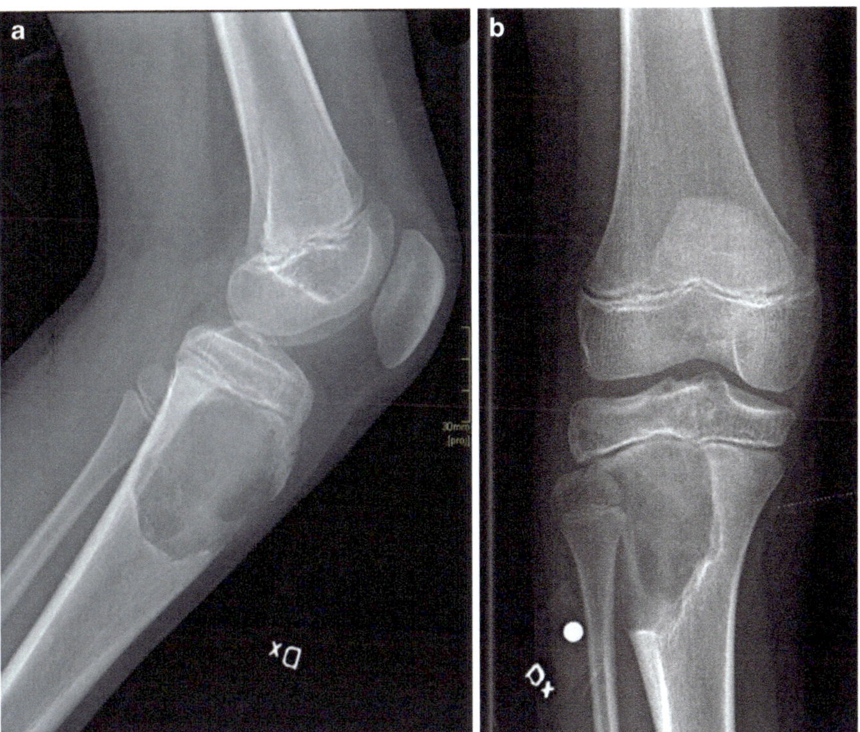

Fig. 15.11 (**a** and **b**) X-ray of the knee

A. a, b, c, d
B. a, b, c
C. a, b, d
D. b, d
E. a, d

42. A 56-year-old patient presents with shoulder pain. MRI was performed (Fig. 15.12). What is the correct answer regarding this patient?
    a. Chondroid matrix mineralization is seen on MRI.
    b. Deep endosteal scalloping is present.
    c. Soft tissue extension is seen

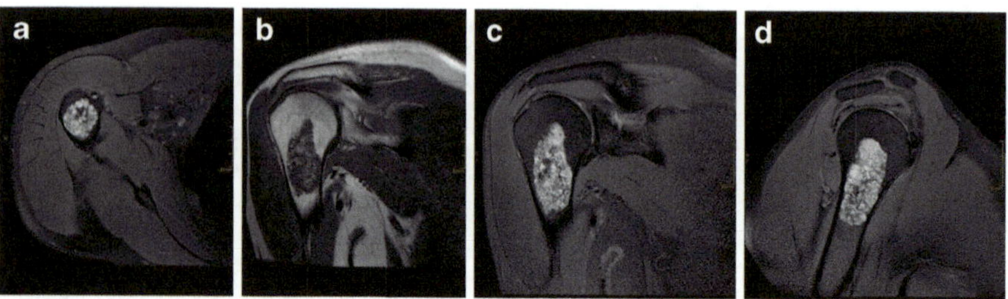

Fig. 15.12 (**a**) T2-weighted image with fat suppression; (**b**) T1-weighted image; (**c**) T2-weighted image with fat suppression; (**d**) T2-weighted image with fat suppression

A. a, b, c
B. a, b
C. b, c
D. a, c
E. a

43. What is the correct option regarding the radiological findings in Fig. 15.13?
    a. permeative growth
    b. soft tissue component
    c. aggressive periosteal reaction

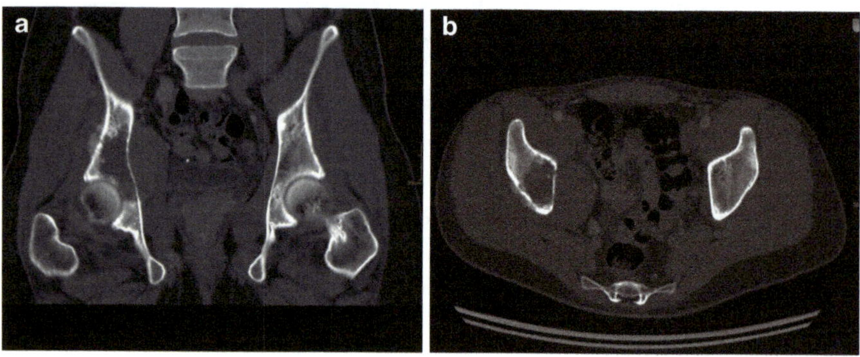

Fig. 15.13 Computed tomography of the pelvis. (**a**) coronal section; (**b**) axial section

A. a, b, c
B. a, b
C. b, c
D. a, c
E. b

44. Regarding the 20-year-old patient from the previous question, what is the most likely diagnosis?
    A. paraosteal osteosarcoma
    B. classical osteosarcoma
    C. aneurysmal bone cyst
    D. Ewing sarcoma
    E. osteomyelitis
45. A 72-year-old patient presents with non-specific back pain, weight loss, fever, and night sweats. No other significant medical history was reported. CT and MRI were performed (Fig. 15.14). Choose the correct option regarding this patient:
    a. Metastases are possible.
    b. Spondylodiscitis is possible.
    c. Lymphoma is possible.
    d. Ewing sarcoma is possible.

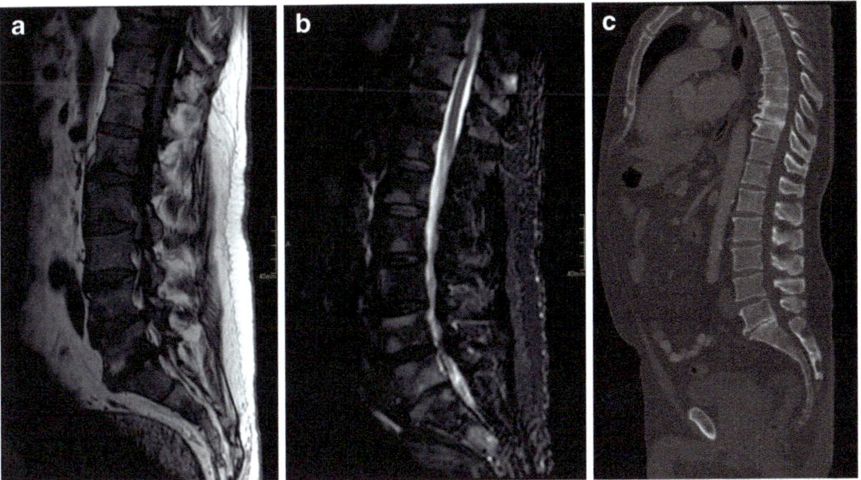

Fig. 15.14 (**a**) T1-weighted image, sagittal section; (**b**) T2-weighted image with contrast, sagittal section; (**c**) computed tomography, sagittal section

A. a, b, c, d
B. a, b, c
C. b, d
D. a, c
E. a, d

46. A 24-year-old patient presents with knee pain after trauma. MRI was performed (Fig. 15.15). Choose the correct option regarding the radiological findings:
    a. Lesion is located eccentrically.
    b. Sclerotic rim is present.
    c. Lesion is not calcified.
    d. Biopsy is indicated.

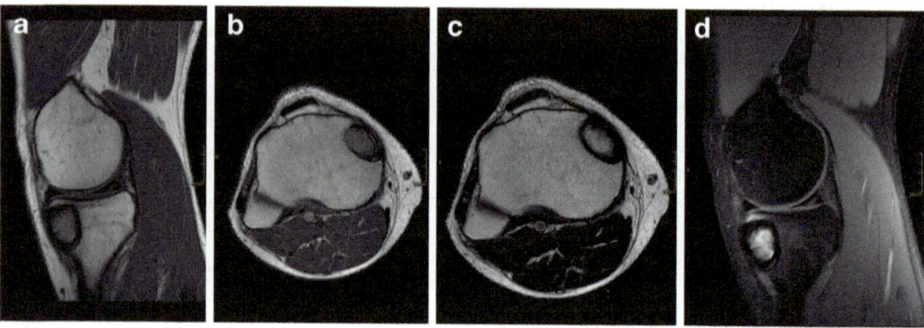

Fig. 15.15 (**a**) T1-weighted image, sagittal section; (**b**) T1-weighted image, axial section; (**c**) T2-weighted image, axial section; (**d**) proton density-weighted image with fat suppression, sagittal section. The lesion is approximately 3.5 cm

A. a, b, c, d
B. a, b, c
C. a, b
D. a, c, d
E. a, b, d

47. What is the most likely diagnosis regarding the patient from the previous question?
    A. non-ossifying fibroma
    B. fibrous cortical defect
    C. osteoid osteoma
    D. cortical desmoid
    E. osteomyelitis
48. A 24-year-old patient presents with fracture after minor trauma. X-ray was done (Fig. 15.16). What is the most likely diagnosis?

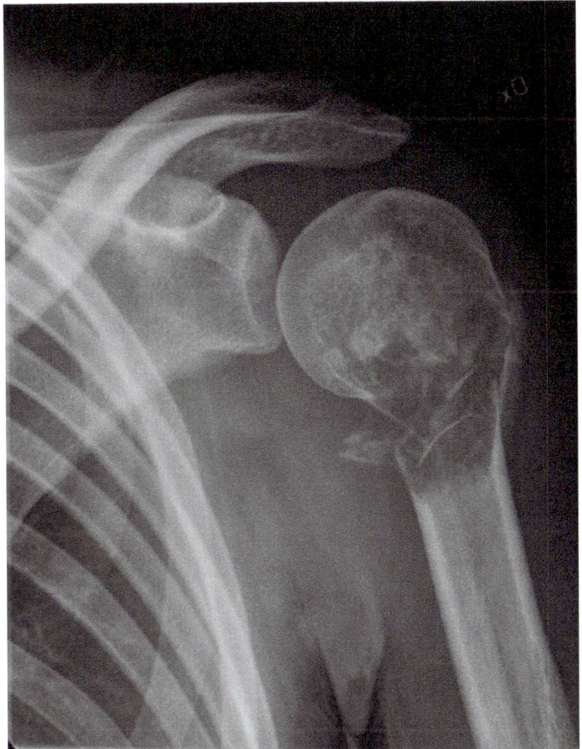

Fig. 15.16 X-ray of the shoulder

    A. non-ossifying fibroma
    B. unicameral bone cyst
    C. aneurysmal bone cyst
    D. giant cell tumour
    E. metastasis

49. A 25-year-old patient presents with painful thoracic scoliosis. CT was done (Fig. 15.17). Choose the correct option regarding this patient:
    a. Periosteal reaction is seen.
    b. The lesion is surrounded by sclerosis.
    c. The lesion showed internal calcifications.
    d. The lesion probably responds well to salicylates.

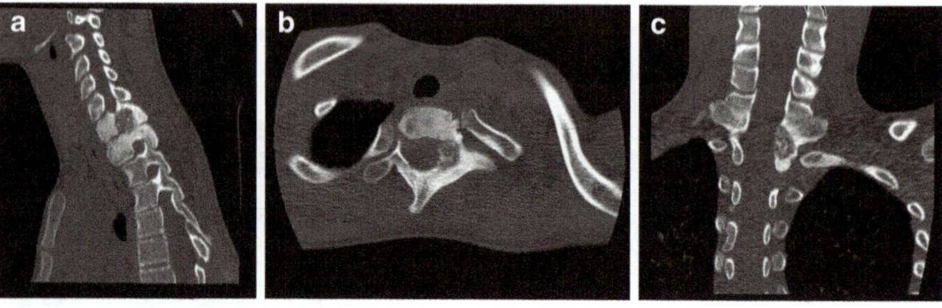

Fig. 15.17 Computed tomography of the cervical spine. (**a**) sagittal section; (**b**) axial section; (**c**) coronal section

    A. a, b, c, d
    B. a, b, c
    C. b, d
    D. a, c
    E. a, d

50. What is the most likely diagnosis regarding the patient from the previous question?
    A. eosinophilic granuloma
    B. aneurysmal bone cyst
    C. giant cell tumour
    D. osteoblastoma
    E. Paget disease

51. Which of the following diagnoses is the most likely based on this X-ray (Fig. 15.18)?

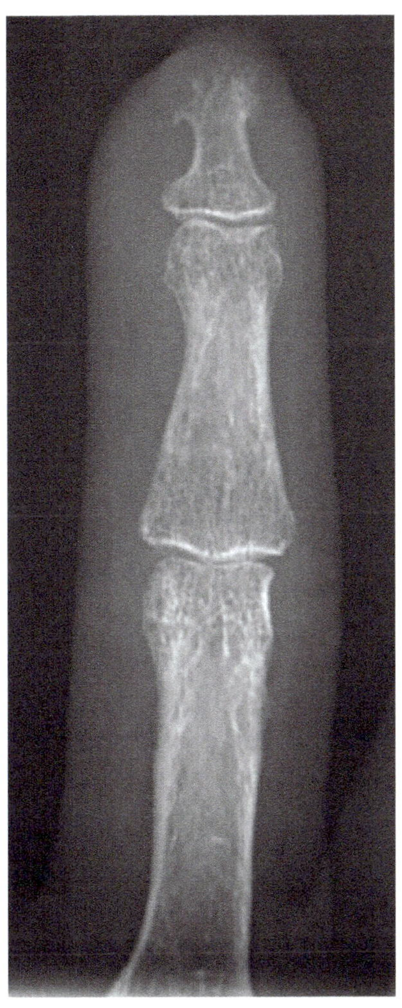

Fig. 15.18 X-ray of the third finger of the hand

A. skeletal manifestation of scleroderma
B. rheumatoid arthritis
C. psoriatic arthritis
D. osteoarthritis
E. gout

52. Choose the correct option regarding changes in hyperparathyroidism and osteopetrosis:
    A. In both cases, lesions are present in the central part of the vertebral body.
    B. In hyperparathyroidism, lesions are present at the endplates, while in osteopetrosis, lesions are in the central part of the vertebral body.
    C. In osteopetrosis, lesions are present at the endplates, while in hyperparathyroidism, lesions are in the central part of the vertebral body.
    D. In both cases, lesions are present at the endplates.
    E. In both cases, step-off deformities in the endplates are present.
53. Choose the most sensitive method for detection of stress fractures:
    A. X-ray
    B. CT without contrast
    C. CT with contrast
    D. ultrasound
    E. MRI
54. Choose the features of Paget disease:
    a. A lytic lesion involving the proximal part, including the proximal end of the tibia in a 65-year-old patient.
    b. Sclerotic and narrowing of the distal phalanx of the hand in a 62-year-old patient.
    c. Pubic bone is enlarged with sclerotic apperance in a 72-year-old patient.
    A. a, b, c
    B. a, b
    C. b, c
    D. a, c
    E. b
55. An avulsion fracture of the fifth metatarsal is caused by:
    A. peroneus longus
    B. peroneus brevis
    C. peroneus tertius
    D. extensor digitorum longus
    E. extensor digitorum brevis

Key to Chapter 15

1. E.
2. A.
3. C.
4. D.
5. C.
6. D.
7. C.
8. C.
9. E.
10. D.

11. C.
12. A.
13. B.
14. B.
15. D.
16. D.
17. B.
18. B.
19. A.
20. B.
21. E.
22. D.
23. A.
24. D.
25. C.
26. B.
27. E.
28. E.
29. B.
30. C.
31. C.
32. C.
33. B.
34. B.
35. B.
36. E.
37. B.
38. D.
39. A.
40. E.
41. C.
42. E.
43. A.
44. D.
45. D.
46. B.
47. A.
48. B.
49. B.
50. D.
51. C.
52. D.
53. E.
54. E.
55. B.

Examination Set 3

16

(One answer is correct, choose one answer from among A, B, C, D, and E)

1. Which nerve passes through the intervertebral foramen of Th11/Th12?
   A. Th10
   B. Th11
   C. Th12
   D. L1
   E. L2
2. Insertion of the tibialis posterior is located on the:
   a. navicular bone
   b. medial cuneiform bone
   c. lateral cuneiform bone
   A. a, b, c
   B. a, b
   C. b, c
   D. a, c
   E. b
3. Which ligament runs horizontally?
   A. deltoid ligament
   B. superomedial ligament
   C. calcaneofibular ligament
   D. posterior talofibular ligament
   E. interosseous talocalcaneal ligament

P. Szaro, *Musculoskeletal Radiology for Residents*,
https://doi.org/10.1007/978-3-030-85182-8_16

4. Choose the correct description of wrist tendons (Fig. 16.1):

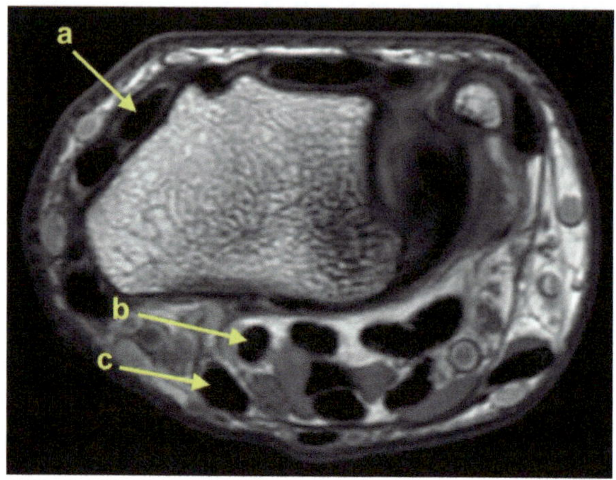

Fig. 16.1 T2-weighted image, axial section

A. a—extensor carpi radialis longus, b—flexor digitorum profundus, c—flexor digitorum superficialis
B. a—extensor carpi radialis longus, b—flexor pollicis longus, c—flexor carpi radialis
C. a—extensor carpi radialis brevis, b—flexor pollicis longus, c—flexor carpi radialis
D. a—extensor carpi radialis brevis, b—flexor carpi radialis, c—flexor pollicis longus
E. a—extensor carpi radialis brevis, b—flexor digitorum profundus, c—flexor digitorum superficialis

5. Which anatomical structure is marked by the arrow in Fig. 16.2?

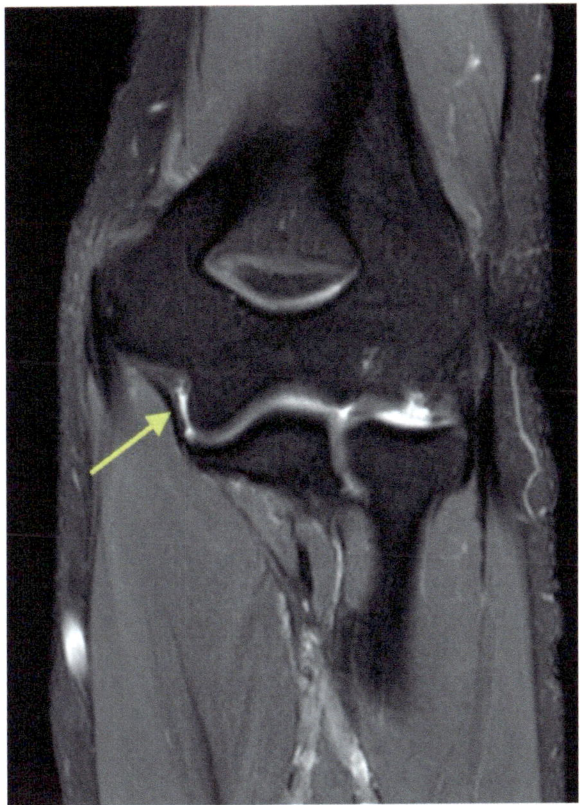

Fig. 16.2 Proton density-weighted image with fat suppression, coronal section

A. the transverse bundle of the ulnar collateral ligament
B. the posterior bundle of the ulnar collateral ligament
C. the anterior bundle of the ulnar collateral ligament
D. the flexor digitorum communis tendon
E. ulnar nerve

6. Which muscles are marked in Fig. 16.3?

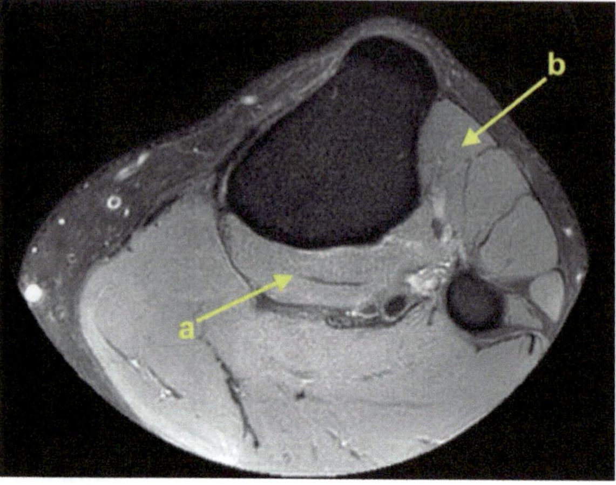

Fig. 16.3 Proton density-weighted image with fat suppression, axial section

A. a—soleus muscle, b—tibialis anterior
B. a—popliteus muscle, b—tibialis anterior
C. a—soleus muscle, b—extensor digitorum
D. a—popliteus muscle, b—extensor digitorum
E. a—flexor digitorum longus, b—extensor hallucis longus

7. Which ligament in the knee joint is located extrasynovially but intracapsularly?
   a. the anterior cruciate ligament
   b. the posterior cruciate ligament
   c. the lateral collateral ligament
   A. a, b, c
   B. a, b
   C. b, c
   D. a, c
   E. c

8. The origin of the rectus femoris is on the:
   A. spina iliaca anterior superior and iliac part of acetabulum
   B. spina iliaca anterior inferior and iliac part of acetabulum
   C. spina iliaca anterior superior
   D. spina iliaca anterior inferior
   E. pubic tuberculum

9. Which nerves run via the infrapiriform foramen?
    a. posterior cutaneous nerve of the thigh
    b. inferior gluteal nerve
    c. pudendal nerve
    d. sciatic nerve
    A. a, b, c, d
    B. a, c
    C. b, d
    D. a, b, c
    E. d
10. Which nerve runs through the tarsal tunnel?
    A. no nerve runs through it
    B. tibial nerve
    C. deep fibular nerve
    D. common fibular nerve
    E. superficial fibular nerve
11. What fibres in the hip joint run circularly?
    A. orbicular zone
    B. ligamentum teres
    C. iliopubic ligament
    D. ischiofemoral ligament
    E. pubofemoral ligament
12. An MRI of the shoulder after anterior dislocation showed detachment of the labrum from the cartilage, with periosteal denudation of the scapula. The scapular periosteum remains intact but is stripped medially. What is the most likely diagnosis?
    A. Perthes lesion
    B. soft tissue Bankart lesion
    C. glenolabral articular disruption
    D. humeral avulsion of the glenohumeral ligament
    E. anterior labroligamentous periosteal sleeve avulsion

13. What structure is marked by the arrows in Fig. 16.4?

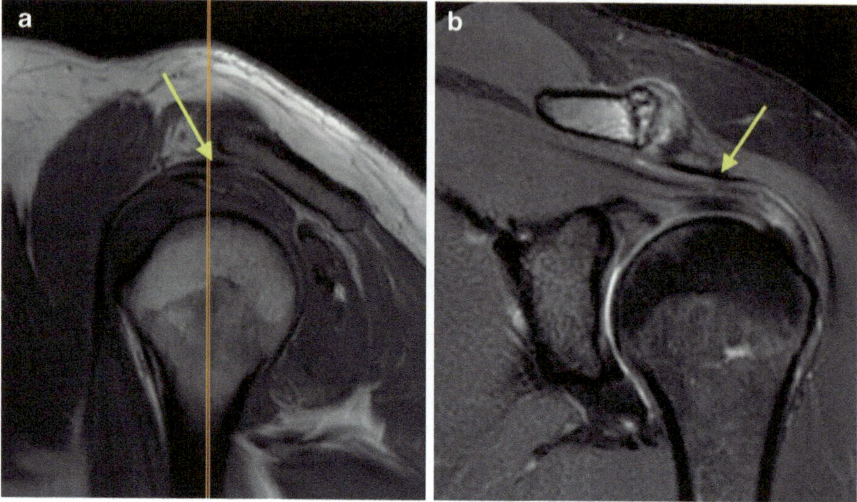

Fig. 16.4 (**a**) T1-weighted image, sagittal section; (**b**) T2-weighted image with fat suppression, coronal section

A. subdeltoid bursa
B. subacromial bursa
C. supraspinatus tendon
D. coracohumeral ligament
E. coracoacromial ligament

14. Choose the typical localisations of the radiographically occult fractures:
    a. neck of femur fracture
    b. scaphoid fracture
    c. radial head fracture
    d. distal radius fracture

    A. a, b, c, d
    B. a, b, c
    C. b, c, d
    D. a, d
    E. b, c

15. Choose the common sites of insufficient fractures:
    a. sacrum
    b. parasymphyseal part of the pubic bone
    c. femoral neck
    d. supraacetabular region
    A. a, b, c, d
    B. a, b, c
    C. b, c, d
    D. a, d
    E. b, c
16. Osteochondritis dissecans:
    a. In the knee, it is most commonly located in the lateral femoral condyle.
    b. In the elbow, it is most commonly located in the posterior part of the capitellum.
    c. In the ankle, it is predominantly located in the superomedial corner of the talus.
    A. a, b, c
    B. a, b
    C. b, c
    D. b
    E. c
17. Choose MRI signs of unstable osteochondritis dissecans on T2-weighted sequences:
    a. when the cystic lesion under the osteochondritis dissecans fragment is greater than 5 mm
    b. when a linear fluid signal intensity surrounds the osteochondritis dissecans fragment
    c. when the defect in overlying cartilage is more than 5 mm
    d. when extensive bone marrow oedema surrounds the osteochondritis dissecans fragment
    A. a, b, c, d
    B. a, b, c
    C. b, c, d
    D. a, d
    E. b, c
18. A 24-year-old weightlifter presents with a painful shoulder. MRI revealed only indentation of the superior surface of the supraspinatus muscle belly at the level of the acromioclavicular joint. Choose the correct answer regarding this patient:
    A. This is a sign of instability.
    B. This is a sign of acromial slope.
    C. Further diagnostic imaging is indicated.
    D. Muscle overdevelopment is the most likely diagnosis.
    E. Acromioclavicular joint degenerative changes is the most likely diagnosis.

19. A 45-year-old swimmer presents with shoulder pain without trauma. What is the most likely diagnosis regarding Fig. 16.5?

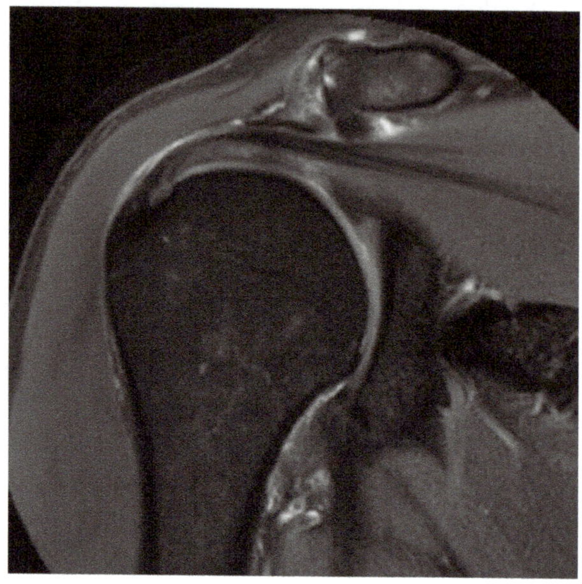

Fig. 16.5 T2-weighted image with fat suppression, coronal section

a. intrasubstance tear
b. bursal side tear
c. articular side tear

A. a
B. b
C. c
D. a, b
E. b, c

20. What is the medial boundary of the rotator interval?
    A. superior glenohumeral ligament
    B. coracohumeral ligament
    C. supraspinatus tendon
    D. coracoid process
    E. acromion

21. What type of anterior labral lesion is presented in Fig. 16.6?

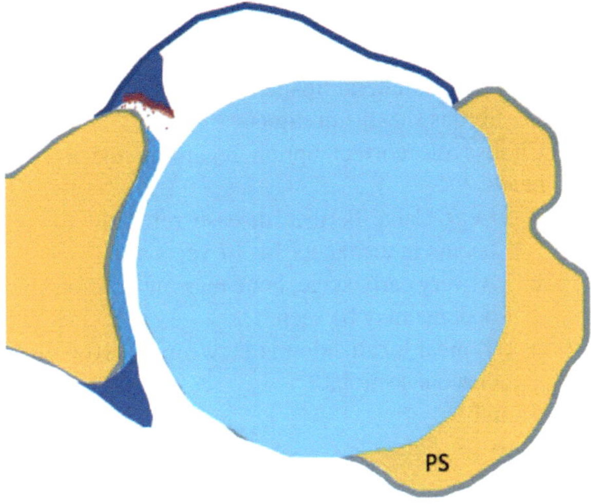

Fig. 16.6 Schematic drawing of the shoulder, axial section

   A. glenolabral articular disruption
   B. soft tissue Bankart lesion
   C. Buford complex
   D. Perthes lesion
   E. Bennet lesion

22. The space between the scaphoid and lunate is increased, and the capitate has migrated proximally. There is osteoarthritis between the scaphoid and radius. What is your diagnosis?
   A. avascular scaphoid necrosis
   B. scapholunate advanced collapse
   C. ulnar impaction syndrome
   D. lunatomalacia
   E. Madelung deformity

23. Choose the correct option regarding the wrist:
   a. Subluxation of the extensor carpi ulnaris can be seen in supination of the wrist.
   b. Tears of the triangular fibrocartilage are associated with lunotriquetral ligament tears.
   c. When the scapholunate ligament is torn, the scaphoid tilts posteriorly while the lunatum tilts anteriorly.
   A. a, b
   B. b, c
   C. c
   D. a
   E. a, b, c

24. The bowstring appearance of the flexor tendons is caused by a tear of the:
    A. pulley
    B. sagittal band
    C. ulnar collateral ligament of interphalangeal joints
    D. radial collateral ligament of interphalangeal joints
    E. fibrous sheaths of digits
25. Choose the correct option regarding the avascular necrosis of the femoral head:
    a. Legg-Calvé-Perthes disease refers to idiopathic avascular necrosis that occurs in teenagers 14–17 years old.
    b. At very early stage, bone marrow oedema similar to transient bone marrow oedema may be seen.
    c. Typical localization is between the 10 o'clock and 2 o'clock positions on coronal sections.
    A. a, b
    B. b, c
    C. a, c
    D. a
    E. a, b, c
26. Choose the conditions which may predispose to slipped capital femoral epiphysis:
    a. obesity
    b. hyperparathyroidism
    c. hyperparathyroidism
    d. radiotherapy
    A. a, b, c, d
    B. a, b, d
    C. a, c, d
    D. a, b, c
    E. a, d
27. A herniation pit is commonly in:
    A. the superior outline of the femoral head
    B. the posterior outline of the femoral head
    C. the anterior outline of the femoral head
    D. the superior outline of the greater trochanter
    E. the medial outline of the femoral neck
28. Choose the correct option regarding an acetabular labrum tear:
    a. Femoroacetabular impingement may be the cause.
    b. It is associated with paralabral cysts.
    c. It is associated with chondral abnormalities.
    A. a, b
    B. b, c
    C. a, c
    D. a
    E. a, b, c

29. The double posterior cruciate ligament sign is seen in:
    A. radial meniscal tear
    B. longitudinal meniscal tear
    C. horizontal meniscal tear
    D. meniscal flounce
    E. meniscal fraying
30. Choose the correct option regarding a discoid meniscus:
    a. It is frequently asymptomatic but more prone to degeneration.
    b. It is often congenital and commonly bilateral.
    c. It may be unstable in the Wrisberg variant.
    A. a, b
    B. b, c
    C. a, c
    D. a
    E. a, b, c
31. Speckled appearance of the anterior horn of the lateral meniscus is:
    A. a normal variant
    B. meniscal flounce
    C. meniscal fraying
    D. vertical tear
    E. radial tear
32. Choose the correct option regarding post-operative anterior cruciate ligament assessment:
    a. Within the first year, the graft may be lax.
    b. Within the first year, the signal on T2-weighted sequences may be higher.
    c. The tibial tunnel should be parallel to the line of the roof of the femoral intercondylar notch.
    A. a, b
    B. b, c
    C. a, c
    D. a
    E. a, b, c
33. A 23-year-old athlete presents with the patellar pain. MRI revealed only oedema in the suprapatellar fat pad. What is your diagnosis?
    A. fat necrosis
    B. impingement
    C. jumper's knee
    D. quadriceps tendinopathy
    E. pigmented villonodular synovitis
34. A 34-year-old patient presents after knee trauma. X-ray showed no fracture. MRI revealed reticular bone marrow oedema in the anterior aspects of the lateral femoral condyle and tibial plateau. This is a pattern seen with:
    A. clip injury
    B. pivot shift
    C. hyperflexion
    D. hyperextension
    E. dashboard injury

35. A thickened proximal portion of the patellar tendon with high intrasubstance signal is diagnostic of:
    A. impingement
    B. jumper's knee
    C. quadriceps tendinopathy
    D. infrapatellar plica syndrome
    E. medial synovial plica syndrome
36. A 33-year-old patient presents after trauma, MRI showed (Fig. 16.7) a:

Fig. 16.7 Proton density-weighted image with fat suppression, axial section

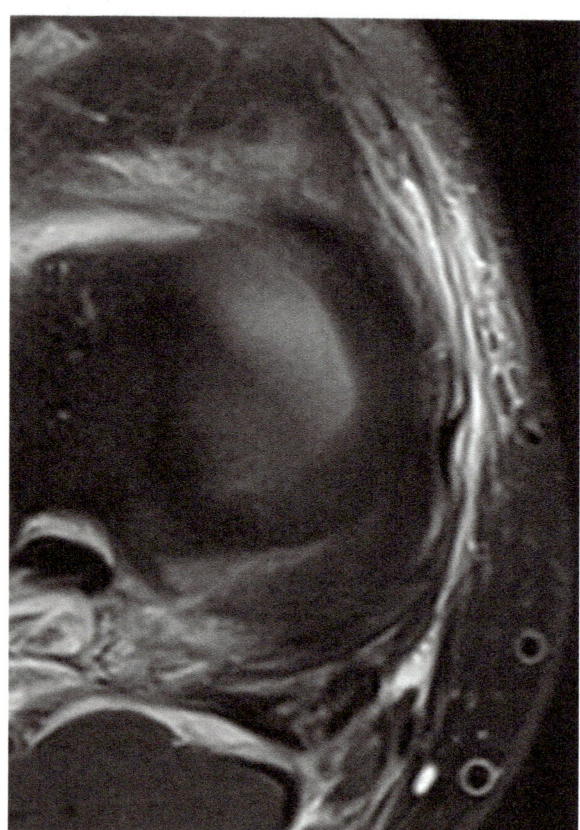

    A. longitudinal meniscal tear
    B. horizontal meniscal tear
    C. radial meniscal tear
    D. bucket handle tear
    E. flipped meniscus

37. Which tendons have a common synovial sheath?
    A. peroneus brevis and peroneus longus
    B. tibialis posterior and flexor digitorum longus
    C. tibialis anterior and extensor digitorum longus
    D. flexor digitorum longus and flexor hallucis longus
    E. extensor digitorum longus and extensor hallucis longus
38. A 42-year-old patient presents after trauma to the thumb. The X-ray in Fig. 16.8 shows the pathological fracture. What is the correct answer regarding this patient?

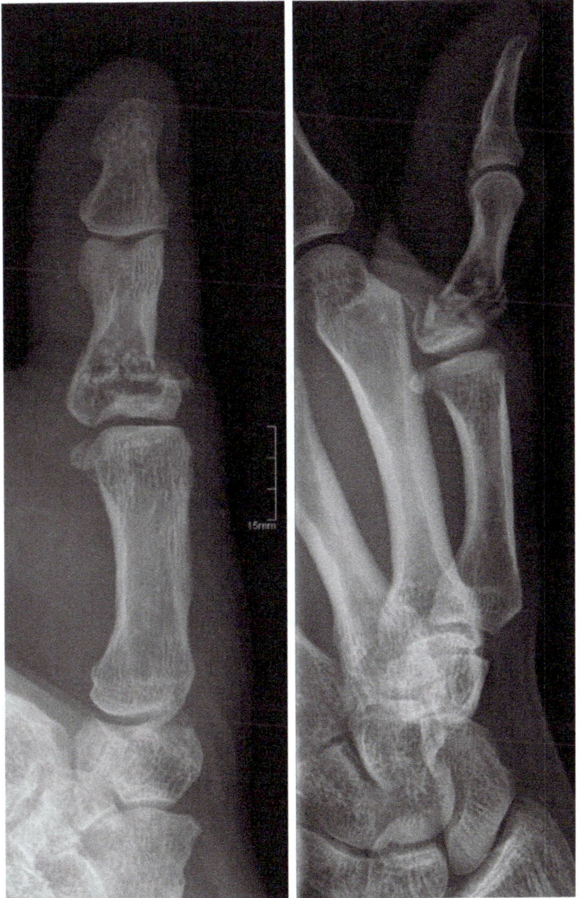

Fig. 16.8 X-ray of the thumb

    A. No further diagnostic imaging is indicated.
    B. CT without contrast is indicated.
    C. CT with contrast is indicated.
    D. Ultrasound is indicated.
    E. MRI with contrast is indicated.

39. What is the most likely diagnosis of the patient in the previous question?
    A. It is an osteosarcoma.
    B. It is an enchondroma.
    C. it is chondrosarcoma.
    D. It is a solitary bone cyst.
    E. It is a paraosteal osteosarcoma.
40. A 32-year-old patient presents with knee pain without trauma. X-ray was performed (Fig. 16.9). What is the most likely diagnosis?

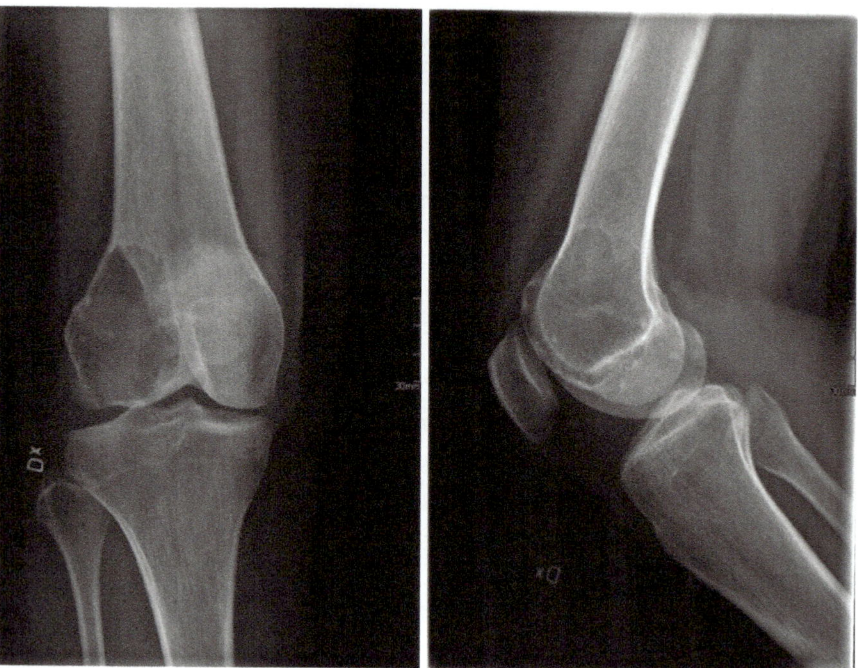

Fig. 16.9 X-ray of the knee

    a. Solitary bone cyst.
    b. Giant cell tumour.
    c. Aneurysmal bone cyst.
    d. Chondromyxoid fibroma.
    e. No further diagnostic imaging is recommended.
    f. MRI is recommended.
    A. b, d, e
    B. a, b, e
    C. b, c, f
    D. a, b, f
    E. a, b, c, e

41. Regarding the patient from the previous question, what is the most likely diagnosis based in Fig. 16.10?
    a. solitary bone cyst
    b. giant cell tumour
    c. chondroblastoma
    d. aneurysmal bone cyst

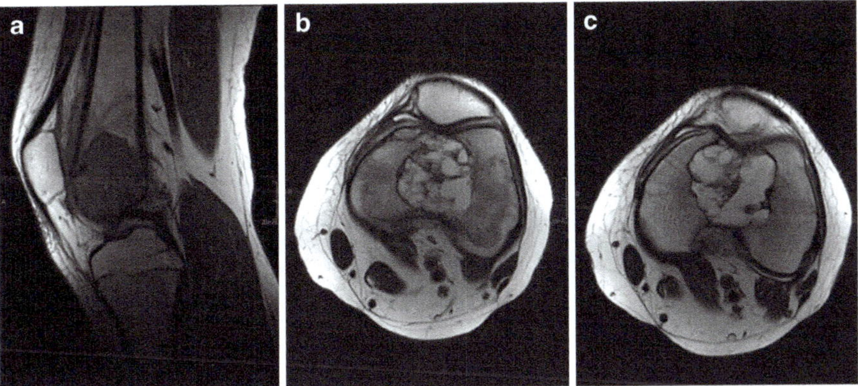

Fig. 16.10 (**a**) T1-weighted image, sagittal section; (**b** and **c**) T2-weighted images, axial sections

A. a, c, and d
B. b, c, and d
C. a and b
D. b and d
E. a, b, c, and d

42. What is the correct answer regarding the radiological findings in Fig. 16.11?
    a. Codman triangle
    b. permeative growth
    c. sunburst periosteal reaction
    d. multi-layered periosteal reaction

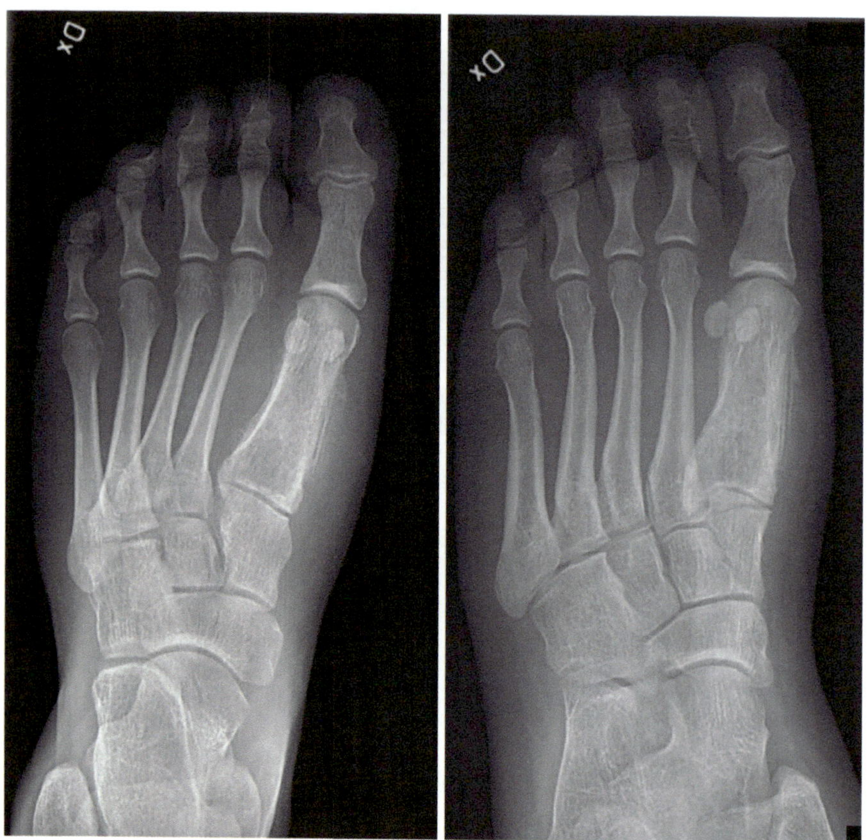

Fig. 16.11 X-ray of the foot

A. a, b, c, d
B. a, b, c
C. b, c, d
D. a, c, d
E. b, d

43. Regarding the patient from the previous question, what is the most likely diagnosis?
    A. paraosteal osteosarcoma
    B. classical osteosarcoma
    C. Ewing sarcoma
    D. osteomyelitis
    E. metastasis
44. A 54-year-old patient presents with abdominal pain. CT revealed a lesion in the left ilium (Fig. 16.12). What is the most likely diagnosis?

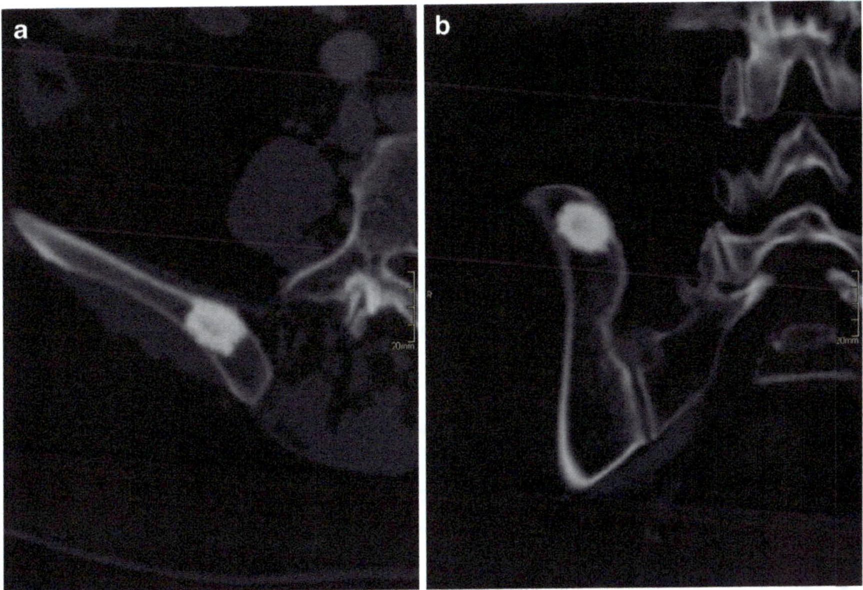

Fig. 16.12 Computed tomography of the pelvis, (**a**) axial section, (**b**) coronal section

A. osteoblastic metastasis
B. sclerotic metastasis
C. osteoid osteoma
D. osteosarcoma
E. bone island

45. A 62-year-old patient presents with sacral pain. CT was performed (Fig. 16.13). What is the most likely diagnosis?

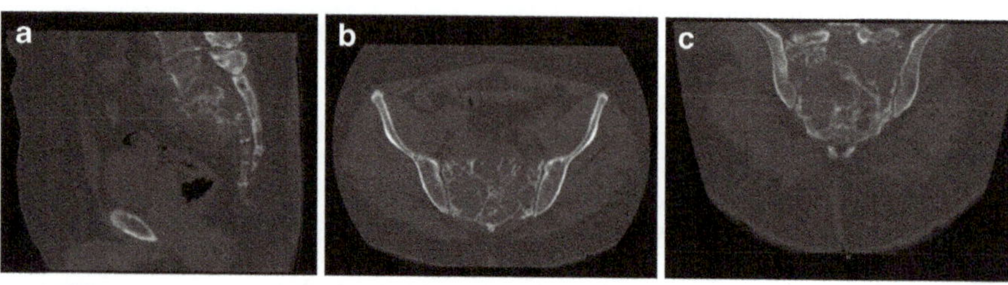

Fig. 16.13 Computed tomography of the pelvis. (**a**) sagittal section, (**b**) axial section, (**c**) coronal section

A. chondrosarcoma
B. giant cell tumour
C. osteomyelitis
D. lymphoma
E. chordoma

46. A 20-year-old patient presents with a swollen and painful knee, with no trauma. X-ray was performed (Fig. 16.14). What is the correct answer regarding the radiological findings?
a. Codman triangle is seen.
b. It is located in the epiphysis.
c. Reactive sclerosis is seen.
d. A wide zone of transition is seen.
e. A lamellated periosteal reaction is seen.

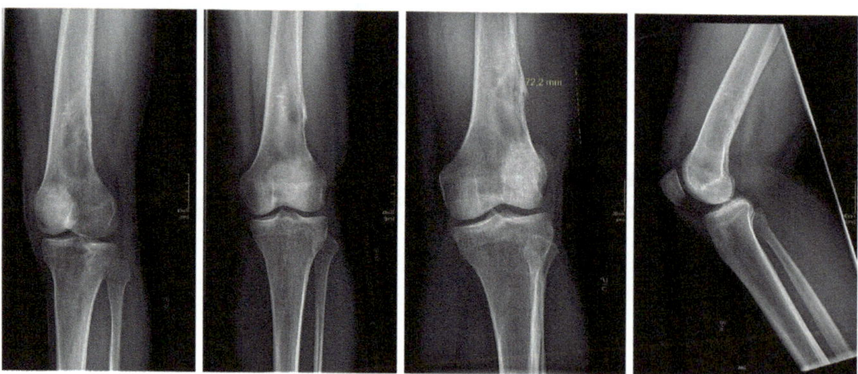

Fig. 16.14 X-ray of the knee

A. a, c, d, e
B. a, c, d
C. c, e
D. d
E. a, b, c, d, e

47. What is the correct option regarding the lesion form the previous question?
    a. Localization in the femur is the common both for osteosarcoma and Ewing sarcoma.
    b. Permeative destruction is common for both osteosarcoma and Ewing sarcoma.
    c. Extension into adjacent soft tissues is more typical for Ewing sarcoma than osteosarcoma.
    d. Calcified matrix is seen more commonly in Ewing sarcoma than osteosarcoma.
    A. a, b, c, d
    B. a, b, c
    C. a, b
    D. b, c, d
    E. c, d
48. A 69-year-old patient presents with bilateral hip pain, somewhat more on the right side. X-ray was performed (Fig. 16.15). Choose the correct option regarding the radiological findings:
    a. Cortical thickening is seen.
    b. Acetabular protrusion is seen.
    c. Prominent trabeculations are present

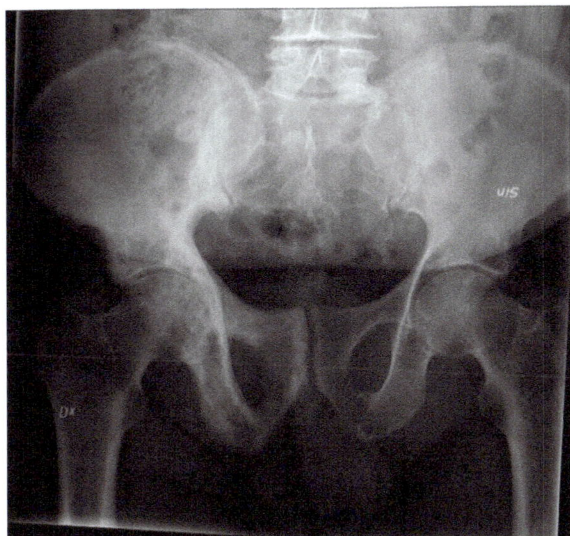

Fig. 16.15 X-ray of the pelvis

    A. a, b, c
    B. a, b
    C. b, c
    D. a, c
    E. c

49. What is the most likely diagnosis regarding the patient from the previous question?
    A. bone haemangioma
    B. fibrous dysplasia
    C. Ewing sarcoma
    D. osteosarcoma
    E. Paget disease
50. A 20-year-old patient presents with knee pain after trauma. X-ray was performed (Fig. 16.16). Choose the correct regarding this patient:
    a. The lesion is multiloculated with a sclerotic rim.
    b. No periosteal reaction or cortical breach is seen.
    c. Biopsy is indicated because the lesion is unclear and symptomatic.
    d. The lesion is located eccentrically in the metaphysis neighbouring the epiphysis.

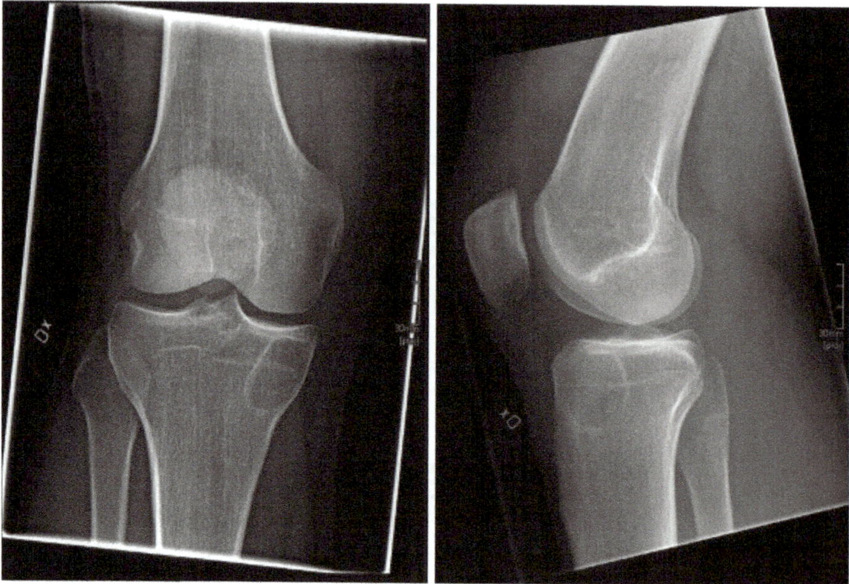

Fig. 16.16 X-ray of the knee

    A. a, b, c, d
    B. a, b, d
    C. a, c
    D. b, d
    E. c, d

51. What is the most likely diagnosis regarding the patient from the previous question?
    A. non-ossifying fibroma
    B. osteoid osteoma
    C. cortical desmoid
    D. osteomyelitis
    E. metastasis

52. A 24-year-old patient presents with foot pain without trauma. X-ray was done (Fig. 16.17). Choose the correct option regarding the X-ray:
    a. No fracture line is seen.
    b. Cortical thickening is seen.
    c. A periosteal reaction is seen.
    d. Female athlete triad is a risk factor for this condition.
    e. MRI is indicated because of a worrisome periosteal reaction

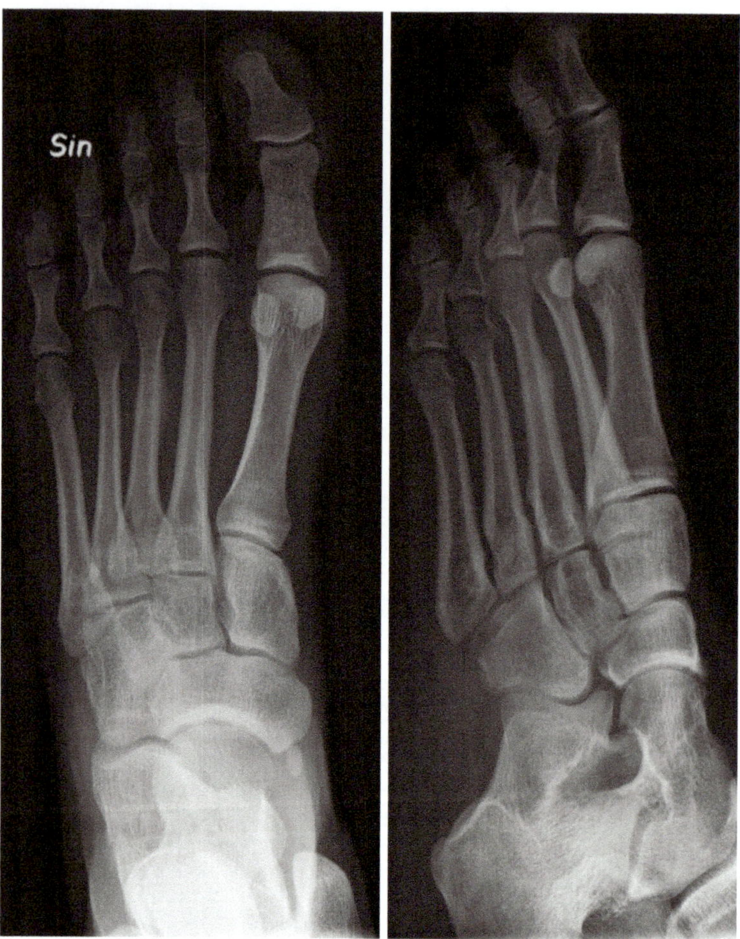

Fig. 16.17 X-ray of the foot

A. a, b, c, d, e
B. a, b, c, d
C. a, c, d
D. d, e
E. a, c

53. Which of the following diagnoses is the most likely based on this X-ray (Fig. 16.18)?

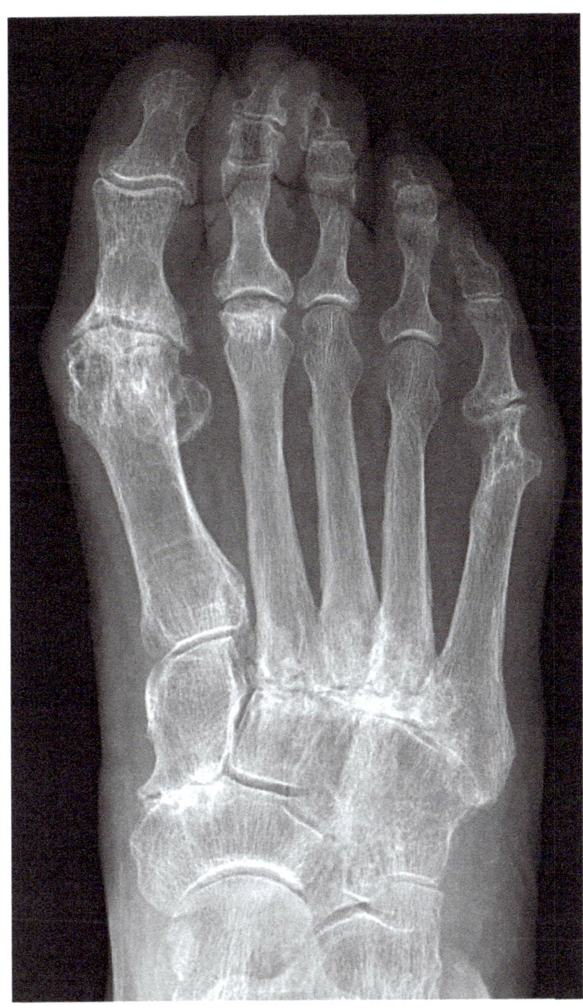

Fig. 16.18 X-ray of the foot

A. skeletal manifestation of scleroderma
B. rheumatoid arthritis
C. psoriatic arthritis
D. osteoarthritis
E. gout

54. The most common benign osseous conditions of the spine include:
    A. eosinophilic granuloma, osteochondroma, and enchondroma
    B. simple bone cyst, giant cell tumour, and osteoblastoma
    C. bony island, fibrosus dysplasia, and brown tumour
    D. enchondroma, osteochondroma, and aneurysmal bone cyst
    E. osteoid osteoma, osteoblastoma, and giant cell tumour
55. Choose the typical features of most common interosseous haemangiomas:
    A. high signal on T1-weighted images and low signal on T2-weighted images
    B. high signal on T1-weighted images and high signal on T2-weighted images
    C. low signal on T1-weighted images and low signal on T2-weighted images
    D. low signal on T1-weighted images and high signal on T2-weighted images
    E. high signal on short tau inversion recovery (STIR)

Key to Chapter 16

1. B.
2. B.
3. D.
4. C.
5. C.
6. B.
7. B.
8. B.
9. A.
10. B.
11. A.
12. A.
13. E.
14. A.
15. A.
16. E.
17. B.
18. D.
19. C.
20. D.
21. D.
22. B.
23. A.
24. A.
25. B.
26. B.
27. C.
28. E.

29. B.
30. E.
31. A.
32. B.
33. B.
34. D.
35. B.
36. A.
37. A.
38. A.
39. B.
40. C.
41. D.
42. A.
43. C.
44. E.
45. D.
46. B.
47. B.
48. D.
49. E.
50. D.
51. A.
52. C.
53. B.
54. E.
55. B.

GPSR Compliance

The European Union's (EU) General Product Safety Regulation (GPSR) is a set of rules that requires consumer products to be safe and our obligations to ensure this.

If you have any concerns about our products, you can contact us on ProductSafety@springernature.com

In case Publisher is established outside the EU, the EU authorized representative is:

Springer Nature Customer Service Center GmbH
Europaplatz 3
69115 Heidelberg, Germany

Batch number: 10370712

Printed by Printforce, the Netherlands